EMQs for Medical Students

Volume 3
Practice Papers

Second Edition

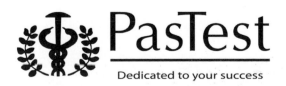

PasTest

Dedicated to your success

EMQs for Medical Students

Volume 3: Practice Papers

Second Edition

Adam Feather FRCP
Charles H Knowles BChir PhD FRCS (Gen Surg)
Paola Domizio BSc MBBS FRCPath
Kevin Hayes MRCOG
John S P Lumley MS FRCS

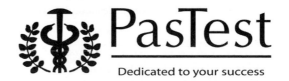

PasTest
Dedicated to your success

© 2008 PASTEST LTD

Egerton Court
Parkgate Estate
Knutsford
Cheshire
WA16 8DX

Telephone: 01565 752000

First Edition 2004
Reprinted 2007

Second Edition 2008
Reprinted 2008, 2010, 2011

ISBN 10: 1 905635 44 3
ISBN 13: 978 1 905635 443

PasTest Revision Books and Intensive Courses

PasTest has been established in the field of postgraduate medical education since 1972, providing revision books and intensive study courses for doctors preparing for their professional examinations. Books and courses are available for the following specialties:

MRCGP, MRCP Parts 1 and 2, MRCPCH Parts 1 and 2, MRCPsych, MRCS, MRCOG Parts 1 and 2, DRCOG, DCH, FRCA, PLAB Parts 1 and 2.

For further details contact:

PasTest, Freepost, Knutsford, Cheshire WA16 7BR
Tel: 01565 752000   Fax: 01565 650264
www.pastest.co.uk   enquires@pastest.co.uk

Typeset by Saxon Graphics Ltd, Derby
Printed and bound in the UK by CPI Antony Rowe

Contents

List of contributors	*vi*
Preface	*vii*
Introduction	*ix*
Glossary	*xi*
Normal values	*xv*
Paper 1	1
Paper 2	33
Paper 3	67
Paper 4	101
Paper 5	135
Paper 6	169
Paper 7	205
Paper 8	239
Paper 9	273
Paper 10	307
Radiology images	343
Index	*357*

List of contributors

Adam Feather FRCS
Senior Lecturer in Medical Education, Barts
and The London Medical School,
Consultant Geriatrician, Newham University Hospital NHS Trust.

Charles H Knowles BChir PhD FRCS (Gen Surg)
Senior Lecturer and Hon Consultant Colorectal Surgeon
Centre for Academic Surgery
Royal London Hospital

Paola Domizio BSc MB BS FRCPath
Professor of Pathology Education
Barts and the London School of Medicine and Dentistry, Queen Mary,
University of London

Kevin Hayes MRCOG
Senior Lecturer/Consultant Obstetrics and Gynaecology
St George's Hospital
London

John S P Lumley MS FRCS
Emeritus Professor of Vascular Surgery, St. Bartholomew's and the Royal
London School of Medicine and Dentistry
Honorary Consultant Surgeon
St. Bartholomew's Hospital, London
Member of Council, Royal College of Surgeons and England,

Preface

This new third volume in the series has been compiled in response to the demand for further questions of this type, a format that is becoming increasingly widely used throughout medical schools in the UK. Whereas in the previous two volumes a systems approach has been used, this volume mixes questions, testing the reader across all disciplines. No excuses are made for the use of some previous option lists with minor modifications or for occasionally repeating a question: this should reassure readers that there is a limit to the number of medical lists that can be thrown at them! It also serves to reinforce important topics.

We are also pleased to point out that the format of the questions is similar to that of the questions in the previous volumes and that the same 'Introduction' has been retained. This, we hope, will also provide reassurance that not everything is changing all the time in medical education.

Each examination is 2 hours in duration. Each correct answer scores 1 mark and there is no negative marking for incorrect answers. Where there is more than one answer for a given scenario, each answer scores 1 mark if they are independent of one another. If they depend on one another to complete a given syndrome or clinical picture, they score the given part of 1 mark, so if there are three answers, each scores a third of a mark.

This new edition also provides exclusive access to all questions from this book online www.pastest.co.uk/onlineextras.

With 'Online Extras' you can take fixed exams to test your knowledge across the syllabus. You can acquire knowledge, analyse your strengths and weaknesses through detailed feedback and develop your revision strategy and exam technique. 'Online Extras' also compares your performance with that of your peers, helping you to see if you are performing at the right level.

Introduction

We have included several innovations within these new editions. The most striking are the inclusion of radiology and other images, and the increased use of 'two step' items. Radiological images will help students remember both 'cause' and 'effect'. As with all data interpretation, one needs to be careful to treat the patient in conjunction with the radiological findings and not one in isolation of the other.

Traditional final and postgraduate examinations consisted of a written essay paper, a clinical examination consisting of long and short cases, and a viva. Although these methods provided excellent doctors for most of the last century, when they were assessed by objective measurements their reliability, reproducibility and validity came into question. Another problem with each of these methods was the limited amount of a curriculum that could be assessed in a single diet of an examination. It could therefore be a lottery as to whether candidates were asked questions on well-known or unfamiliar material or whether examiners were just asking for obscure details of their own specialty.

Continuous assessment of a course ensures matching of the training and assessment of its content. However, this is only possible for internal examinations.

Many techniques have been introduced to extend the area covered by a single examination and to standardise its marking system. The objective structured clinical examination (OSCE) has so far proved to be the most reproducible and reliable of the new systems. The written paper has received a great deal of attention: although the traditional free-response essay allows a candidate to demonstrate extensive knowledge, it covers an extremely small area of the course. When questions are set around the core of the curriculum, as is appropriate in a valid and reliable examination, these questions are easily spotted. Also, poor organisation of facts and illegible handwriting can contribute to failure as much as a lack of basic knowledge. Short answer and short-essay questions widen the area of assessment, and also reduce the reliance on technique. The MCQ has retained an important place in medical examinations for 30 years. The technique allows examination across a wide field, but clinical options are rarely totally right or wrong and well-constructed questions, even when set by a group of examiners, can still mislead well-prepared candidates.

The extended matching question (EMQ) is able to cover a wide area of the curriculum and assess the candidate's knowledge of clinically relevant information. It also goes beyond a simple recall of factual information, and assesses a candidate's ability to interpret data drawn from realistic, often existing, clinical problems.

Each EMQ in these books has a theme, a list of options, an introductory statement and a series of stems or scenarios. A quick look at any of the subsequent questions will provide an idea of its format. The chosen themes cover a wide range of topics that are all relevant and important in clinical practice. They include the anatomy of tissues and organs, symptoms, abnormal signs, normal and abnormal investigations, and specific diseases. They are organised by system and are listed in the contents at the beginning of each volume.

All options are feasible answers and are clustered around the chosen theme. They usually provide an extensive cover of the topic, and serve as revision aids, but are not necessarily all-inclusive. The larger the number of options, the less likely a correct answer can be obtained by chance, elimination or exclusion. However, the number also relates to the topic, the design of the question and the maximum number of feasible alternatives. Rare conditions are occasionally included, both as options and correct answers, providing a broad exposure to the field. There are 8–12 options for each theme, although the range can be extended to 5–20, depending on the topic. The options are listed alphabetically, unless amore appropriate order exists.

The introductory statement must be read carefully because it tells the reader what is expected of them. Usually, one option has to be chosen to answer each stem or scenario. The stems or scenarios determine the standard of a question, and must be pitched at the appropriate level for any examination. At an undergraduate level, scenarios are rich in uninterpreted symptoms, signs and investigations, but in more advanced examinations a clinical summary might be given without the need to sort out basic information. Key diagnostic criteria might be deliberately excluded in order to avoid making an answer too easy, or to stimulate the reader to think more deeply around a topic.

The scenarios must be sufficiently detailed that they only match the intended option from the list. However, in a few cases, where this increases understanding and clinical reasoning, more than one option has been identified: this is stated clearly within the introductory statement. Options provide a whole range of alternatives, including isolated facts, encouraging recognition and recall, but emphasis is given to clinical decision-making and interpretation of material, focusing on clinical scenarios. There are usually five scenarios per theme, but the number varies in different sections.

In the past, most EMQ vignettes required the students to derive an answer that was one of the items included in the alphabetical list. A two step item differs in that it requires the student to derive a fact or series of facts from the vignette (step one), and then link this with the items and theme of the vignette (step two). For example in a series where the theme is ECG rhythm strips (so all the items are rhythm strips) the first vignette implies that the patient is in fast AF. The student must be able to make the first answer of fast AF (first step) and then recognise the correct rhythm strip (second step). This two step approach is now commonly used in the later stages of the medical curriculum, to assess clinical diagnostic reasoning rather than straightforward factual recall.

The second half of each book gives the answers to each question, together with an extended explanation, providing an overview of the topic and a revision aid for each theme. It is not necessarily comprehensive, but should identify gaps and direct further reading.

The time allowed for an EMQ examination differs from that of an MCQ examination because each scenario can be quite complex, reflecting clinical practice, and time is needed to consider all options. In general, 120–160 scenarios can be answered in 2 hours, and not more than 200 should be included in a 3-hour examination. The scoring is 1 mark for each correct answer: if more than one option is correct, a mark or a proportion of the mark can be scored. There is no negative marking in EMQ assessment.

Ten practice examinations are listed in the prelim section of the book, drawing questions from across the syllabus: each is intended as a 2-hour examination.

Glossary

FP	Alpha-fetoprotein
AAFB	Acid- and alcohol-fast bacilli
ABPI	Ankle–brachial pressure index
ACE	Angiotensin-converting enzyme
ACTH	Adrenocorticotrophic hormone
ADH	Antidiuretic hormone
AIDS	Acquired immunodeficiency syndrome
AIHA	Autoimmune haemolytic anaemia
ALL	Acute lymphoblastic leukaemia
ALT	Alanine aminotransferase
AMA	Antimitochondrial antibody
AML	Acute myeloid leukaemia
AMTS	Abridged mental test score
ANA	Antinuclear antibody
ANCA	Antineutrophil cytoplasmic antibody
APCKD	Adult polycystic kidney disease
APTT	Activated partial thromboplastin time
ASD	Atrial septal defect
ASOT	Antistreptolysin-O titre
AST	Aspartate aminotransferase
AV	Atrioventricular
AVSD	Atrioventricular septal defect
βhCG	Beta-human chorionic gonadotrophin
BMI	Body mass index
BMR	Best motor response
BP	Blood pressure
BPH	Benign prostatic hypertrophy
bpm	beats per minute
BVR	Best vocal response
c-ANCA	cytoplasmic ANCA
CIN	Cervical intraepithelial neoplasia
CLL	Chronic lymphocytic leukaemia
CLO	*Campylobacter*-like organism
CML	Chronic myeloid leukaemia
CMV	Cytomegalovirus

CNS	Central nervous system
COPD	Chronic obstructive pulmonary disease
COX	Cyclo-oxygenase
CREST	Calcinosis, Raynaud's, oesophageal dysmotility, sclerodactyly and telangiectasia
CRF	Chronic renal failure
CRH	Corticotrophin-releasing hormone
CRP	C-reactive protein
CSF	Cerebrospinal fluid
CT	Computed tomography
CVP	Central venous pressure
DC	Direct current
DDAVP®	Des-amino-D-arginine vasopressin
DIC	Disseminated intravascular coagulation
DMARD	Disease-modifying agents of rheumatoid disease
DNA	Deoxyribonucleic acid
dsDNA	Double-stranded DNA
DVT	Deep venous thrombosis
EBV	Epstein–Barr virus
ECG	Electrocardiography (or -gram)
EEG	Electroencephalography (or -gram
EMG	Electromyelography (or –gram)
EMU	Early-morning urine
ENA	Extractable nuclear antigen
ERCP	Endoscopic retrograde cholangiopancreatography
ESR	Erythrocyte sedimentation rate
ESRF	End-stage renal failure
Fab	Fragment antigen binding
FAP	Familial adenomatous polyposis
FBC	Full blood count
Fc	Fragment crystallisable
FEV_1	Forced expiratory volume in 1 second
FNAC	Fine-needle aspiration cytology
FSH	Follicle-stimulating hormone
fT3	free Tri-iodo-thyronine
fT_4	Free thyroxine
FTA	Fluorescent *Treponema* absorption
FVC	Vital capacity during forced expiration
G6PD	Glucose-6–phosphate dehydrogenase
γGT	Gamma-glutamyltransferase
GCA	Giant-cell arteritis
GCS	Glasgow coma scale
GCSF	Granulocyte colony-stimulating factor
GnRH	Gonadotrophin-releasing hormone
GORD	Gastro-oesophageal reflux disease
GP	General Practitioner
GVHD	Graft-versus-host disease
Hb A_{1c}	Glycosylated haemoglobin
HBV	Hepatitis B virus
hCG	Human chorionic gonadotrophin
HDL	High-density lipoprotein

HHV	Human herpesvirus
HIV	Human immunodeficiency virus
HLA	Human leucocyte antigen
HMGCoA	Hydroxymethyl glutaryl co-enzyme A
HNPCC	Hereditary non-polyposis colorectal cancer (syndrome)
HOCM	Hypertrophic obstructive cardiomyopathy
HONK	Hyperosmolar non-ketotic acidosis
HPV	Human papillomavirus
HSMN	Hereditary sensory and motor neuropathy
HSP	Henoch–Schönlein purpura
IAPP	Islet amyloid polypeptide
IBD	Inflammatory bowel disease
IBS	Irritable bowel syndrome
IDDM	Insulin-dependent diabetes mellitus
Ig	Immunoglobulin
IGT	Impaired glucose tolerance
IHD	Ischaemic heart disease
IL1	Interleukin 1
INO	Internuclear ophthalmoplegia
INR	International normalised ratio
IVU	Intravenous urography/gram
IVP	Intravenous pyelography/gram
JVP	Jugular venous pressure
LDH	Lactate dehydrogenase
LDL	Low-density lipoprotein
LEMS	Lambert–Eaton myasthenic syndrome
LFT	Liver function test
LH	Luteinising hormone
LKM	Liver, kidney-microsomal
LVF	Left ventricular failure
LVH	Left ventricular hypertrophy
MALT	Mucosa-associated lymphoid tissue
MCHC	Mean corpuscular haemoglobin concentration
MCV	Mean corpuscular volume
MEN	Multiple endocrine neoplasia
MGUS	Monoclonal gammopathy of unknown significance
MHC	Major histocompatibility complex
MI	Myocardial infarction
MIBG	Metaiodobenzylguanidine
MLF	Medial longitudinal fasciculus
MND	Motor neurone disease
MODS	Multiorgan dysfunction syndrome
MRI	Magnetic resonance imaging
MSU	Mid-stream urine
NADPH	Nicotinamide adenine dinucleotide phosphate
NEP	Nucleotide excision pathway
NK	Natural killer (cell)
NSAID	Non-steroidal anti-inflammatory drug
OGD	Oesophagastroduodenoscopy
OGTT	Oral glucose tolerance test
PAN	Polyarteritis nodosa

pANCA	perinuclear ANCA
PAS	Periodic acid–Schiff
PBC	Primary biliary cirrhosis
PCKD	Polycystic kidney disease
PCOS	Polycystic ovary syndrome
PCR	Polymerase chain reaction
PCV	Packed cell volume
PDA	Patent ductus arteriosus
PEA	Pulseless electrical activity
PID	Pelvic inflammatory disease
PLE	Protein-losing enteropathy
PND	Paroxysmal nocturnal dyspnoea
PSA	Prostate-specific antigen
PT	Prothrombin time
PTH	Parathyroid hormone
PTT	Partial thromboplastin time
PUO	Pyrexia of unknown origin
RNA	Ribonucleic acidt
rT_3	Reverse tri-iodothyronine
RTA	Road traffic accident
SACD	Subacute combined degeneration of the cord
SARS	Severe acute respiratory syndrome
SCBU	Special Care Baby Unit
SHBG	Sex hormone-binding globulin
SIADH	Syndrome of inappropriate ADH secretion
SIRS	Systemic inflammatory response syndrome
SLE	Systemic lupus erythematosus
SSRI	Selective serotonin reuptake inhibitor
TB	Tuberculosis
TMRP	Transmembrane regulator protein
TNF-α	Tumour necrosis factor alpha
TPHA	*Treponema pallidum* haemagglutination assay
TSH	Thyroid-stimulating hormone
TT	Thrombin time
TURP	Transurethral resection of the prostate
U&Es	Urea and electrolytes
UTI	Urinary tract infection
UV	Ultraviolet
VDRL	Venereal Disease Research Laboratory
VER	Visual-evoked response
VMA	Vanillyl mandelic acid
V/Q	Ventilation-perfusion (scan)
VSD	Ventricular septal defect
vWF	von Willebrand factor
WCC	White cell count
WHO	World Health Organisation

Normal values

Blood, serum and plasma

Haematology

Haemoglobin
  Males   13.5–17.5 g/dl
  Females   11.5–15.5 g/dl
MCV   76–98 fl
Haematocrit   0.35–0.55
WCC $4–11 \times 10^9/l$
  Neutrophils $2.5–7.58 \times 10^9/l$
  Lymphocytes $1.5–3.5 \times 10^9/l$
Platelets $150–400 \times 10^9/l$

ESR   0–10 mm in the 1st hour

PT   10.6–14.9 s
PTT   23.0–35.0 s
TT   10.5–15.5 s
Fibrinogen   125–300 mg/dl

Vitamin B_{12} 160–900 pmol/l
Folate   1.5–10.0 mg/l
Ferritin
  Males   20–250 µg/l
  Females   10–120 µg/l

Immunoglobulins

IgM   0.5–2.0 g/l
IgG   5–16 g/l
IgA   1.0–4.0 g/l

Biochemistry

Na^+ 135–145 mmol/l
K^+ 3.5–5.0 mmol/l
Urea   2.5–6.5 mmol/l
Creatinine   50–120 µmol/l
ALT   5 30 IU/l
AST   10–40 IU/l
Bilirubin   2–17 µmol/l

Alkaline phosphatase	30–130 IU/l
Albumin	35–55 g/l
γGT	5–30 IU/l
α-FP	10 kU/l
Corrrected Ca^{2+}	2.20–2.60 mmol/l
$PO_3^-{}_4$	0.70–1.40 mmol/l
Creatine kinase	23–175 IU/l
LDH	100–190 IU/l
Amylase	200 U/l
Lactate	0.5–2.2 mmol/l
Mg^{2+}	0.75–1.00 mmol/l
Urate	0.1–0.4 mmol/l
CRP	0–10 mg/l
Troponin	0.1 ng/l

Diabetes

Glucose	
Random	3.5–5.5 mmol/l*
Fasting	<7 mmol/l
Hb A_{1c}	<7.0%

* If >5.5 mmol/l, then OGTT at 2 hours:
<7.8 mmol/l = normal
7.8–11.0 = IGT
>11.1 mmol/l = diabetes mellitus

Endocrinology

TSH	0.17–3.2 μU/l
fT_4	11–22 pmol/l
fT_3	3.5–5 pmol/l
Cortisol	
9 am	140–500 nmol/l
Midnight	50–300 nmol/l
Growth hormone	<10 ng/ml
Cholesterol	<5.2 mmol/l
Triglycerides	0–1.5 mmol/l
LDL	<3.5 mmol/l
HDL	>1.0 mmol/l
Total/HDL	<5.0
FSH	1–25 U/l
LH	1–70 U/l
Prolactin	<400 mU/l

Blood gases

pH	7.35–7.45
$PaCO_2$	4.6–6.0 kPa
PaO_2	10.5–13.5 kPa
HCO_3^-	24–30 mmol/l
Base excess	−2 to +2.0 mmol/l

CSF

Protein	<0.45 g/l
Glucose	2.5–3.9 mmol/l (two-thirds plasma value)
Cells	<5 (WCC) mmol/l
Opening pressure	6–20 cmH$_2$O

PAPER 1

Paper 1 Questions

1. THEME: UREA, ELECTROLYTES AND CREATININE

	Na⁺ (mmol/l)	K⁺ (mmol/l	Urea (mmol/l	Creatinine (μmol/l)
A	105	1.0	0.8	29
B	113	4.9	4.8	89
C	115	6.9	6.8	91
D	127	4.0	1.8	57
E	128	8.9	13.3	139
F	129	3.9	24.8	101
G	132	5.9	32.8	809
H	136	4.4	4.3	86
I	139	2.0	4.7	87
J	156	5.1	28.7	155
K	183	5.9	54.8	369

The following patients have all presented with conditions leading to derangement of their urea and electrolytes (U&Es). Please choose the most appropriate set of results from the above list. You may use each option once, more than once or not at all.

1. A 64-year-old lifelong smoker presents to his GP with weight loss, increasing weakness and a recent cough associated with episodic fresh haemoptysis. On examination, he is unwell with obvious cushingoid features.

2. A 28-year-old Asian woman presents to her GP with a 3–week history of a cough productive of thick, green sputum with occasional dark-red blood mixed into it. She also admits to having night sweats and weight loss.

3. A 61-year-old man with a long history of alcohol abuse presents to his local Emergency Department with a large fresh haematemesis (>500 ml). His subsequent U&Es confirm that he has had an occult upper gastrointestinal bleed for some time prior to the haematemesis. ☐

4. A 42-year-old woman with long-standing, poorly controlled type 1 diabetes is admitted to hospital with diabetic ketoacidosis. The FY1 doctor who takes her initial bloods is rung by the laboratory technician to tell her that the U&Es sample needs to be repeated as the original sample looks as if it has been taken proximal to an intravenous infusion. ☐

5. A 71-year-old man with ischaemic cardiomyopathy presents to his GP with increasing weakness and malaise. The doctor notes that he has recently had losartan added to his ramipril. ☐

2. THEME: ANAEMIA

A   Anaemia of chronic disease
B   Aplastic anaemia
C   Autoimmune haemolytic anaemia
D   Vitamin B$_{12}$ deficiency
E   Iron deficiency
F   Myelodysplasia
G   Pancytopenia secondary to multiple myeloma
H   Sickle-cell disease
I   Sideroblastic anaemia
J   Thalassaemia trait

The following patients have all presented with anaemia. Please choose the most appropriate cause from the above list. Each option may be used once, more than once or not at all.

1. A 73-year-old woman presents to her GP with lethargy and malaise. Of note, she has recently been placed on clopidogrel for the treatment of unstable angina. Her routine blood tests show: haemoglobin 6.8 g/dl, mean corpuscular volume (MCV) 68 fl, white cell count (WCC) 9.2 × 10^9/l, platelets 491 × 10^9/l; Na$^+$ 136 mmol/l, K$^+$ 3.9 mmol/l, urea 4.7 mmol/l, creatinine 88 μmol/l.

2. A 79-year-old man, who has recently been started on phenytoin after neurosurgery, is re-admitted under the physicians with a severe pneumonia and is noted to have bleeding gums and 'heavy' bruising over his limbs. Investigations reveal: haemoglobin 4.9 g/dl, MCV 88 fl, WCC 2.2 × 10^9/l, platelets 11 × 10^9/l. The blood film shows 'pancytopenia with few reticulocytes seen'; a bone marrow trephine shows 'hypocellularity with increased fat spaces'.

3. A 67-year-old woman is admitted to hospital with severe lumbar back pain associated with recurrent chest infections and general malaise. Investigations show: haemoglobin 3.9 g/dl, MCV 98 fl, WCC 1.9 × 10^9/l, platelets 27 × 10^9/l; Na$^+$ 130 mmol/l, K$^+$ 5.9 mmol/l, urea 24.4 mmol/l, creatinine 412 μmol/l; erythrocyte sedimentation rate (ESR) 122 mm/h; corrected Ca^{2+} 3.37 mmol/l.

4. A 51-year-old Asian woman is seen in the pre-operative assessment clinic prior to her planned breast lumpectomy. Routine investigations reveal: haemoglobin 10.3 g/dl, MCV 58 fl, WCC 5.5 × 10^9/l, platelets 369 × 10^9/l, ferritin 92 μg/l.

5. An 83-year-old woman is admitted to hospital with a severe community-acquired pneumonia. Investigations reveal: haemoglobin 7.9 g/dl, MCV 102 fl, WCC 3.2 × 10^9/l, platelets 254 × 10^9/l. The blood film shows 'significant reticulocytosis'. 'Cold' IgM antibodies are later shown to be responsible.

3. THEME: RESPIRATORY FAILURE

A   Asbestosis
B   Asthma
C   Chronic obstructive pulmonary disease (COPD)
D   Guillain–Barré syndrome
E   Idiopathic pulmonary fibrosis
F   *Legionella* pneumonia
G   *Mycoplasma* pneumonia
H   Pickwickian syndrome
I   Pulmonary embolism
J   Pulmonary oedema

The following patients have all presented with respiratory failure. Please choose the most appropriate cause from the above list. Each option may be used once, more than once, or not at all. (The arterial blood gases have all been taken on room air.)

1. A 71-year-old retired boiler lagger is referred to Medical Out-patients with a 6-month history of worsening exertional dyspnoea. On examination, he is dyspnoeic at rest but does not have finger clubbing or cyanosis. Auscultation reveals bibasal fine inspiratory crepitations. His chest radiograph shows pleural and diaphragmatic plaques with diffuse lower-zone changes. The arterial blood gases show: pH 7.39, $PaCO_2$ 4.1 kPa, $PaCO_2$ 7.9 kPa, oxygen saturation 91%, HCO_3^- 25 mmol/l, base excess 1.9 mmol/l.

2. An obese 61-year-old man presents to his GP with exertional dyspnoea, early-morning headaches and daytime somnolence. Spirometry reveals an obstructive problem and the arterial blood gases show: pH 7.37, $PaCO_2$ 7.9 kPa, $PaCO_2$ 7.3 kPa, oxygen saturation 87%, HCO_3^- 34 mmol/l, base excess 6.9 mmol/l. He improves with overnight nasal ventilation.

3. A 49-year-old woman presents in the Emergency Department with acute shortness of breath. On examination, she is peripherally 'shutdown', clammy, tachycardic and hypotensive. The arterial blood gases show: pH 7.13, $PaCO_2$ 3.5 kPa, $PaCO_2$ 7.9 kPa, oxygen saturation 89%, HCO_3^- 15 mmol/l, base excess −7.3 mmol/l. Her chest radiograph shows alveolar shadowing in a 'bat-wing' configuration.

4. A 35-year-old woman becomes acutely unwell, with shortness of breath and a dry, non-productive cough. Investigations reveal: Na^+ 127 mmol/l, K^+ 4.9 mmol/l, urea 7.4 mmol/l, creatinine 122 µmol/l. Her chest radiograph is relatively unremarkable but the arterial blood gases show: pH 7.33, $PaCO_2$ 3.7 kPa, $PaCO_2$ 6.3 kPa, oxygen saturation 82%, HCO_3^- 20 mmol/l, base excess 2.9 mmol/l. The diagnosis is later confirmed by urine antigen testing.

5. A 56-year-old man presents to his GP with a 4-month history of increasing exertional dyspnoea. On examination, he has marked clubbing of the fingernails and is short of breath on relatively mild exertion. Auscultation of his chest reveals fine inspiratory crepitations. Subsequent investigations confirm a restrictive pattern on spirometry.

4. THEME: ASCITES

A   Alcoholic cirrhosis
B   Chronic hepatitis B infection
C   Colonic carcinoma
D   Constrictive pericarditis
E   Ischaemic cardiomyopathy
F   Ovarian carcinoma
G   Pericarditis
H   Peritoneal mesothelioma
I   Renal-cell carcinoma
J   Tuberculosis

The following patients have all presented with ascites. Please choose the most appropriate cause from the above list. Each diagnosis may be used once, more than once or not at all.

1. A 51-year-old woman presents to her GP with increasing abdominal swelling. Subsequent investigations reveal a grossly elevated Ca-125. Her chest radiograph is unremarkable but there are adenocarcinoma cells in the ascitic fluid.

2. A 49-year-old woman presents in the Emergency Department with increasing exertional dyspnoea and swelling of her abdomen and ankles. On examination, she has tar-stained fingers on her right hand, her pulse is 120 beats per minute (bpm) regular, and her blood pressure (BP) is 105/70 mmHg. Her jugular venous pressure (JVP) is elevated to the angle of her jaw but Kussmaul's sign is negative. Her apex beat is grossly displaced into the posterior axillary line and she has a marked pansystolic murmur which is clearly heard throughout the praecordium. Her electrocardiogram (ECG) shows sinus rhythm 120 bpm, left axis deviation, and deep Q-waves in leads V_1-V_4.

3. A 71-year-old retired docker presents to his GP with increasing abdominal swelling, lethargy and malaise. On examination, he is clinically anaemic and has gross ascites but no organomegaly, masses or lymphadenopathy. Abdominal computed tomography (CT) shows infiltration of the peritoneum and ascites. The diagnosis is later confirmed by laparoscopy and biopsy.

4. A 57-year-old man presents to his GP with night sweats, increasing exertional dyspnoea, lethargy and abdominal swelling. Subsequent investigations reveal: haemoglobin 6.4 g/dl, MCV 79 fl, WCC 12.2×10^9/l, platelets 494×10^9/l. His chest radiograph confirms multiple large, round lesions throughout both lung fields.

5. A 29-year-old Asian woman presents to her GP with acute abdominal pains and diarrhoea. She is admitted to hospital, where colonoscopy is unremarkable, as are her chest radiograph and ECG. Subsequent CT scan of the abdomen with contrast confirms terminal ileitis with associated para-aortic and coeliac lymphadenopathy.

5. THEME: HEADACHE

A Benign intracranial hypertension
B Cervical spondylosis
C Giant-cell arteritis
D Bacterial meningitis
E Viral meningitis
F Sagittal sinus thrombosis
G Staphylococcal abscess
H Subarachnoid haemorrhage
I Subdural haemorrhage
J Tension headache

The following patients have all presented with a headache. Please choose the most appropriate cause from the above list. The options may be used once, more than once or not at all.

1. A 23-year-old woman who has recently been started on the oral contraceptive pill presents in the Emergency Department with a sudden, severe headache that is radiating across the top of her head. Fundoscopy reveals papilloedema but a CT head scan and lumbar puncture are relatively normal. A repeat CT with contrast confirms the diagnosis, showing a 'positive delta sign'.

2. A 19-year-old woman with a body mass index (BMI) of 34 kg/m^2 presents to her GP with a 6-month history of intermittent headaches associated with visual blurring. She is referred to a neurologist but routine investigations including ESR, CT head scan and lumbar puncture are normal. Her symptoms improve with weight loss and diuretics.

3. A 21-year-old man presents in the Emergency Department with a 12-hour history of severe headache. On examination he is unwell, distressed and photophobic. He has marked meningism and cannot tolerate fundoscopy. There is no rash and no other clinical signs. Cerebrospinal fluid (CSF) examination reveals a raised lymphocyte count, and normal protein and glucose concentrations.

4. A 64-year-old man presents to his GP with a 24-hour history of right-sided weakness associated with a 3–4-day history of a worsening headache. On examination, he has a grade 3/5 right hemiparesis but nothing else of note. A CT head scan shows an isodense, concave rim over the left frontal and parietal lobes with significant mass effect to the right.

5. A 71-year-old woman presents to her GP with severe headaches over the forehead, associated with pain in her shoulders. Her cervical spine radiographs show mild osteoarthritic changes but her ESR is 110 mm/h.

6. THEME: EPONYMOUS SIGNS

A   Cullen's sign
B   de Musset's sign
C   Duroziez's sign
D   Chvostek's sign
E   Grey Turner's sign
F   Nikolsky's sign
G   Quinke's sign
H   Romberg's sign
I   Troisier's sign
J   Trousseau's sign

Each of the following presentations are associated with an eponymous sign or signs. Please choose the most appropriate from the above list. The options may be used once, more than once or not at all.

1. A 48-year-old Bengali woman presents in the Emergency Department with lethargy and several tonic-clonic seizures. Routine investigations show: corrected Ca^{2+} 1.83 mmol/l, PO_4^{3-} 2.10 mmol/l, alkaline phosphatase 498 IU/l.

2. A 38-year-old Somalian woman presents in the Emergency Department with severe shortness of breath on exercise. On examination, she has 'titubation of her head' and a loud early diastolic murmur that is heard best with patient leaning forwards in expiration. There are no features of infective endocarditis.

3. A 61-year-old man presents to his GP with a 3-month history of weight loss, lethargy and abdominal fullness on eating. On examination he has a large epigastric mass and is clinically anaemic.

4. A 37-year-old alcohol abuser is admitted to hospital with severe upper abdominal pains. He has marked abdominal tenderness and investigations show an amylase of 1080 IU/l and a marked metabolic acidosis.

5. A 63-year-old woman is seen by her GP with a severe blistering rash involving the upper and lower limbs, truncal areas and the mucous membranes of her mouth. While examining apparent normal areas of skin, firm pressure leads to shearing off of the skin.

7. THEME: ILIAC FOSSA MASSES

A   Appendix mass
B   Caecal carcinoma
C   Crohn's disease
D   Iliac artery aneurysm
E   Iliac lymphadenopathy
F   Ovarian cancer
G   Ovarian cyst
H   Pelvic kidney
I   Psoas abscess
J   Tuberculous ileitis
K   Undescended testis

The following are descriptions of patients who have presented with masses in their iliac fossae. Please select the most appropriate diagnosis from the above list. Each diagnosis may be used once, more than once or not at all.

1. A 19-year-old man presents with a 3-day history of right iliac fossa pain with nausea, anorexia and fever. On examination, he is pyrexial (temperature 38.2 °C) and has a tender, indistinct mass in the right iliac fossa associated with guarding.

2. A 25-year-old woman is seen in the Emergency Department with a 3-day history of severe, colicky right iliac fossa pain and diarrhoea. On questioning, she admits to having had several previous (though less severe) episodes over a 2-year period and weight loss of over 7 kg during this time. On examination there is a tender, indistinct mass in the right iliac fossa.

3. A 32-year-old man complains of weight loss, night sweats and dull abdominal pain over a period of several months. More recently, he has noticed a swelling in his left groin. On examination of this swelling, you also find a moderate-sized, indistinct mass in the left iliac fossa. There is no history of foreign travel.

4. A 66-year-old woman presents to her GP because she has noticed a large mass in her abdomen. Other than a dull lower abdominal ache and a slight decrease in appetite, she has had no other symptoms. On observation of the abdomen, there is a large left iliac fossa mass which, on palpation, has an easily defined upper border but which you cannot get below.

5. A 72-year-old man is referred to the clinic with anaemia (haemoglobin 9.4 g/dl, MCV 69.6 fl). He is otherwise asymptomatic. On examination, you feel a distinct, hard, mobile mass in the right iliac fossa.

8. THEME: NIPPLE DISCHARGE

A	Carcinoma of the breast
B	Fibrocystic disease of the breast (fibroadenosis)
C	Intraduct papilloma
D	Lactating breast
E	Mammary duct ectasia
F	Mammary duct fistula
G	Paget's disease of the nipple
H	Prolactinoma

The following patients have all presented with nipple discharge. Please select the most appropriate diagnosis from the above list. Each diagnosis may be used once, more than once or not at all.

1. A 35-year-old woman presents with a 2-month history of unilateral painless, serosanguinous nipple discharge. Examination is unremarkable, with no lumps palpable in either breast.

2. A 65-year-old woman presents with a 2-month history of cheese-like nipple discharge from her right breast and nipple retraction. Breast examination reveals a slit-like retraction of her right nipple, with no lumps palpable in her breast.

3. A 27-year-old woman is referred from the Fertility Clinic with a history of watery, whitish discharge from her breasts over several months. She also complains about recent problems with her vision. Examination of her breasts is unremarkable but she has bitemporal hemianopia.

4. A 66-year-old woman has been referred by her GP with unilateral heavily bloodstained nipple discharge.

5. A 40-year-old woman presents with a green–brown watery discharge from both nipples. She has a long history of mastalgia.

9. THEME: HAEMATURIA

A   Anticoagulant therapy
B   Catheter trauma
C   Cystitis
D   Glomerulonephritis
E   Polycystic kidney disease
F   Prostate carcinoma
G   Pyelonephritis
H   Renal-cell carcinoma
I   Squamous-cell carcinoma of bladder
J   Transitional-cell carcinoma of bladder
K   Urethritis
L   Urolithiasis

The following patients have all presented with haematuria. Please select the most appropriate diagnosis from the above list. Each option may be used once, more than once or not at all.

1. An obese, 70-year-old man attends his GP for a routine check-up. Apart from the backache that he has suffered for many years, he is also complaining of increasing dyspnoea. On examination, he is hypertensive, with a BP of 195/115 mmHg. Urinalysis shows: blood ++, protein +. Subsequent investigation reveals: haemoglobin 19.8 g/dl, corrected Ca^{2+} 3.0 mmol/l.

2. A 'miserable-looking' 12-year-old boy is accompanied by his concerned mother to the children's Emergency Department with lethargy, joint pain and puffiness around the eyes. On examination he has peri-orbital oedema. Two weeks before, the child was given penicillin for treatment of a recurrent sore throat. Urinalysis shows: blood +, protein +++.

3. A 65-year-old man with past medical history of recurrent urinary tract calculi attends his GP with a 6-month history of painless haematuria and recent weight loss. On examination, the patient looks thin and clinically anaemic. Urinalysis shows: blood +++, protein trace, nitrites negative. Other investigations show: haemoglobin 10.2 g/dl, WCC 9.0 × 10⁹/l; urea 7.2 mmol/l, creatinine 90 μmol/l; prostate-specific antigen (PSA) 2 ng/ml.

4. A 35-year-old woman visits her GP with a short history of painless haematuria. Three weeks before this visit, she was admitted to hospital for treatment of a pulmonary embolism after spending a holiday in Australia. Examination is unremarkable. Investigations show: haemoglobin 11.8 g/dl, WCC 8.9 × 10⁹/l; urea 3.2 mmol/l, creatinine 59 μmol/l. Urinalysis results: blood ++, protein trace, nitrites negative.

5. A 33-year-old man presents with a short history of severe right-sided abdominal pain that is radiating to the groin. He is writhing around, unable to sit or lie still. He has microscopic haematuria but an abdominal radiograph is normal.

10. THEME: GENITAL TRACT INFECTIONS

A   Bacterial vaginosis
B   *Candida albicans*
C   *Chlamydia trachomatis*
D   *Haemophilus ducreyi*
E   Herpes simplex virus
F   Human papillomavirus
G   *Neisseria gonorrhoeae*
H   *Sarcoptes scabei*
I   *Treponema pallidum*
J   *Trichomonas vaginalis*

From the above list please choose the infection or infectious agent most likely to cause the clinical picture described. Each organism may be used once, more than once or not at all.

1. A 30-year-old woman presents with a grey–white, offensive vaginal discharge. Microscopy of the discharge reveals 'clue cells' and the vaginal pH is raised.

2. A 28-year-old woman has a flu-like illness, followed shortly afterwards by the appearance of several painful vulval blisters. She has had no recent foreign travel. On examination she has bilateral tender inguinal lymphadenopathy.

3. Following a vaginal delivery by an asymptomatic woman, a baby develops ophthalmia neonatorum. Gram staining of the ophthalmic discharge reveals Gram-negative intracellular diplococci.

4. A 27-year-old woman has lower abdominal pain and on examination is found to have a temperature of 38 °C and cervical excitation on vaginal examination. Her partner is currently being treated for non-specific urethritis.

5. A 32-year-old woman presents with offensive, creamy-yellow vaginal discharge. Examination confirms this and microscopy of the discharge reveals motile, flagellated protozoa.

11. THEME: NEOPLASMS

A   Adenocarcinoma
B   Adenoma
C   Chondroma
D   Fibroadenoma
E   Lymphoma
F   Malignant melanoma
G   Malignant mesothelioma
H   Meningioma
I   Osteosarcoma
J   Squamous-cell carcinoma

From the above list, please select the neoplasm which each of the following patients is most likely to have. Each tumour may be used once, more than once or not at all.

1. A 65-year-old man presents with a 6-week history of rectal bleeding and altered bowel habit. Investigations show a mass in the sigmoid colon. Biopsy of the mass reveals a malignant tumour composed of glandular cells.

2. A 35-year-old woman attends for a routine cervical smear. This shows severely dyskaryotic cells and highly keratinised cells suspicious of malignancy. Colposcopy shows a 3-cm polypoid mass on the ectocervix which bleeds on contact. Biopsy confirms an invasive malignant tumour.

3. A 74-year-old man with Paget's disease of bone presents with a 2–month history of pain around the left hip joint. Radiographs of the hip and pelvis show a partly calcified lytic lesion in the left pelvic bone.

4. A 72-year-old man who had worked in a shipyard as a young man presents with a 6–month history of worsening dyspnoea. A radiograph and CT scan of the chest show a mass in the right pleural cavity. Biopsy shows a malignant biphasic tumour.

5. A 22-year-old woman presents with a 3-cm mobile breast lump which is solid and has well-defined margins on ultrasound examination. Fine-needle aspiration cytology (FNAC) shows benign cells.

12. THEME: RELATIONSHIPS IN THE MEDIASTINUM

A   Aortic arch
B   Azygos vein
C   Body of the fourth thoracic vertebra
D   Body of the seventh thoracic vertebra
E   Descending thoracic aorta
F   Inferior vena cava
G   Left vagus nerve
H   Oesophagus
I   Right phrenic nerve
J   Superior vena cava

For each of the following descriptions, please choose the most appropriate structure from the above list. The options may be used once, more than once or not at all.

1. Lies at the level of the xiphisternal joint. ☐

2. Lies wholly within the superior mediastinum. ☐

3. Has a lateral relationship to the right atrium. ☐

4. Passes through the diaphragm at the level of the tenth thoracic vertebra. ☐

5. Lies in the groove between the trachea and the oesophagus. ☐

13. THEME: CUTANEOUS INNERVATION OF THE UPPER LIMB

A   Anterior interosseous nerve
B   Axillary nerve
C   Lateral cutaneous nerve of forearm
D   Medial cutaneous nerve of forearm
E   Median nerve
F   Posterior cutaneous nerve of arm
G   Posterior cutaneous nerve of forearm
H   Posterior interosseous nerve
I   Radial nerve
J   Ulnar nerve

For each of the following cutaneous areas please choose the nerve that innervates it from the above list. The nerves may be used once, more than once or not at all.

1. Nail bed of the index finger.   ☐

2. Skin over the distal attachment of brachioradialis.   ☐

3. Skin over the pisiform bone.   ☐

4. Skin over the distal attachment of the deltoid muscle.   ☐

5. Skin over the common flexor origin.   ☐

14. THEME: CHEST RADIOGRAPHS – CLINICAL SCENARIOS

*Using the radiographic images **A–J on pages 345–347** please match the scenarios described below to the correct image. You may use each image once, more than once or not at all.*

1. A 38-year-old man presents to the Emergency Department with a 3–day history of a worsening cough productive of green sputum and right-sided, pleuritic chest pain. On auscultation of his chest your hear coarse crackles in the right axilla.

2. A 69-year-old man is brought into the Emergency Department by ambulance after being involved in a serious road traffic accident. Twenty minutes after arriving into the resuscitation area he becomes increasingly distressed, with severe chest pain and shortness of breath, and he rapidly becomes hypoxic, hypotensive and bradycardic.

3. A 48-year-old woman is seen in Emergency Department with a 3-month history of weight loss, night sweats and increasingly frequent episodes of frank haematuria. On examination, she is cachectic and clinically anaemic and has a ballotable mass in her left loin.

4. A 61-year-old woman who has been a lifelong smoker presents to the Emergency Department with weight loss, haemoptysis and generalised weakness. On examination, she appears to be cushingoid but is also cachectic and unwell. Investigations show: Na^+ 133 mmol/l, K^+ 2.0 mmol/l, urea 8.4 mmol/l, creatinine 77 μmol/l.

5. A 26-year-old woman with a previous history of 'severe' Epstein–Barr virus (EBV) infection as a teenager presents to her GP with increasing lethargy and malaise. On examination, she looks unwell and has large, firm lymphadenopathy in the neck and axilla. Further investigations confirm that she has Hodgkin's lymphoma.

Paper 1 Answers

1. UREA, ELECTROLYTES AND CREATININE

The blood urea and electrolytes (U&Es) and creatinine give us information about sodium and potassium metabolism and about basic renal function. In some laboratories, serum chloride and bicarbonate are also included in the 'U&Es' but with the advent of 'near patient testing', a basic U&Es screen usually comprises sodium, potassium, urea and creatinine. Sodium and potassium metabolism are intimately related and should be reviewed with respect to one another. The urea and creatinine are a reflection of basic renal function and need to be considered in light of the patient's clinical presentation. There are several common patterns of derangement which we have included in these examples but, as with many other things in medicine, basic principles are often useful in working out complex derangement.

1. **I – Na^+ 139 mmol/l, K^+ 2.0 mmol/l, urea 4.7 mmol/l, creatinine 87 μmol/l**
    This patient has presented with features of an adrenocorticotrophic hormone (ACTH-) secreting lung tumour. The cushingoid features and severe (often rapid-onset) hypokalaemia are both features of the steroid excess, and the weakness is a classic presentation of hypokalaemia. Other causes of hypokalaemia include loop and thiazide diuretics, potassium loss secondary to chronic diarrhoea, vomiting and renal causes such as renal tubular acidosis types 1 and 2.

2. **B – Na^+ 113 mmol/l, K^+ 4.9 mmol/l, urea 4.8 mmol/l, creatinine 89 μmol/l**
    This patient has pulmonary tuberculosis and this in turn has caused hyponatraemia secondary to syndrome of inappropriate antidiuretic hormone secretion (SIADH). To diagnose SIADH one must exclude other causes of hyponatraemia such as hypothyroidism, Addison's disease and drugs (eg diuretics). Before making a diagnosis of SIADH in a patient, they must be shown to be normotensive, euvolaemic and euthyroid, with normal renal function. Once these have been confirmed or corrected, patients should have a paired serum and urinary sodium test. SIADH is confirmed when the patient has hyponatraemia associated with an 'inappropriately (but relatively) concentrated urine with measurable urinary sodium'.

3. **F – Na^+ 129 mmol/l, K^+ 3.9 mmol/l, urea 24.8 mmol/l, creatinine 101 μmol/l**
    This scenario, an occult upper gastrointestinal bleed, causes an exaggeration of the normal pattern produced by pre-renal impairment. One can differentiate pre-renal from renal and obstructive renal impairment by looking at the urea:creatinine ratio. In pre-renal impairment, the distal convoluted tubule still retains a degree of functionality, which means that it is able to reabsorb urea. In pre-renal impairment, therefore, the rise in urea is far greater than the rise in creatinine. In renal impairment, this absorption can no longer occur so, in relative terms, the rise in creatinine is greater than the rise in urea. When they rise in equal proportions this usually infers a greater degree of renal impairment. In an upper gastrointestinal bleed, the blood tracking down the gastrointestinal tract forms a large protein meal. This is absorbed

and metabolised to urea, which is then excreted and reabsorbed in the kidney. The rise in urea is therefore often massive (as in this case) compared with the relatively normal creatinine. Any patient presenting with this derangement of their U&Es should have a rectal examination and be placed on a stool chart to exclude melaena.

4. **A – Na+ 105 mmol/l, K+ 1.0 mmol/l, urea 0.8 mmol/l, creatinine 29 μmol/l**
    When results really make no sense at all (as in this case) they are usually wrong! This also reinforces the old adage about treating the patient, not investigation results. All the values in this set of U&Es are literally 'watered down' and make no sense whatsoever. They need to be repeated, ensuring the same mistake does not happen again. Turning a drip off for a few minutes will be enough to allow a proximal sample to be taken if no other veins are available.

5. **E or G – Na+ 128 mmol, K+ 8.9 mmol/l, urea 13.3 mmol/l, creatinine 139 μmol/l (or Na+ 132 mmol, K+ 5.9 mmol/l, urea 32.8 mmol/l, creatinine 809 μmol/l)**
    Both results reflect a patient with impaired renal function, hyperkalaemia and hyponatraemia. These are common findings in patients on angiotensin-converting enzyme (ACE) inhibitors, angiotensin II-receptor blockers or potassium-sparing diuretics, especially in sick elderly patients who have poor functional renal reserve.

2. ANAEMIA

1. **E – Iron deficiency**
   This patient has been started on clopidogrel, which is one of the newer antiplatelet treatments used in ischaemic heart disease and in cerebrovascular disease. Like aspirin, it causes upper gastrointestinal inflammation and subsequent occult or frank upper gastrointestinal blood loss. The blood results show a microcytic anaemia compatible with iron-deficiency secondary to the blood loss.

2. **B – Aplastic anaemia**
   This patient has developed aplastic anaemia secondary to his phenytoin therapy. this is thankfully a relatively uncommon side-effect of a number of medications which are remembered by the fact that most are an 'anti' treatment – antibiotic (sulphonamides and chloramphenicol), antiepileptic (phenytoin), anti-inflammatory (indometacin and gold therapy), antithyroid (propylthiouracil, carbimazole), antiemetic (prochlorperazine), anti-cancer (all chemotherapeutic agents) and anti-hyperglycaemics (chlorpropamide).

3. **G – Pancytopenia secondary to multiple myeloma**
   This patient has developed a pancytopenia secondary to her multiple myeloma. She also has renal failure, hypercalcaemia and a grossly elevated erythrocyte sedimentation rate (ESR), all in keeping with the diagnosis. Other investigations should include plasma electrophoresis, looking for monoclonal gammopathy with associated immunoparesis, urinary Bence Jones protein and skeletal radiographs (in this patient's case, of the lumbar spine) looking for lytic bone lesions. (**NB**: Lytic bone lesions do not show up on a radioisotope bone scan.)

4. **J – Thalassaemia trait**
   This patient has a microcytic anaemia but if one compares the MCV in this patient with that of the patient in questions 1 we can see that there is a grossly reduced MCV in proportion to the degree of anaemia. This, and the normal ferritin are highly suggestive of anaemia secondary to thalassaemia trait. The diagnosis should be confirmed on haemoglobin electrophoresis and the patient's relatives should also be screened.

5. **C – Autoimmune haemolytic anaemia**
   This woman has developed a Coombs-positive haemolytic anaemia secondary to her pneumonia, the most likely cause of which is an atypical infection with an organism such as *Mycoplasma*. Coombs-positive haemolytic anaemias are subdivided into 'warm' and 'cold' types, on the basis of whether the autoantibodies produced attach to the red cells at body temperature (warm) or at 4 °C (cold). Warm antibodies are principally IgG and IgA and are often idiopathic. They can be associated with haematological malignancies such as lymphoma and leukaemia, carcinoma and, classically, with the antihypertensive drug methyldopa. Cold antibodies (IgM) can also be idiopathic but are produced in association with Epstein–Barr virus (EBV) and *Mycoplasma* infections as well as lymphomas.

3. RESPIRATORY FAILURE

1. **A – Asbestosis**
   This man has developed asbestosis secondary to his previous employment. The asbestos fibres cause an inflammatory response over the pleural, pericardial and diaphragmatic surfaces, leading to the formation of asbestos 'plaques'. These are signs of asbestos exposure but not of asbestosis. Asbestosis is the pneumoconiosis associated with asbestos exposure and this causes a basal fibrosis (unlike the other pneumoconioses, which predominantly cause upper-zone/apical fibrosis). They can all progress to cause overwhelming pulmonary fibrosis and 'honeycomb' lung. Initially, patients develop a type-I respiratory failure, as in this case, but later on, with more diffuse disease, the patient can develop a type-II picture. Other complications include the development of mesothelioma, which can occur 30 or more years after the exposure.

2. **H – Pickwickian syndrome**
   This obese man with chronic obstructive pulmonary disease (COPD) has developed Pickwickian syndrome. His early-morning headaches and daytime somnolence result from his nocturnal hypoventilation, hypercapnia and intermittent episodes of sleep apnoea and waking. Patients classically have episodes of snoring followed by episodes of upper-airway obstruction and apnoea. They should be treated as for any patient with COPD but should be encouraged to lose weight and might benefit from non-invasive ventilation at , which maintains the patency of the upper airway and thus oxygenation, while avoiding the apnoea and hypercapnia.

3. **J – Pulmonary oedema**
   This woman has developed pulmonary oedema, as shown by the classic 'bat-wing' appearance on the chest radiograph. Her arterial blood gases reveal a type-I respiratory failure and a metabolic acidosis secondary to a lactic acidosis due to tissue hypoxia. She should be treated with 60–100% oxygen, should sit upright and should be given diuretics. If she remains hypotensive she will need intravenous inotropic support.

4. **F – *Legionella* pneumonia**
   This woman has developed a dry, non-productive cough, type-I respiratory failure, hyponatraemia and mild renal impairment. This picture is highly suggestive of an atypical pneumonia and in particular of *Legionella pneumophila* infection. This diagnosis is confirmed, as in this case, by the presence of urinary antigens.

5. **E – Idiopathic pulmonary fibrosis**
   This man has developed signs and symptoms suggestive of a fibrotic lung condition, in particular idiopathic pulmonary fibrosis or cryptogenic fibrosing alveolitis. This is a basal fibrotic disease which has no identifiable cause. A very similar condition is seen in rheumatoid arthritis and in other connective tissue diseases. The patients have type-I respiratory failure and show a restrictive picture on spirometry. They can develop a more diffuse fibrotic picture over time and go on to develop type-II failure.

4. ASCITES

1. **F – Ovarian carcinoma**
    A middle-aged woman presenting with ascites but with no history of liver disease or alcohol excess should be assumed to have ovarian carcinoma until proved otherwise. The Ca-125 is a marker of ovarian carcinoma, although it is better employed as a treatment marker rather than as a diagnostic tool. The diagnosis can be confirmed by ascitic cytology, ultrasound scan of the pelvis or laparoscopy and biopsy.

2. **E –Ischaemic cardiomyopathy**
    This chronic smoker (as evidenced by her tar-stained fingers) has signs consistent with gross primarily right-sided heart failure. Her signs of right heart failure include her peripheral oedema, ascites, raised jugular venous pressure (JVP) and tricuspid regurgitation. Her electrocardiogram (ECG) suggests an old anterior myocardial infarct. This is the clinical picture of chronic ischaemic cardiomyopathy.

3. **H – Peritoneal mesothelioma**
    This retired docker has signs suggestive of peritoneal mesothelioma. Prolonged asbestos exposure can lead to pleural, pericardial and diaphragmatic plaques, pulmonary fibrosis (asbestosis) and pleural and peritoneal mesothelioma. This relatively rare malignancy has a poor prognosis and at present the only treatments available are palliative.

4. **I – Renal-cell carcinoma**
    This man has night sweats, lethargy, a microcytic anaemia and cannon-ball metastases on his chest radiograph. The diagnosis of renal-cell carcinoma can be confirmed on urine cytology, renal ultrasound scan or a computed tomographic (CT) scan of the abdomen. Depending on the tumour stage and the histology, patients (if well enough) might be offered nephrectomy, chemotherapy and radiotherapy.

5. **J – Tuberculosis**
    White people with this presentation and these CT findings would be assumed to have Crohn's disease or backwash ileitis of ulcerative colitis. Asian people, however, rarely develop inflammatory bowel disease and this is a typical presentation of tuberculous ileitis and secondary peritoneal tuberculous infection. The patient should be treated with a 6-month course of antituberculous treatment and might need nutritional supplements and, more rarely, bowel resection.

5. HEADACHE

1. **F – Saggital sinus thrombosis**
   This patient has developed saggital sinus thrombosis secondary to her oral contraceptive pill. Similar in pathogenesis to deep vein thrombosis and pulmonary embolism, saggital sinus thrombosis can occur in females or males with thrombophilic tendencies. Risk factors include dehydration, malignancy, the oral contraceptive pill (in females), thrombocytosis and the congenital coagulopathies, including antiphospholipid syndrome, factor V Leiden deficiency, protein C and protein S deficiency and antithrombin III deficiency.

2. **A – Benign intracranial hypertension**
   This obese woman has developed 'benign' intracranial hypertension. This is a diagnosis of exclusion and is not truly benign as it can lead to blindness. Patients should be encouraged to lose weight (if overweight) and often improve with diuretics.

3. **E – Viral meningitis**
   This patient has developed viral meningitis, as evidenced by the normal cerebrospinal fluid (CSF) glucose and protein levels and lymphocytosis. The clinical picture can be very similar to that of bacterial or tuberculous meningitis, but it is rarely fatal and primarily requires symptomatic relief with analgesia, antiemetics and intravenous fluids. Patients should be nursed in a quiet darkened side room until the diagnosis is confirmed.

4. **I – Subdural haemorrhage**
   This man has a left-sided frontoparietal subdural haemorrhage with significant mass effect to the right. The haematoma has caused a similar clinical picture to that of a stroke with hemiparesis. The patient should be referred for an urgent neurosurgical opinion and evacuation of the subdural haemorrhage.

5. **C – Giant-cell arteritis**
   This patient has frontal headaches associated with shoulder pains and an ESR of 110 mm/h. This is the typical picture of giant-cell arteritis. The patient should be started immediately on steroids (prednisolone 30–40 mg a day) and an attempt to confirm the diagnosis (by temporal artery biopsy) should be made within 48 hours of the initiation of steroids.

6. EPONYMOUS SIGNS

Despite the facts that eponymous disorders or signs were rarely described first by their namesake, that they often have little clinical significance, and that they merely confuse the overstressed (and underprepared) student, we make no apologies for including a few historical facts about the eponymous signs in this question.

1. **D, J – Chvostek's and Trousseau's signs**
    This patient has developed osteomalacia and subsequent marked hypocalcaemia, confirmed by Chvostek's and Trousseau's signs. Chvostek's sign (Franz Chvostek, 1835–1884, Viennese physician): this sign is positive when the seventh (facial) nerve is lightly tapped below the ear, producing ipsilateral hemifacial spasm. Trousseau's sign (Armand Trousseau, 1801–1867, Parisian physician): in this sign, the hand goes into a characteristic spasm (*main d'accoucher*) when a blood pressure cuff is inflated for several minutes above systolic blood pressure.

2. **B, C, G – de Musset's, Duroziez's and Quinke's signs**
    This patient has signs consistent with significant aortic regurgitation. There are several eponymous signs associated with this disorder, many of which relate to the significant 'collapsing' wave of blood back through the regurgitant valve. Alfred De Musset was a relatively famous nineteenth-century French poet who had significant aortic regurgitation; his (less famous) brother, a physician, described the associated nodding or titubation of the head. Duroziez's sign (Paul Duroziez, 1826–1897, French physician) is the most significant clinical sign of aortic regurgitation. It is a diastolic and systolic bruit heard over the femoral pulse while attempting to occlude the pulse distal to the stethoscope with the fingers (thus attempting to stop the regurgitant wave travelling back towards the heart). Quinke's sign (Heinrich Quinke, German neurologist, 1842–1922) is also known as the 'lighthouse sign' and consists of flushing of the capillary bed when the fingernail is pressed distally.

3. **I – Troisier's sign**
    This patient has signs of gastric carcinoma. This can be associated with Troisier's sign and with Sister Joseph's nodule. Troisier's sign (Charles Emile Troisier, 1844–1919, professor of pathology, Paris): a left supraclavicular fossa lymph node, eponymously known as 'Virchow's node'. Sister Joseph's nodule was described by Sister Joseph to Dr William Mayo (of the Mayo Clinic and also of salad dressing fame), and is a metastatic deposit within the umbilicus.

4. **A, E, J – Cullen's, Grey Turner's and Trousseau's signs**
    This man has developed acute severe pancreatitis. This is associated with signs of peritonism and, more rarely, with Grey Turner's sign (bruising in the flanks, named for George Grey Turner, an English surgeon) or with Cullen's sign (peri-umbilical haematoma or 'umbilical black eye'), which was first described by Thomas Cullen (1869–1953, professor of obstetrics) in relation to a ruptured ectopic pregnancy. Severe, acute pancreatitis is also associated with hyopocalcaemia.

5. **F – Nikolsky's sign**
    Nikolsky's sign (Pyotr Nikolsky, b. 1858, a dermatologist who worked in Russia and Poland) is commonly seen in pemphigus and other blistering conditions such as dermatitis herpetiformis and drug eruptions. Firm pressure is applied to 'apparently' normal skin, which then shears away.

7. ILIAC FOSSA MASSES

1. **A – Appendix mass**
   In a young man, an appendix mass tops the list of likely diagnoses (tubo-ovarian causes are probably most common in females of this age). The history is characteristic of acute appendicitis, in this case complicated by mass formation. It is caused by adherence of omentum or other adjacent viscera to a severely inflamed or locally perforated appendix, and can have an abscess component. Depending on the clinical state of the patient, and to some extent the size of the mass, treatment can be surgical or conservative (intravenous antibiotics).

2. **C – Crohn's disease**
   The preceding history should alert you to this diagnosis in a patient who might otherwise have an acute history and findings compatible with a diagnosis of appendicitis. The management depends on the patient's overall clinical condition, but surgery should ideally be avoided and the patient with acute Crohn's disease should be treated medically and the disease assessed further by appropriate imaging.

3. **E – Iliac lymphadenopathy**
   The history here suggests a diagnosis of lymphoma, although tuberculosis (TB) might also be a possibility had there been a history of exposure. The patient has presented with inguinal lymph nodes but he also has an iliac node mass.

4. **F – Ovarian cancer**
   A mass of this size in a woman strongly suggests this diagnosis. Other symptoms can include weight loss, vaginal bleeding from hormone disturbance or endometrial invasion, and unilateral leg swelling resulting from lymphatic or venous compression. In addition to a palpable mass, there might be ascites. The patient might also be anaemic and have lymphadenopathy. (The classification of ovarian tumours and their treatment is covered elsewhere.)

5. **B – Caecal carcinoma**
   With a microcytic anaemia in a patient of this age (ie an age in which cancer is prevalent) you should strongly consider bleeding into the gastrointestinal tract as a result of neoplasia to be a possibility (the urogenital tract being the other major contender). Of the gastrointestinal malignancies, caecal carcinoma is the commonest cause of asymptomatic anaemia because other more distal colonic sites of malignancy tend to cause other symptoms such as diarrhoea or rectal bleeding, and gastric cancer is less common than colorectal cancer. Colonoscopy (ideally) or barium enema is indicated.

8. NIPPLE DISCHARGE

There are five common causes of nipple discharge: breast cancer, fibrocystic disease of the breast, intraduct papilloma, mammary duct ectasia and lactation. The main points in to consider in the diagnosis are whether discharge is unilateral or bilateral and whether it is bloodstained.

1. **C – Intraduct papilloma**

   This should be suspected from the age of the patient (younger than carcinoma) and the solitary symptom of recurrent bloodstained nipple discharge without the finding of a discrete lump. A true papilloma is usually single and occurs in a major duct in the subareolar area. The tumour consists of hyperplastic columnar epithelium with a rich blood supply (hence the presentation). They are entirely benign. Mammography might show a dilated duct behind the papilloma, although there is usually no visible abnormality. Treatment is excision of the involved duct (microdochectomy).

2. **E – Mammary duct ectasia**

   Symptomatic duct ectasia is best considered as an aberration of normal breast involution. Duct ectasia principally affects older women and presents as a slit-like retraction of the nipple or with nipple discharge (brown-green or cheese-like). No special treatment is required unless the discharge becomes troublesome, when a microdochectomy (excision of one duct) or subareolar resection (of multiple ducts) can be performed.

3. **H – Prolactinoma**

   Prolactinomas are benign tumours of the anterior pituitary. They are four times more common in women than in men and usually present in young women in their second and third decades with a history of amenorrhoea (fertility problems) and galactorrhoea (as in this case). Tumours <1 cm in diameter are called 'microadenomas' and if they are >2 cm, 'macroadenomas'. The latter can extend into the suprasellar region, causing optic chiasma compression and visual failure. Treatment is usually by trans-sphenoidal resection.

4. **A – Carcinoma of the breast**

   In a patient of this age with unilateral bloodstained nipple discharge, this diagnosis should be considered before all others, regardless of other clinical findings.

5. **B – Fibrocystic disease of the breast (fibroadenosis)**

   The bilaterality and colour of the discharge, in association with mastalgia, point to this diagnosis. This is a diffuse and painful benign condition of the breast that occurs in women aged 25–45. The condition is characterised by exacerbations and remissions that are usually cyclical with the menses. The disorder is probably caused by abnormal expression of physiological proliferative and involutionary changes. There are four main pathological processes: adenosis, epitheliosis, fibrosis and cyst formation. The diagnosis is made on the basis of the history and examination and mammography/ultrasound, with or without cyst aspiration and cytological examination.

9. HAEMATURIA

1. **H – Renal-cell carcinoma**
   The textbook description of a 'classic triad' of findings in renal-cell carcinoma (haematuria, loin pain and abdominal mass) can in practice be obscured in an obese, elderly patient with chronic back pain. However, other less common but well-recognised paraneoplastic effects – hypertension, polycythaemia and hypercalcaemia (secondary to ectopic production of renin, erythropoietin and parathyroid hormone, respectively) – and effects of lung secondaries (dyspnoea) should alert you to the possibility of this diagnosis. Genitourinary tumours (renal, testicular and ovarian) commonly cause cannonball pulmonary metastases.

2. **D – Glomerulonephritis**
   The patient has developed a post-streptococcal (and therefore usually proliferative) glomerulonephritis. This condition usually develops 2–3 weeks after the streptococcal infection and presents with features of the nephrotic syndrome (generalised oedema, hypoproteinaemia, proteinuria). Investigations include throat swab for microscopy, culture and sensitivity and antistreptolysin-O titre (ASOT) serology. Treatment is mainly supportive, with elimination of the *Streptococcus* infection itself. The prognosis in terms of progression to renal failure is excellent.

3. **J – Transitional-cell carcinoma of bladder**
   Painless haematuria in this age group should be considered indicative of this diagnosis because it is more common than renal-cell carcinoma. While squamous-cell carcinoma of bladder is weakly associated with chronic urolithiasis, this is still a very uncommon tumour in Western populations (in whom schistosomiasis is not endemic).

4. **A – Anticoagulant therapy**
   Warfarin treatment is a common iatrogenic cause of haematuria (the other being urethral trauma from catheterisation). The international normalised ratio (INR) (or partial thromboplastin time, PTT) should be checked and the dose adjusted if required. Patients might still require cystoscopy to exclude a bleeding lesion.

5. **L – Urolithiasis**
   This patient has ureteric colic, which is caused by calculus obstruction of the right ureter. The appearance of a patient unable to get comfortable in any position is classic for this condition, which causes acute, very severe, colicky pain, which can be felt in the abdomen or loin and classically radiates to the groin or even to the tip of the penis. The finding of blood in the urine in a male invariably indicates pathology and is consistent with this diagnosis. The abdominal radiograph is normal because a proportion of ureteric stones are radiolucent. The confirmatory investigation is an intravenous urogram (IVU), provided this is not contraindicated (asthma/allergy).

10. GENITAL TRACT INFECTIONS

1. **A – Bacterial vaginosis**
   Bacterial vaginosis is a polymicrobial disturbance of the vaginal flora that is characterised by a lack of lactobacilli and overgrowth of anaerobic bacteria. The vaginal discharge is homogenous, grey in colour and offensive (due to anaerobic byproducts). 'Clue' cells are epithelial cells coated with anaerobes ('iron filings') and the raised vaginal pH (>4.5) is likely to be the underlying cause of the bacterial imbalance – together with the characteristic discharge and a positive amine test with potassium hydroxide, these cells are diagnostic of bacterial vaginosis. *Trichomonas* is the only other likely cause of offensive discharge but this does not fulfil the other criteria.

2. **E – Herpes simplex virus**
   Primary herpes simplex virus (HSV) infection is characterised by viraemic symptoms followed by multiple painful vulval ulcers and tender lymphadenopathy. Syphilitic ulcers (chancres) are classically single and non-painful and are not usually preceded by a flu-like illness. *Haemophilus ducreyi* (chancroid) also tends to cause single lesions without systemic upset, and foreign travel is nearly always involved.

3. **G – *Neisseria gonorrhoeae***
   Ophthalmia neonatorum is transmitted to the fetus via contact with infected endocervical secretions during vaginal delivery in women with asymptomatic *Neisseria gonorrhoeae* or, more commonly, *Chlamydia trachomatis* organisms. *N. gonorrhoeae* are Gram-negative intracellular diplococci and are commonly seen on Gram staining of infected secretions. Though intracellular, *C. trachomatis* are not visible on microscopy of Gram stained preparations.

4. **C – *Chlamydia trachomatis***
   Acute pelvic inflammatory disease is characterised by lower pelvic pain plus at least two of the following: temperature >38 °C, pulse >90 bpm, peritonism, cervical excitation and adnexal tenderness and a raised WCC. Pelvic inflammatory disease is caused by *Chlamydia* organisms commonly and by *Neisseria gonorrhoeae* less commonly. 'Non-specific urethritis' is an umbrella term for urethritis before a causative organism is found (or not), the commonest cause being *Chlamydia*. Infection with *N. gonorrhoeae* in men is usually picked up at the time of presentation with symptoms using Gram staining of urethral discharge, and would therefore be very unlikely to be labelled as 'non-specific urethritis'.

5. **J – *Trichomonas vaginalis***
   Trichomonas vaginalis and bacterial vaginosis both cause offensive vaginal discharge but *Trichomonas* is a motile, flagellated protozoon that can be seen when discharge is placed in a spot of saline on a microscopy slide.

11. NEOPLASMS

1. **A – Adenocarcinoma**
    An adenocarcinoma is a malignant tumour originating in glandular epithelium; an adenoma is the benign counterpart. Adenocarcinoma is the most common malignant tumour of the large intestine and is increasing in frequency, accounting for up to 15% of cancer-related deaths in industrialised countries. Rectal bleeding and altered bowel habit are typical presenting features of adenocarcinomas arising in the left side of the colon, while caecal and right-sided tumours more frequently present with anaemia.

2. **J – Squamous-cell carcinoma**
    The main differential diagnosis of a malignant tumour of the cervix lies between squamous-cell carcinoma and adenocarcinoma. Squamous-cell carcinomas are more common than adenocarcinomas, accounting for about 80% of all cervical malignancies. Well-differentiated squamous-cell carcinoma produces keratin and this can be seen on a cervical smear as atypical keratinised cells.

3. **I – Osteosarcoma**
    This is the typical presentation of an osteosarcoma arising on a background of Paget's disease of the bone. Osteosarcoma is a malignant tumour of osteoblasts (bone-forming cells) and has a bimodal age distribution. So-called 'primary' osteosarcoma occurs predominantly in teenage boys and most commonly around the knee. 'Secondary' osteosarcomas develop as a complication of Paget's disease of the bone and therefore occur in the elderly. In this setting the most common sites of origin are the pelvis, femur and humerus. The malignant osteoblasts produce varying amounts of osteoid, some of which becomes mineralised, and this can be seen radiologically.

4. **G – Malignant mesothelioma**
    Malignant mesothelioma is a tumour of mesothelial cells that arises most commonly in the visceral or parietal pleura. Approximately 50% of patients with malignant mesothelioma have a history of exposure to asbestos, usually related to their occupation. Shipyard workers, miners and insulators are at greatest risk. The latent period for developing this tumour is long, often 25–40 years after initial exposure. Malignant mesothelioma is a biphasic tumour, with both sarcomatoid and epithelioid elements. In this scenario, the differential diagnosis lies between malignant mesothelioma, squamous-cell carcinoma and adenocarcinoma. The location of the tumour in the pleural cavity is strongly suggestive of mesothelioma but it is only the biphasic nature of the tumour that distinguishes it from a squamous-cell carcinoma or an adenocarcinoma.

5. **D – Fibroadenoma**
    Fibroadenoma is the commonest benign tumour of the breast and occurs most frequently in young women. Fibroadenomas arise from the breast lobule and are mixed tumours containing both glandular epithelium and connective tissue stroma. Like areas of fibrocystic change, the epithelium of a fibroadenoma is hormonally responsive and there can therefore be a slight increase in size during the second half of the menstrual cycle. Unlike fibrocystic change, however, fibroadenomas are well circumscribed and solid, with a lobulated macroscopic appearance. Fibroadenomas are not tethered to the surrounding breast tissue and this accounts for their mobility on palpation.

12. RELATIONSHIPS IN THE MEDIASTINUM

1. **C – Body of the fourth thoracic vertebra**
   The line from the sternal angle to the middle of the body of the fourth thoracic vertebra separates the superior mediastinum above from the anterior, middle and posterior mediastinum below. The sternal angle is also the marking for the second costal cartilage and this is a useful marker when counting ribs.

2. **A – Aortic arch**
   The aortic arch is formed from the ascending aorta and becomes the descending aorta. It lies within the superior mediastinum, giving off its innominate, left common carotid and left subclavian arterial branches. It arches over the hilum of the left lung.

3. **I – Right phrenic nerve**
   The right phrenic is also in a lateral relationship with the inferior vena cava and with the superior vena cava. It pierces the central dome of the diaphragm and innervates the right half from its undersurface.

4. **H – Oesophagus**
   The oesophagus pierces the right crus of the diaphragm at this level. The inferior vena cava pierces the central tendon at the level of the eighth thoracic vertebra and the aorta passes between the right and left crura at the level of the body of the twelfth thoracic vertebra.

5. **G – Left vagus nerve**
   The vagi contribute to the pulmonary and cardiac plexuses before uniting as the oesophageal plexus around the lower oesophagus. They then form the anterior and posterior vagal trunks, which pass with the oesophagus into the abdomen as the anterior and posterior gastric nerves.

13. CUTANEOUS INNERVATION OF THE UPPER LIMB

1. **E – Median nerve**
   The median nerve supplies the lateral aspect of the palm, the palmar aspect of the thumb and adjacent two and a half fingers, and their nailbeds.

2. **C – Lateral cutaneous nerve of forearm**
   This nerve is a continuation of the musculocutaneous nerve. The radial nerve overlaps its innervation over the snuffbox and also supplies a limited area over the dorsolateral aspect of the hand.

3. **J – Ulnar nerve**
   The ulnar nerve supplies the cutaneous innervation of the medial aspect of the palm and one and a half fingers through its palmar branch and, through its dorsal branch, the dorsal surface of the medial three and a half fingers.

4. **B – Axillary nerve**
   This is through its upper lateral cutaneous nerve of arm branch and has important clinical implications because it is a convenient way to test the integrity of the axillary nerve after shoulder dislocation, pain making it difficult to confirm associated paralysis of the deltoid muscle.

5. **D – Medial cutaneous nerve of forearm**
   This nerve pierces the deep fascia in the mid upper arm with the basilic vein. It supplies the skin over the medial aspect of the cubital fossa and forearm to the wrist.

14. CHEST RADIOGRAPHS – CLINICAL SCENARIOS

1. **(P1–P2) C – Right middle lobe pneumonia**
   This man has symptoms and signs suggestive of a right middle lobe pneumonia. Other signs of consolidation include dullness to percussion, increased tactile and vocal fremitus, and bronchial breathing.

2. **(P1–P2) J – Right-sided tension pneumothorax**
   This man has developed a tension pneumothorax secondary to the trauma of his road traffic accident. He requires immediate insertion of a chest drain, oxygen via a mask and, once stabilised, needs to be admitted to a high-dependency area within the hospital.

3. **(P1–P2) F – Cannonball metastases**
   This patient has signs consistent with a left-sided renal tumour, which in turn might be associated with cannonball metastases. Renal tumours are one of the commonly forgotten differential diagnoses of the causes of night sweats, fevers and weight loss.

4. **(P1–P2) E – Right lower zone primary**
   This patient has presented with a bronchogenic carcinoma associated with ectopic ACTH secretion, in turn producing the cushingoid features and the marked hypokalalaemia. Ectopic ACTH secretion is most commonly associated with small-cell and carcinoid tumours.

5. **(P1–P2) G – Bilateral hilar lymphadenopathy**
   This patient has developed Hodgkin's lymphoma following an EBV infection several years earlier. As well as a chest radiograph, staging should be undertaken, with chest, abdomen and pelvic CT scans. EBV is strongly implicated in the development of Burkitt's lymphoma, a non-Hodgkin's lymphoma, particularly in African children who have previously had chronic malaria. However, EBV is also associated with the development of Hodgkin's lymphoma and even more closely with nasopharyngeal carcinoma.

IMAGES: pages 345–347

PAPER 2

Paper 2 Questions

1. THEME: HEART SOUNDS

A   Early diastolic murmur
B   Early systolic murmur
C   Ejection systolic click
D   Fourth heart sound
E   Late systolic murmur
F   Mid-diastolic murmur
G   Mid-systolic click
H   Opening snap
I   Pansystolic murmur
J   Third heart sound

The following patients have all presented with added heart sounds on auscultation. Please choose the most appropriate options from the above list. The options may be used once, more than once, in combination or not at all.

1. A 64-year-old man presents in the Emergency Department with increasing angina and two episodes of collapse on exertion. Of note, his BP is 110/100 mmHg and his ECG shows the voltage criteria of left ventricular hypertrophy (LVH).

2. A 71-year-old woman attends the Emergency Department with acute shortness of breath. On examination, she is cold and clammy with a BP of 80/40 mmHg, and is tachycardic with a pulse of 120 bpm. No murmurs are heard. Her ECG confirms a large anterior myocardial infarction.

3. A 32-year-old Somalian woman is admitted to hospital with heart failure. On examination she is noted to have a collapsing pulse, de Musset's sign and a grossly displaced, hyperdynamic apex beat.

4. A 69-year-old man with a previous history of rheumatic fever is admitted for a valve replacement. He is noted to have a low-volume radial pulse, atrial fibrillation (rate 70–80 bpm) and a BP of 120/70 mmHg, and has a 'tapping', undisplaced apex beat.

5. A 19-year-old woman is reviewed by an anaesthetist prior extraction of a wisdom tooth. She notes that the patient has an 'innocent' murmur consistent with a floppy mitral valve. The ECG reveals anterolateral T-wave inversion.

2. THEME: FULL BLOOD COUNT

	Haemoglobin (g/dl))	MCV (fl)	WCC (cells 10⁹/l)	Differential WCC (cells × 10⁹/l)	Platelets (cells × 10⁹/l)	Other information
A	4.9	124	4.8	Normal	75	
B	7.8	87	7.2	Normal	312	
C	7.9	85	1.8	Neutrophils 0.7	38	Blood film shows rouleaux
D	8.3	65	7.4	Normal	343	
E	10.5	89	146.5	Lymphocytes 136.8	128	
F	11.1	55	6.8	Normal	288	
G	12.9	82	7.9	Normal	2809	
H	13.9	83	6.6	Normal	365	
I	14.6	90	8.0	Normal	18	
J	18.9	80	13.8	Neutrophils 11.9	406	Haematocrit 0.58

The following patients have all presented with signs and symptoms secondary to abnormalities of their full blood count (FBC). Please choose the most likely abnormal FBC profile responsible from the above list. The options may be used once, more than once or not at all.

1. A 39-year-old woman presents to her GP with increasing lethargy and malaise. The GP finds she that she is clinically anaemic and has vitiligo on her left forearm. Her blood film demonstrates hypersegmented neutrophils.

2. A 76-year-old woman presents to the Emergency Department with increasing malaise and painless swelling of the lymph nodes in her neck and under her arms. Her blood film confirms the presence of large numbers of 'smudge cells'.

3. A 54-year-old man presents to his GP with a 3-month history of weight loss, increasing early satiety on eating and general malaise. He is weighed, which shows that he has lost 8 kg over a period of 6 months, he has a palpable, large, firm, left supraclavicular lymph node and an epigastric fullness.

4. A 67-year-old woman presents to her GP with pains in her arms, legs and lumbar spine. On further questioning, she admits that she has been unwell for several months with recurrent 'coughs and colds', weight loss and general malaise. Initial investigations show an ESR of 110 mm/h and a corrected Ca^{2+} of 3.43 mmol/l.

5. A 69-year-old woman presents to her GP with headaches, itching, particularly when going to the sauna in her gym, and night sweats. On examination, she is obviously plethoric and has splenomegaly 6 cm below the left costal margin. The diagnosis is confirmed by her FBC and by measuring the total red cell volume, which is shown to be 39 ml/kg.

3. THEME: CHEST PATHOLOGY

A   Empyema
B   Haemothorax
C   Lobar collapse
D   Pleural effusion
E   Pneumothorax
F   Pulmonary consolidation
G   Pulmonary embolism
H   Pulmonary fibrosis
I   Pulmonary oedema
J   Tension pneumothorax

The following patients have all presented with chest 'problems'. Please choose the most appropriate cause from the above list. Each option may be used once, more than once or not at all.

1. A 23-year-old man re-presents 2 weeks after being admitted with a spontaneous pneumothorax. On examination, he is unwell, tachypnoeic and pyrexial. On examination of his chest, he has decreased expansion on the left (the side of his previous pneumothorax), there is dullness to percussion with reduced breath sounds and tactile vocal fremitus on the left.

2. A 47-year-old man being investigated for weight loss and haemoptysis is admitted with increasing exertional dyspnoea. He has a right-sided Horner's syndrome and, on examination of his chest, he has dullness to percussion extending up to the mid-zone on the right associated with quiet breath sounds and reduced tactile vocal fremitus. Whispering pectoriloquy is also reduced.

3. A 57-year-old previous pipe lagger and boiler fitter presents to his GP with a 6-month history of increasing exertional dyspnoea. On examination, he has clubbing of the fingernails and marked fine inspiratory basal crepitations, which are unchanged with coughing. His chest radiograph shows multiple pleural and diaphragmatic shadows.

4. A 29-year-old woman presents in the Emergency Department with acute shortness of breath. On examination she is obviously distressed and tachypnoeic. She is apyrexial and her oxygen saturation is 98% on air. Examination of her chest reveals her trachea to be in the midline and a hyper-resonant percussion note on the right associated with markedly reduced breath sounds and vocal fremitus.

5. A previously fit and well, 21-year-old man presents in the Emergency Department with a 4-day history of increasing shortness of breath, pleuritic chest pain and a productive cough. On examination, he looks unwell, he is tachypnoeic and pyrexial. Examination of his chest reveals reduced expansion on the right, secondary to pain, and dullness to percussion associated with bronchial breathing and increased vocal fremitus in the right axilla.

4. THEME: ORAL AND GLOSSAL LESIONS

A Aphthous ulceration
B Atrophic glossitis
C Candidiasis
D Geographic tongue
E Kaposi's sarcoma
F Lichen planus
G Perifollicular haemorrhages
H Oral hairy leukoplakia
I Snail track ulceration
J Tonsillitis

The following patients have all presented with oral and/or glossal lesions. Please choose the most appropriate cause from the above list. Options may be used once, more than once, in combination or not at all.

1. A 29-year-old Malawian man presents in the Emergency Department with weight loss and a 4-day history of confusion and left-sided paresis. On examination, he is noted to have multiple violaceous lesions over his chest and palate.

2. A 34-year-old HIV-positive man is admitted to hospital with *Pneumocystis carinii* pneumonia (PCP). On examination, he is obviously unwell and is noted to have white, plaque-like lesions on his tongue, covering the right border more than the left border. These do not scrape away with a tongue spatula.

3. A 21-year-old woman is admitted to hospital for investigation of 6 months of increasing weight loss and steatorrhoea. Examination is remarkable only for the facts that she is thin and clinically anaemic. She is clinically euthyroid and has no lymphadenopathy. The diagnosis is confirmed with positive antiendomysial antibodies (anti-EMA) and subtotal villous atrophy on duodenal biopsy.

4. A 31-year-old man is incidentally noted by his dentist to have bilateral white papular lesions over the buccal mucosa and the dorsum of the tongue. He tells the dentist that these have been present for more than 18 months and are not associated with any other symptoms.

5. A 48-year-old homeless woman is brought into the Emergency Department by the police, having been found unconscious. On examination, she is dishevelled and pyrexial and has signs of a right lower lobe pneumonia. Among other nutritional deficiencies, she is confirmed to have vitamin A and vitamin C deficiencies.

5. THEME: GAIT DISTURBANCE

A   Antalgic gait
B   Cerebellar ataxia
C   Festinating gait
D   Hemiparetic/circumducting gait
E   Hysterical gait
F   Scissoring gait
G   Sensory ataxia
H   Spastic gait
I   Trendelenburg gait
J   Waddling gait

The following patients have all presented with an abnormal gait. Please choose the most appropriate cause from the above list. The options may be used once, more than once, in combination or not at all.

1. A 69-year-old woman who has had osteoarthritis of both hips for 4–5 years is referred to Orthopaedic Out-patients by her GP with increasing pain and immobility. On examination, she has severely decreased abduction and internal and external rotation of both hips, the right worse than the left, and her gait shows her left hip 'giving way'. When asked to stand on her right leg only, her left hip is seen to 'sag down'.

2. A 64-year-old man with Dupuytren's contracture and gynaecomastia is seen in the Out-patient Department with falls. On examination has dysdiadochokinesia and past-pointing.

3. A 37-year-old woman presents to her GP with falls. On examination, she has a high-stepping gait and is clinically anaemic.

4. A 64-year-old man presents to his GP with increasing instability and falls. On examination, he has a resting tremor, cogwheel rigidity and 'mask-like' facies.

5. A 61-year-old woman on long-term steroids presents to her GP with increasing falls and 'weakness'. On examination, she has difficulty standing from a sitting position and the GP finds that she is unable to maintain her arms in abduction when he pushes lightly down on them.

6. THEME: LYMPHADENOPATHY

A   Acute lymphoid leukaemia
B   Cytomegalovirus
C   Epstein–Barr virus
D   Human immunodeficiency virus (HIV)
E   Hodgkin's lymphoma
F   Non-Hodgkin's lymphoma
G   Sarcoidosis
H   Syphilis
I   Toxoplasmosis
J   Tuberculosis

The following patients have all presented with lymphadenopathy. Please choose the most appropriate cause from the above list. The diagnoses may be used once, more than once or not at all.

1. A 17-year-old schoolboy attend his GP with fevers, severe malaise and increasingly tender cervical lymphadenopathy. A Paul–Bunnell test is negative but an IgM immunofluorescent antibody test (IgM-IEA) confirms the diagnosis.

2. A 24-year-old woman presents to her GP with increasing shortness of breath on exertion associated with a rash over her anterior shins. Apart from the rash, examination is relatively unremarkable, but her chest radiograph shows bilateral hilar lymphadenopathy and her serum ACE and corrected Ca^{2+} levels are elevated.

3. A 29-year-old woman presents to her GP with increasing malaise and predominantly right-sided 'massive cervical lymphadenopathy'. On examination, she is noted to have firm, 'rubbery' lymph nodes in the neck, axillae and inguinal regions. Her chest radiograph confirms bilateral hilar lymphadenopathy. The diagnosis is confirmed on lymph-node biopsy, which shows 'large abnormal predominant B-cell lymphocytes'.

4. A 15-year-old girl presents to her GP with flu-like illness for 2 weeks associated with pharyngitis and tender cervical lymph nodes. Her peripheral blood film shows atypical monocytes and the diagnosis is confirmed by increasing titres of specific IgM.

5. A 31-year-old black Zimbabwean woman presents in the Emergency Department with a non-productive cough, fever and weight loss. She looks very ill, has widespread lymphadenopathy and florid oral candidiasis. Routine investigations reveal a relatively normal chest radiograph but her peripheral blood film shows 'marked lymphopenia with atypical lymphocytes and thrombocytopenia'.

7. THEME: NAUSEA AND VOMITING

A Appendicitis
B Central neuronal causes
C Cholecystitis
D Drug therapy
E Infective gastroenteritis
F Metabolic
G Gastric outflow obstruction
H Obstruction of the large intestine
I Obstruction of the small intestine
J Pancreatitis

The following patients have all presented with vomiting. Please select the most appropriate cause from the above list. Each option may be used once, more than once or not at all.

1. A 67-year-old woman with a 5-month history of dyspepsia, nausea, early satiety and weight loss is admitted with a 4-day history of vomiting followed by an episode of coffee-ground vomiting. On examination, the patient is anaemic, severely dehydrated and has a distended abdomen with a succussion splash. Investigations show: haemoglobin 9.7 g/dl, WCC 10.8 × 10^9/l, platelets 368 × 10^9/l; Na$^+$ 135 mmol/l, K$^+$ 2.9 mmol/l, urea 17.7 mmol/l, creatinine 180 μmol/l.

2. A 25-year-old man returns from holiday with a 24-hour history of severe, lower abdominal, cramp-like pain, with watery, brown, offensive diarrhoea. He has felt generally unwell with flu-like symptoms for the preceding 2–3 days and is now vomiting. On examination, he is clinically dehydrated and febrile (38.2 °C) with a pulse of 100 bpm. Blood tests show: haemoglobin 15.4 g/dl, WCC 14.8 × 10^9/l.

3. A 92-year-old woman presents with a 3-day history of colicky central abdominal pain and bilious vomiting. On examination, the abdomen is distended and tympanic but non-tender. She has a small, tender swelling in the groin.

4. An 80-year-old man is brought to the Emergency Department with confusion. He has been found at home lying in a pool of vomit, which his son describes as brown and smelling of faeces. On examination, he has a Glasgow Coma Scale (GCS) score of 14/15 and is clinically severely dehydrated. The abdomen is hugely distended and tympanic but not obviously tender. He has no surgical incisions and there are no hernias. His son adds that his father has had several months of abdominal pain, reduced appetite and weight loss.

5. A 38-year-old man with a history of attending the Emergency Department with injuries sustained while drunk presents with a 2-day history of increasing epigastric and left-sided upper abdominal pain radiating to the back. He is retching continuously in the Department and is clinically dehydrated. There is upper abdominal tenderness and guarding.

8. THEME: AUDITORY CONDITIONS

A Acoustic neuroma
B Acute middle ear effusion
C Acute suppurative otitis media
D Cholesteatoma
E Chronic serous middle ear effusion (glue ear)
F Foreign body in the ear
G Ménière's disease
H Otitis externa
I Otosclerosis
J Referred pain
K Wax

The following patients have all presented with otalgia, discharge from the ear or deafness. Please select the most appropriate diagnosis from the above list. The options may be used once, more than once or not at all.

1. A 59-year-old woman presents with a 1-year history of progressive hearing loss and ringing in her right ear. On examination, she has an absent right corneal reflex and a partial lower motor neurone facial nerve palsy. Audiometry reveals a right sensorineural deafness.

2. A 3-year-old child presents to his GP with a history of bilateral otalgia and poor speech development. On examination, both eardrums are dull and indrawn. Acoustic impedance testing gives a flat trace.

3. A 40-year-old man presents with unilateral loss of hearing for 6 weeks. On examination, the tympanic membrane is indrawn and dull. Acoustic impedance testing shows a flat trace. Audiometry reveals conductive deafness. On examination, there is cervical lymphadenopathy in the upper posterior triangle and examination of the postnasal space shows an ulcerated infected lesion.

4. A 25-year-old man is referred by his GP with recurrent right-sided otalgia without deafness or discharge. He has been treated unsuccessfully on several occasions for otitis media. On examination, the external canal and tympanic membranes are normal but there is tenderness on palpation over the angle of the mandible. Dental examination shows that the right lower third molar tooth is not present. An orthopantomogram of the mandible shows an unerupted and impacted lower third molar (wisdom tooth).

5. A 55-year-old man is referred with an episode of acute vertigo associated with nausea and vomiting that gradually subsided over 24 hours. This left him 'unsteady' for 3 weeks. On direct questioning, he had noticed hearing loss and tinnitus in his left ear before the vertigo, and the tinnitus had increased shortly before the attack. After the attack he noticed that his hearing had also worsened. On examination, the only abnormal finding is a left-sided sensorineural hearing loss, confirmed on audiometry.

9. THEME: HEAD INJURY AND THE GLASGOW COMA SCALE (GCS)

A GCS 3
B GCS 4
C GCS 5
E GCS 7
F GCS 8
G GCS 10
H GCS 11
I GCS 12
J GCS 13
K GCS 14
L GCS 15

The following patients have all sustained head injuries. Please select the appropriate Glasgow Coma Scale (GCS) score from the above list. The scores may be used once, more than once, or not at all.

1. A 34-year-old man is hit on the vertex of the skull with a hammer by a mugger who steals his mobile phone. There is a large boggy swelling over the left high-parietal region. There was a momentary loss of consciousness but he is now alert and orientated.

2. A 33-year-old builder falls from low scaffolding, hitting his head. At the scene he was alert and orientated. On arrival in the Emergency Department, he has a localised right temporoparietal boggy swelling. Approximately 1 hour later, while waiting for further assessment, he suddenly collapses in the waiting room. At this time his speech is confused, he has eye opening to and localisation of pain.

3. An 18-year-old French student is hit by a bus after looking the wrong way before crossing a road. He has severe external injuries to the scalp and facial skeleton and other internal injuries. He has no eye opening, verbal or motor responses. After appropriate, sustained resuscitation, a CT head scan demonstrates multiple vault and facial fractures and loss of the brain sulcal pattern with poor grey–white differentiation. There are small brain contusions but no focal space-occupying lesion.

4. A 19-year-old girl falls from a height and sustains multiple injuries, including a blunt injury to the head. She is deeply unconscious on arrival in the Emergency Department and there are no responses other than extension to pain on the right-hand side.

5. A 24-year-old is attacked after leaving his bar one night after closing. On examination, he has multiple facial injuries and scalp lacerations, bilateral black eyes and a left subconjunctival haemorrhage. Blood mixed with a clear fluid is leaking from his nose. He has eye opening to verbal commands and obeys some commands, but is only mumbling occasional, inappropriate words.

10. THEME: INFERTILITY

A Azoospermia
B Endometriosis
C Genital tract agenesis/dysgenesis
D Hypothalamic dysfunction
E Oligospermia
F Pelvic adhesions
G Pelvic inflammatory disease (PID)
H Polycystic ovary syndrome (PCOS)
I Prolactinoma
J Sexual dysfunction

The couples below have all recently been diagnosed with primary infertility by their GP. From the above list please choose the condition most likely to cause the clinical picture described. The options may be used once, more than once or not at all.

1. A 30-year-old woman has a long history of oligomenorrhoea and hirsutism. Her 29-year-old partner has no medical history of note. On examination, she has a BMI of 32 kg/m² and some male-pattern hair distribution. Her routine investigations reveal: follicle-stimulating hormone (FSH) 3.1 U/l, luteinising hormone (LH) 8.7 U/l, testosterone high-normal and sex hormone-binding globulin (SHBG) reduced.

2. A married couple are seen by their GP. The husband has no medical history of note and routine examination and investigations are all normal. His 26-year-old wife has secondary amenorrhoea but no other gynaecological or medical history of note. Her BMI is 17 kg/m² but examination is otherwise unremarkable. Investigations reveal: FSH 1.3 U/l, LH 1.2 U/l, testosterone and SHBG normal, prolactin is 375 mU/l. Her pelvic ultrasound is also normal.

3. A 36-year-old woman has a regular menstrual cycle but describes severe dysmenorrhoea and deep dyspareunia. She has no other gynaecological, medical or surgical history of note. On examination, she has a fixed, retroverted uterus. Her 35-year-old partner has no medical history of note.

4. A 20-year-old woman has primary amenorrhoea, short stature, a webbed neck and appears 'young' for her age. Her LH and FSH are found to be grossly elevated and her oestradiol levels very low. Testosterone and SHBG levels are normal and the prolactin is 275 mU/l. Her 22-year-old partner has no medical history of note.

5. A couple with infertility are seen by their GP. The 36-year-old woman has regular cycles with no other gynaecological or medical history of note. Her hormone profile and pelvic ultrasound are normal. Her 45-year-old partner has long-standing type 1 diabetes mellitus and has evidence of systemic vasculopathy and neuropathy. He is reluctant to provide a semen sample when requested.

11. THEME: PATHOGENS IN THE IMMUNOCOMPROMISED PATIENT

A   Aspergillus flavus
B   *Candida albicans*
C   *Cryptococcus neoformans*
D   *Cryptosporidium parvum*
E   Cytomegalovirus
F   Human papillomavirus
G   *Leishmania donovani*
H   *Mycobacterium avium intracellulare*
I   *Pneumocystis carinii*
J   *Toxoplasma gondii*

From the above list, please select the pathogen with which each of the following patients is most likely to be infected. The organisms may be used once, more than once or not at all.

1. A 32-year-old man who is receiving chemotherapy for high-grade lymphoma presents with a 2-week history of dysphagia. Endoscopy reveals white plaques on the oesophageal mucosa. Biopsy of the plaques shows fungal hyphae and yeast forms on the mucosal surface.

2. A 35-year-old, HIV-positive woman develops shortness of breath accompanied by a dry cough. A chest radiograph shows bilateral reticulonodular shadowing. Sputum culture is negative. Transbronchial biopsy shows alveoli filled with a foamy eosinophilic material and numerous boat-shaped organisms that stain positively with a silver stain.

3. A 40-year-old man with established AIDS develops abdominal pain, bloody diarrhoea and low-grade pyrexia. Sigmoidoscopy shows a friable ulcerated mucosa. Rectal biopsies show severe active chronic proctitis with 'owl's eye' intranuclear inclusions in endothelial and epithelial cells.

4. A 54-year-old woman who had a renal transplant 3 years ago presents with several warty nodules on both hands. On examination, she has two similar lesions on the ectocervix. Excision biopsy of one of the cervical lesions shows a condyloma acuminatum with cervical intraepithelial neoplasia grade 2 (CIN 2).

5. A 36-year-old, HIV-positive man presents with severe watery diarrhoea, anorexia and malabsorption. Duodenal biopsy shows numerous small cysts adherent to the surface epithelium.

12. THEME: PATHOLOGICAL PROCESSES

A   Apoptosis
B   Atrophy
C   Dysplasia
D   Embolism
E   Fibrosis
F   Hyperplasia
G   Hypertrophy
H   Infarction
I   Metaplasia
J   Thrombosis

From the above list, please select the pathological process occurring in each of the following scenarios. The options may be used once, more than once or not at all.

1. A 75-year-old woman who is taking tamoxifen for breast carcinoma develops post-menopausal vaginal bleeding. An endometrial aspirate shows closely packed glands with obvious proliferative activity.

2. A 45-year-old man who has been a heavy smoker for 30 years develops haemoptysis. His chest radiograph shows signs suggestive of a bronchial neoplasm. Biopsies of the suspicious area taken at bronchoscopy show stratified squamous epithelium lining the bronchial wall.

3. A 35-year-old woman suffers complications after a colectomy for toxic megacolon and is bed-bound on the Intensive Care Unit for several weeks. On recovery, her legs are weak and both quadriceps are visibly wasted.

4. A 72-year-old man suffers a right-sided 'stroke'. A CT scan shows a necrotic lesion with associated oedema in the left cerebral hemisphere.

5. A 65-year-old man with long-standing emphysema develops right-sided cardiac failure. An echocardiogram shows a thickened right ventricular free wall.

13. THEME: CHEST RADIOGRAPHS – CLINICAL SCENARIOS

*Using the radiographic images **A–J on pages (345 – 347)**, please match the scenarios described below to the correct image. You may use each image once, more than once or not at all.*

1. A previously fit and well, 43-year-old man presents to his GP with a 2-week history of a flu-like illness associated with increasing shortness of breath. On examination, his peripheral pulses and apex beat are very difficult to palpate and, on auscultation, his heart sounds are poorly heard. His JVP is grossly elevated but he does not have any other signs of heart failure.

2. A 78-year-old woman with a previous history of rheumatic fever attends a pre-admission clinic for an anaesthetic review prior to undergoing a left total hip replacement. On examination, she is noted to have 'ruby-red' cheeks but otherwise looks well. Her JVP is grossly elevated and on auscultation the FY2 doctor thinks she can hear a low rumbling diastolic murmur at the apex.

3. A 52-year-old lifelong smoker presents to the Emergency Department with a 3-hour history of severe central chest pain. His ECG confirms an acute anterior ST-elevation myocardial infarction (STEMI) but he cannot be given thrombolytic therapy because he has recently been diagnosed with a duodenal ulcer. Six hours after admission he becomes increasingly distressed, dyspnoeic and clammy.

4. A 59-year-old man presents to his GP with a 2–3-year history of a worsening cough associated with daily production of large volumes of greenish sputum and occasional haemoptysis.

5. A 71-year-old woman with a history of diabetes, hypertension and peripheral vascular disease presents in the Emergency Department with an 8-hour history of increasingly severe, central chest pain which radiates through to her back, between the scapulae. The blood pressure in the right upper limb is 80/60 mmHg and in the left upper limb, 110/70 mmHg.

14. THEME: INNERVATION OF THE MUSCLES OF THE UPPER LIMB

A   Anterior interosseous nerve
B   Axillary nerve
C   Long thoracic nerve
D   Lower subscapular nerve
E   Medial cutaneous nerve of forearm
F   Median nerve
G   Musculocutaneous nerve
H   Posterior interosseous nerve
I   Radial nerve
J   Ulnar nerve

For each of the following muscles please choose the nerve that innervates it from the above list. Each nerve may be used once, more than once or not at all.

1.   Serratus anterior.

2.   Biceps.

3.   Extensor carpi radialis longus.

4.   Pronator teres.

5.   Flexor carpi ulnaris.

Paper 2 Answers

1. HEART SOUNDS

1. **B, C, D – Early systolic murmur, ejection systolic click and fourth heart sound**
    This man has presented with symptoms and signs suggestive of significant aortic stenosis. He has worsening angina due to obstruction of the coronary sinuses and exertional collapses. He has a narrow pulse pressure and a slow-rising pulse. The murmur of aortic stenosis (an ejection systolic or 'crescendo–decrescendo' murmur) might or might not be preceded by an ejection click and associated with a fourth heart sound, occurring in late diastole. A fourth heart sound reveals the pressure overload being experienced by the left ventricle. Other causes of a fourth heart sound include severe systemic hypertension, coarctation of the aorta and ischaemic heart disease leading to a poorly compliant left ventricle.

2. **D, J – Fourth and third heart sounds**
    This woman has developed acute cardiogenic shock associated with heart failure, secondary to her anterior myocardial infarction. Such infarcts can be associated with a loud systolic murmur due to acute rupture of the mitral valve's chordae or the ventricular septum, leading to acute mitral regurgitation or a ventricular septal defect. No murmurs are heard in this case and so auscultation reveals the normal heart sounds plus a third and possible fourth heart sound. The early diastolic third heart sound signifies volume overload of the left ventricle, leading to a 'gallop' rhythm. A fourth heart sound occurs late in diastole and is caused by the poorly compliant left ventricle associated with the acute infarct. It is more commonly associated with pressure overload of the ventricle, when the ventricle has to contract against increased resistance.

3. **A, F – Early diastolic murmur and mid-diastolic murmur**
    This woman has signs consistent with significant aortic regurgitation. The murmur of aortic regurgitation is an early diastolic murmur that is heard loudest at the left sternal edge with the patient sitting forwards in expiration. There can be an associated mid-diastolic murmur, known as the 'Austin Flint murmur'. This murmur is supposedly caused by the regurgitant jet of blood hitting the mitral valve in diastole.

4. **F, H – Mid-diastolic murmur and opening snap**
    This man has signs consistent with significant mitral stenosis, as evidenced by his low-volume pulse in atrial fibrillation and the tapping, undisplaced apex beat. Mitral stenosis causes a low, rumbling, mid-diastolic murmur best heard at the apex using the bell of the stethoscope (the 'L' of be**LL** and the '**L**' of **L**ow rumbling murmur). It can be preceded by an early diastolic opening snap. The time interval between the second heart sound and the opening snap determines the significance of the mitral stenosis – the closer the two sounds, the more significant the lesion.

5. **E, G – Late systolic murmur and mid-systolic click**
   This patient has a floppy mitral valve, which is characterised by a mid-systolic click and a late systolic murmur. If the prolapse of the valve leaflets becomes significant there can be regurgitation and cardiac failure and this might require valve replacement. As with this patient, all patients identified as having a floppy valve require endocarditis prophylaxis when undergoing any procedure associated with significant bacteraemia.

2. THEME: FULL BLOOD COUNT

When considering the full blood count (FBC), start with the five major components – the haemoglobin and the mean corpuscular volume (MCV), the white cell count (WCC) and its differential, and the platelets. The other elements, including the mean corpuscular haemoglobin concentration (MCHC), the red-cell distribution width (RDW), the haematocrit and the blood film are also useful when differentiating possible underlying causes. The absolute values of the haemoglobin and the WCC are almost useless without knowing the paired MCV and white cell differential results and these should always be sought. A haemoglobin of 5.0 g/dl might be 'impressively low', but if the MCV is 124 fl as opposed to 67 fl, the causes and management are likely to be very different. Likewise, a WCC of $6.5 \times 10^9/l$ is 'impressively normal' but if all these cells are lymphocytes, or indeed blast cells, then the patient might in fact be unwell or at risk.

1. **A – Haemoglobin 4.9 g/l, MCV 124 fl, WCC $4.8 \times 10^9/l$, differential normal, platelets $75 \times 10^9/l$**
   This patient has developed a megaloblastic anaemia with characteristic hypersegmented neutrophils. Megaloblastosis is the dysfunctional production of erythrocytes, which are larger than normal red cells and have a higher nuclear to cytoplasmic ratio (normoblastic cells). Hypersegmented neutrophils have multilobulated nuclei (defined as more than five lobes) and are characteristic of vitamin B_{12} and folate deficiency and, less commonly, chronic infection. Vitamin B_{12} and folate are essential in the production of cellular DNA and deficiencies lead to reduced and abnormal synthesis in all three blood cell lines. Megaloblastic anaemias can therefore be associated with a marked pancytopenia. Of note, vitamin B_{12} deficiency is most commonly due to pernicious anaemia, an autoimmune disorder, and so it is commonly associated with other autoimmune diseases, in this case vitiligo. Very few conditions other than these deficiencies cause such a marked macrocytosis (often the MCV is >120 fl). Other causes of macrocytosis, with or without anaemia, include multiple myeloma, reticulocytosis, alcohol excess, drugs (eg phenytoin, which can also cause a folate deficiency) and hypothyroidism.

2. **E – Haemoglobin 10.5 g/l, MCV 89 fl, WCC $146.5 \times 10^9/l$, lymphocytes $136.8 \times 10^9/l$, platelets $128 \times 10^9/l$**
   Chronic lymphocytic leukaemia (CLL) is a malignant proliferation of B-cell lymphocytes. It is a disease which is unusual before the age of 50 and is more common in men than women (approximately 2:1). Common presentations range from incidental identification on an FBC of asymptomatic patients to patients with lymphadenopathy (which is classically painless), splenomegaly (which is relatively common) and hepatomegaly (less common). The FBC typically shows a lymphocytosis and the peripheral blood film might show 'smudge' cells, which probably represent damaged lymphocytes – these lyse during processing and so appear as 'smudges' on the film. They are common in several conditions but are often present in relatively large numbers in CLL. Because the lymphocyte proliferation produces dysfunctional cells, patients are particularly prone to viral infections, including herpes zoster and respiratory tract infections. Treatment is based on the lymphocyte count, the patient's symptoms and co-morbidities. Treatments include steroids, oral and intravenous chemotherapy, blood transfusions and other supportive care.

3. **D – Haemoglobin 8.3 g/l, MCV 65 fl, WCC 7.4 × 10⁹/l, differential normal, platelets 343 × 10⁹/l**

    This man presents with signs and symptoms suggestive of a large gastric carcinoma and associated Virchow's node and anaemia. Menstruation and gastrointestinal pathologies are the commonest causes of iron-deficiency anaemia and this is characterised by a microcytic anaemia. Other causes of a microcytosis include sideroblastic anaemia, anaemia of chronic disease and some of the haemoglobinopathies (thalassaemia trait). Thalassaemia trait is common in Asian and Mediterranean people and should be excluded in such patients prior to subjecting them to invasive procedures such as upper and/or lower gastrointestinal endoscopy. Characteristically, thalassaemia causes a significant microcytosis with a relatively normal haemoglobin (see results profile F).

4. **C – Haemoglobin 7.9 g/l, MCV 85 fl, WCC 1.8 × 10⁹/l, neutrophils 0.7 × 10⁹/l, platelets 38 × 10⁹/l; rouleaux on the film**

    This patient has presented with several features of myeloma. Her bony pain is due to multiple lytic bony lesions, she has hypercalcaemia and a very high ESR. Of note, her FBC shows pancytopenia with a neutropenia, and this makes her very susceptible to severe and often life-threatening sepsis. Her blood film shows characteristic rouleaux which is due to the stacking of red cells into long chains. This stacking occurs in the presence of increased serum proteins, particularly globulins (as in this case) and fibrinogen (associated with inflammation and sepsis). These chains of cells sediment more readily and so lead to the very high ESR seen in myeloma and inflammatory conditions (eg vasculitis).

5. **J – Haemoglobin 18.9 g/l, MCV 80 fl, WCC 13.8 × 10⁹/l, neutrophils 11.9 × 10⁹/l, platelets 406 × 10⁹/l; haematocrit 0.58**

    Polycythaemia rubra vera (PRV) is one of the myeloproliferative disorders; these include essential thrombocytosis and myelofibrosis. It results in abnormal erythropoiesis and this in turn causes an increase in the total erythrocyte count, haemoglobin concentration and the total red blood cell volume and total blood volume. Recently it has been found that a genetic mutation is present in about 80% of patients with the disorder. The mutation of the *JAK2* gene is thought to cause a hypersensitivity to erythropoietin. Included in the diagnostic criteria are:

    - An elevated red blood cell mass (>25% more than the mean normal predicted value – this is often taken to be a red cell mass greater than 36 ml/kg for men and greater than 32 ml/kg for women)
    - Haemoglobin >18.5 g/dl in men or >16.5 g/dl in women (or greater than the 99th percentile of method-specific reference range for age, sex, and altitude of residence)
    - No cause of a secondary erythrocytosis – the principal cause of this is chronic hypoxaemia, seen with chronic respiratory conditions and living at high altitude for prolonged periods.
    - Splenomegaly
    - Thrombocytosis greater than 400 × 10⁹/l
    - WCC greater than 12 × 10⁹/l
    - Low serum erythropoietin levels.

3. CHEST PATHOLOGY

1. **A – Empyema**
   This man has developed an empyema secondary to the insertion of a chest drain for his spontaneous pneumothorax. The signs are similar to those of a pleural effusion or haemothorax but the history and the pyrexial illness are more suggestive of an empyema. Treatment should include aspiration and/or drainage of the empyema, intravenous broad-spectrum antibiotics, which should include an agent to cover *Staphylococcus*, appropriate analgesia and antipyretics.

2. **D – Pleural effusion**
   This man has signs and symptoms suggestive of a malignancy in the chest. He has now developed a malignant pleural effusion and a Horner's syndrome, suggesting an apical tumour. He should have the effusion drained and fluid sent for cytological examination to confirm the diagnosis. He might also require a bronchoscopy and staging CT scan of the chest and abdomen. The treatment will depend on the histology, the stage of the tumour and the patient's wishes.

3. **H – Pulmonary fibrosis**
   This man has developed basal pulmonary fibrosis due to asbestosis. The fine inspiratory crepitations that are 'fixed' (ie they do not change with coughing) are very typical of this disorder. The chest radiograph confirms asbestos exposure by the presence of the pleural and diaphragmatic plaques but it is only when the patient has signs confirmed radiologically and by respiratory function tests that one can diagnose fibrotic lung disease (ie asbestosis). Other complications of asbestos exposure include pleural and peritoneal mesothelioma.

4. **E – Pneumothorax**
   This patient has developed a right-sided pneumothorax. The diagnosis should be confirmed on a chest radiograph and she should be treated by initial attempts to aspirate the free air using a large syringe, needle and three-way tap. If this fails to re-inflate the affected lung, you should site an intercostal chest drain in the fifth intercostal space in the mid-axillary line.

5. **F – Pulmonary consolidation**
   This young man has developed right middle lobe consolidation as evidenced by the dullness to percussion, bronchial breathing and increased vocal fremitus in the right axilla. The radiological sign associated with this condition is loss of the right heart border due to overlying consolidation. The patient should be treated with analgesia and intravenous amoxicillin or cefuroxime and clarithromycin.

4. ORAL AND GLOSSAL LESIONS

1. **E – Kaposi's sarcoma**
   This man has developed an AIDS-related illness with an intracranial lesion, due possibly to toxoplasmosis, to non-Hodgkin's lymphoma or to an abscess. The violaceous lesions are consistent with Kaposi's sarcoma, which can produce lesions over the upper chest, back, palate, and the face, as well as intrapulmonary and gastrointestinal tract lesions.

2. **H – Oral hairy leukoplakia**
   This man has developed white, plaque-like lesions over the border of his tongue which do not scrape away with a spatula. In view of his HIV status this is most likely to be to oral hairy leukoplakia. Any part of the oral mucosa and tongue can be involved and there can be malignant transformation. In the absence of HIV-related disease, it can be related to viral infection or to smoking.

3. **A and B – Aphthous ulceration and atrophic glossitis**
   This young woman has signs, symptoms and investigations suggestive of coeliac disease. This can be associated with aphthous ulceration and atrophic glossitis due to the associated malabsorption of vitamin B_{12} and folate.

4. **F – Lichen planus**
   This patient has developed lichen planus, which characteristically forms white linear lesions at areas of trauma. In the mouth this trauma occurs in the bite areas around the inner cheek and produces the classical white, lacy pattern that does not scrape away. Other commonly affected areas include the ankles and wrists and, to a lesser extent, the scalp, nails and genitalia. It is one of the skin conditions which exhibits the 'Koebner phenomenon'.

5. **B and G – Atrophic glossitis and perifollicular haemorrhages**
   This malnourished patient has developed scurvy due to vitamin C deficiency and this, together with the associated vitamin K deficiency, has lead to severe bleeding of the gums. With this degree of malnutrition she will also almost certainly have vitamin B_{12} and folate deficiencies, leading to atrophic glossitis.

5. GAIT DISTURBANCE

1. **A, I – Antalgic gait and Trendelenburg gait**
   This patient has developed a Trendelenburg gait as a result of her severe osteoarthritis around the hips. The abductors of the hip weaken with the chronic arthritis and this leads to the hip 'giving way' when standing on the affected side. If asked to stand only on the affected leg, the abductors are unable to hold the contralateral hip up and the raised leg then 'drops down' – this is known as a positive Trendelenburg test. She might also have an antalgic gait.

2. **B – Cerebellar ataxia**
   This man has signs of chronic liver disease and cerebellar disease as evidenced by the dysdiadochokinesia and past-pointing. Patients classically have a wide-based, ataxic gait.

3. **G – Sensory ataxia**
   This patient has developed a high-stepping gait that is consistent with sensory ataxia due to peripheral sensory neuropathy. The patient is described as anaemic, which suggests possible vitamin B_{12} deficiency with associated sensory neuropathy or subacute combined degeneration of the cord (SACD).

4. **C – Festinating gait**
   This patient has parkinsonism with associated festinating gait. The most likely cause is idiopathic Parkinson's disease but secondary causes, including vascular parkinsonism, iatrogenic parkinsonism and the parkinsonism-plus syndromes can also present in a similar manner.

5. **J – Waddling gait**
   This patient has been on long-term steroids which has caused secondary Cushing's and proximal myopathy, as evidenced by the weakness of the upper limbs in abduction and inability to stand from a sitting position. Proximal myopathy leads to a 'waddling' gait.

6. LYMPHADENOPATHY

1. **I – Toxoplasmosis**

   This young man has developed toxoplasmosis, which can present in a very similar manner clinically to EBV and cytomegalovirus (CMV) infections in the immunocompetent patient. It is caused by an intracellular protozoan, *Toxoplasma gondii*, and can either be congenital or can be acquired by the ingestion of the cysts through infected lamb or pork meat or foods infected by cat faeces. The major clinical features associated with this illness are lymphadenopathy and fever and, less commonly, meningism, rashes, hepatosplenomegaly, eye problems and myocarditis. In most cases the disorder is a mild condition and is self-limiting, requiring no active treatment.

2. **G – Sarcoidosis**

   This young woman has developed pulmonary sarcoid, as evidenced by the respiratory symptoms, probable erythema nodosum, bilateral hilar lymphadenopathy on her chest radiograph and raised serum ACE and hypercalcaemia. The diagnosis can be confirmed by bronchoscopy and bronchoalveolar lavage (BAL), which shows inflammatory cells with T-helper cells.

3. **F – Non-Hodgkin's lymphoma**

   This patient has developed non-Hodgkin's lymphoma, as evidenced by the non-tender, firm, rubbery lymphadenopathy. The classification of this disorder is based on its division into high-grade and low-grade tumours. High-grade tumours are characterised by rapidly dividing, highly malignant blast cells. Both types of tumour can also be subdivided into B-cell and T-cell lines, although most non-Hodgkin's lymphoma tumours are B cell in origin.

4. **C – Epstein–Barr virus**

   This young girl has developed an EBV infection, or infectious mononucleosis, characterised by tender lymphadenopathy, pharyngitis, malaise, fever and lethargy. In the peripheral blood there are atypical mononuclear cells (hence its name) and specific EBV IgM antibodies. These are responsible for the diagnostic Paul–Bunnell reaction.

5. **D – HIV**

   This patient has presented with widespread or generalised non-tender lymphadenopathy, a dry cough, fever and oral candidiasis and looks unwell. Her peripheral blood film shows lymphopenia with typical lymphocytes in keeping with new-onset HIV infection. After counselling, an HIV test should be performed, along with a CD4 count and viral load estimation.

7. NAUSEA AND VOMITING

A complete overview of all the causes of vomiting (not possible in one EMQ – one recent review listed 150!) should broadly include:

- Central – intracranial and labyrinthine
- Metabolic and endocrine, eg uraemia, pregnancy, diabetes
- Iatrogenic, eg cancer chemotherapy, digoxin, opiates
- Obstructive (any level)
- Mucosal, eg appendicitis, gastritis, cholecystitis.

1.   G – Gastric outflow obstruction

Gastric outflow obstruction, in this case is most probably caused by pyloric carcinoma of the stomach (the other possible diagnosis in this age group is pyloric obstruction secondary to peptic inflammation). Treatment includes resuscitation with correction of electrolyte disturbances, nasogastric drainage, then surgery (either palliative bypass or curative resection).

2.   E – Infective gastroenteritis

This can be caused by bacteria, enteroviruses or parasites. This patient probably has bacterial enteritis, as evidenced by the history of foreign travel and the symptoms and signs. A preceding flu-like 'prodrome' is also common before diarrhoea and vomiting start. Common causative infective agents include *Escherichia coli* strains, *Salmonella*, *Shigella* and *Campylobacter*. More common causes of vomiting-predominant enteritis are *Staphylococcus aureus* and *Bacillus cereus* food poisoning.

3.   I – Obstruction of the small intestine

This is the classic clinical description of a patient presenting with small-bowel obstruction: colicky central abdominal pain, distension, nausea and vomiting (eventually bile-stained). In this woman's case, the cause is probably a femoral hernia.

4.   H – Obstruction of the large intestine

In this case the obstruction is probably due to an obstructing colonic carcinoma. It should be noted that faeculant vomiting is not vomiting of faeces (which only occurs in rare cases of gastrocolic fistula) but of small-intestinal content that has stagnated and been altered by bacteria. This can therefore also occur with distal small-bowel obstruction but in this case no common cause for this is suggested in the scenario (eg adhesions, hernia).

5.   J – Pancreatitis

This diagnosis is evidenced by the history of alcoholism and the clinical presentation. The other possibility would be alcoholic gastritis but the severe abdominal pain is more characteristic of pancreatitis. The diagnosis can be confirmed by blood biochemistry.

8. AUDITORY CONDITIONS

1. **A – Acoustic neuroma**
   These represent 80% of cerebellopontine angle tumours and 8% of all intracranial tumours. They arise from the neurilemmal cells of a cranial nerve, virtually always in the internal auditory meatus. They are slow-growing, benign tumours but exert pressure effects on surrounding structures in the fixed space bounded the bony cranium. The history of progressive loss of hearing and tinnitus (eighth nerve compression) should always prompt you to consider this diagnosis. The accompanying finding of adjacent cranial nerve dysfunction (the ophthalmic branch of the fifth nerve) and of facial nerve dysfunction is pathognomonic. Large tumours can also cause cerebellar signs and raised intracranial pressure.

2. **E – Chronic serous middle ear effusion (glue ear)**
   This very common condition occurs in one in five children between the ages of 1 year and 7 years. The cause is chronic obstruction of the eustachian tube and the condition is therefore often associated with adenoid enlargement, and is commoner in children with allergic rhinitis. If left untreated, 50% resolve spontaneously within 6 months. Surgical intervention comprises drainage followed by grommet insertion. Adenoidectomy decreases the likelihood of recurrence.

3. **B – Acute middle ear effusion**
   This patient has an acute middle ear effusion caused by blockage of the eustachian tube at its opening in the nasopharynx. Acute middle ear effusions usually follow flu and upper respiratory tract infections, when mucosal oedema causes the obstruction. In children, acute suppurative otitis media can occur. In such cases the tympanic membrane can bulge outwards. However, in all other middle ear effusions (acute and chronic) the drum is retracted. In an adult (as in this case) a nasopharyngeal carcinoma must always be excluded by examination.

4. **J – Referred pain**
   Dental and temporomandibular joint dysfunction are common causes of pain referred to the ear (mandibular branch of the fifth cranial nerve). For this reason, any patient in whom no intrinsic auditory cause of otalgia can be found should undergo oral and dental examination, not least because carcinomas of the oropharynx can present in this way.

5. **G – Ménière's disease**
   Prosper Ménière (1799–1862) was a French ear, nose and throat specialist, assistant of Baron Dupuytren, and friend of Balzac and Victor Hugo. The condition he described is characterised by **d**eafness, **d**izziness and tinnitus (**d**in), the three 'd's (as in this patient). All patients presenting with vertigo should have imaging investigations to exclude an acoustic neuroma and testing for syphilis, because neurosyphilis can present in this way and should be treated.

9. HEAD INJURY AND THE GLASGOW COMA SCALE (GCS)

BMR = best motor response
BVR = best vocal response
BER = best eye response
EO = eyes open

1. **L – GCS 15**

   This patient probably has a depressed skull fracture (evidenced by the causative weapon and the clinical findings) and, despite his intact GCS, should have a CT head scan to exclude brain injury (which is 400× the risk of a patient without a skull fracture!) and to further assess the fracture morphology.

2. **H – GCS 11**

   BER = EO to pain = 2, BMR = localisation = 5, BVR = confused speech = 4. This patient probably also has an extradural haematoma on the basis of the description of a 'lucid interval' before a rapid decline in neurological status due to cerebral compression from arterial bleeding – the so-called 'talk and die' scenario.

3. **A – GCS 3**

   There are no responses. The CT findings are those of diffuse axonal injury (the most severe type of diffuse brain injury, less severe types being defined as mild concussion and cerebral concussion).

4. **B – GCS 4**

   BER = 1, BMR = 2, BVR = 1. In many ways this is the worst GCS to have because it almost always implies severe brain injury with decerebration/decortication (a GCS of 3 can also be due to drugs, alcohol, hypoxia or fitting).

5. **I – GCS 12**

   BER = EO to speech = 3, BMR = obeys commands = 6, BVR = inappropriate words = 3. This patient probably has a base of skull fracture, as evidenced by some of the characteristic clinical signs described. These can include 'panda' or 'racoon' eyes, subconjunctival haemorrhage, otorrhoea or blood in the external auditory meatus and CSF rhinnorhoea.

10. INFERTILITY

1. **H – Polycystic ovary syndrome (PCOS)**
   This is by far the commonest cause of oligomenorrhoea and hirsutism. It is diagnosed by on the basis of ultrasound findings and the clinical features, which include obesity (body mass index, or BMI > 30 kg/m²), hirsutism and acne, oligo/amenorrhoea and, sometimes, hypertension and type 2 diabetes. The ratio of luteinising hormone (LH) to follicle-stimulating hormone (FSH) is classically around 3 : 1 but this can vary enormously. Testosterone levels are usually at the top end of the normal range but the sex hormone-binding globulin (SHBG) level is low, meaning that the free androgen fraction is raised.

2. **D – Hypothalamic dysfunction**
   There are several causes for secondary amenorrhoea. Her very low BMI suggests that PCOS is unlikely as these patients are usually obese (but need not be so). Her prolactin level is normal, ruling out a prolactinoma. With a very low BMI, the most likely cause is anorexia nervosa or excessive exercising, which tend to switch off hypothalamic gonadotrophin-releasing hormone (GnRH) production, leading in turn to switching off of the hypothalamic–pituitary–ovarian axis (hence the low FSH and LH levels) and therefore secondary amenorrhoea.

3. **B – Endometriosis**
   This woman's symptoms of severe dysmenorrhoea and deep dyspareunia suggest intrapelvic pathology. Her fixed, retroverted uterus and age (30–40 years) are features of the classic presentation of endometriosis. Pelvic inflammatory disease is more common under the age of 30 and pelvic adhesions will often result from previous pelvic surgery (which she has no history of). Although pelvic adhesions will often be present in a woman with endometriosis and pelvic rigidity, these are a secondary phenomenon and result from the primary disease process (ie the endometriosis).

4. **C – Genital tract agenesis/dysgenesis**
   Primary amenorrhoea has several causes and this woman has the classic features of Turner's syndrome (XO). In Turner's syndrome there is only rudimentary development of the ovaries (streak ovaries). Sometimes menarche does occur, although secondary amenorrhoea is inevitable, but the syndrome commonly presents with primary amenorrhoea. As a result, the hormonal profile is the same as it is in menopausal ovarian function – low oestradiol and high gonadotrophins – as efforts are made to try and stimulate the non-functioning ovaries.

5. **J – Sexual dysfunction**
   The regular cycles and lack of gynaecological symptoms give no obvious indication of anovulation or gynaecological disease, though these cannot be completely ruled out. Men with long-standing type 1 diabetes mellitus can develop neurovascular impotence, which is commonly not talked about due to embarrassment. The semen characteristics are unlikely to be abnormal with type 1 diabetes mellitus alone.

11. PATHOGENS IN THE IMMUNOCOMPROMISED PATIENT

1. **B – *Candida albicans***
   The finding of fungal hyphae in this patient's biopsy is diagnostic of fungal oesophagitis. The differential diagnosis lies between aspergillosis, caused by *Aspergillus* species, and candidiasis caused by *Candida* species, usually *Candida albicans*. The fact that yeast forms were also present rules out *Aspergillus* as this is not a yeast-forming fungus. In addition, the endoscopic appearance of white plaques on the mucosal surface is typical of candidiasis. This disease is common in immunosuppressed patients such as those on chemotherapy or with AIDS.

2. **I – *Pneumocystis carinii***
   Pneumocystis carinii is a ubiquitous organism, now classified as a fungus. It does not cause disease in normal individuals but can cause a severe pneumonia in immunosuppressed patients. The organism cannot be grown in culture, so diagnosis requires cytological or histological identification. Useful cytological preparations include bronchial washings or lavage. Transbronchial biopsy shows foamy eosinophilic material in the alveolar spaces. On both cytology and histology, silver staining outlines the boat-shaped or cup-shaped organisms.

3. **E – Cytomegalovirus**
   The 'owl's eye' intranuclear inclusions are characteristic of CMV infection. Infected cells are strikingly enlarged and show basophilic intranuclear inclusions that are separated from the nuclear membrane by a clear halo. Over 50% of the adult population have serological evidence of infection with CMV, though the infection is usually asymptomatic. As with other herpesviruses, CMV persists for life, becoming latent in leucocytes, which are the major reservoir. In patients with HIV and AIDS, the latent virus becomes reactivated and can be a cause of considerable morbidity, particularly in the later stages of the disease. The major problems encountered are colitis, retinitis, oesophageal ulceration, pneumonitis and encephalitis.

4. **F – Human papillomavirus**
   Warts are benign tumours of squamous epithelium known as 'squamous-cell papillomas'. They arise not only in keratinised squamous epithelium, such as the skin, but also in non-keratinised squamous epithelium such as that lining the ectocervix, where they are called 'condylomata acuminatum'. All warts are caused by human papillomavirus (HPV), of which there are many serotypes. Genital warts are sexually transmitted and are caused by HPV types 6 and 11. Other serotypes, notably types 16, 18 and 31 have been implicated in the development of high-grade cervical intraepithelial neoplasia (CIN) and invasive cervical carcinoma. In immunosuppressed patients, HPV-associated warts are slow to respond to treatment, recur repeatedly and progress to dysplasia and malignancy more rapidly than in normal individuals.

5. **D – *Cryptosporidium parvum***

The two organisms on this list that commonly cause diarrhoea are cytomegalovirus and *Cryptosporidium parvum*. The typical features of CMV infection have been described above. *C. parvum* causes a self-limiting acute diarrhoea in normal individuals but in HIV-infected patients it causes severe, watery diarrhoea associated with anorexia, nausea, vomiting and abdominal pain. Cysts attach to the surface epithelium of the small intestine and cause malabsorption and secretion of fluid into the intestinal lumen. The cysts are readily identified on duodenal biopsy and can also be seen on stool microscopy using a special stain.

12. PATHOLOGICAL PROCESSES

1. F – Hyperplasia

Hyperplasia is an increase in the number of cells in a given cell population. In contrast, hypertrophy is an increase in size of cells without an increase in number. Hyperplasia is usually hormonally driven, while hypertrophy occurs in response to an increased workload. The decrease in oestrogen levels that occurs at the menopause causes atrophy of the post-menopausal endometrium with widely spaced glands that lack mitotic activity. In contrast, this patient's endometrium has closely packed glands with obvious proliferation, indicating hyperplasia. Hyperplasias of the endometrium occur in response to excess oestrogen. This can be endogenous (eg from an oestrogen-secreting ovarian tumour) or exogenous, as a result of oestrogen therapy. Tamoxifen is an oestrogen antagonist in the breast, hence its widespread use in the treatment of breast carcinoma, but in the endometrium it acts as a partial oestrogen agonist and endometrial hyperplasia is therefore common in women on tamoxifen.

2. I – Metaplasia

Metaplasia is a change in cell type from one fully differentiated form to another fully differentiated form. It is usually a protective response to chronic irritation or cell damage, the new cell type being more able to withstand the irritating agent than the original. The respiratory tract is normally lined by ciliated, pseudostratified columnar epithelium. This type of epithelium cannot easily withstand the injury caused by cigarette smoke so metaplasia occurs to stratified squamous epithelium, which is better able to withstand the damage. Like many other metaplastic conditions, squamous metaplasia of the bronchus is prone to developing dysplasia and so is associated with an increased risk of malignancy.

3. B – Atrophy

Atrophy is a decrease in the size of cells, tissues or organs, often leading to a loss of function. Lack of use of striated muscles, as often occurs in patients who are bed-bound, leads to shrinkage in the size of myocytes and to loss of muscle bulk. This is known as 'disuse atrophy'.

4. H – Infarction

A stroke is defined as a neurological deficit that lasts more than 24 hours. Infarction is defined as necrosis of tissue caused by interruption of its blood supply. The vast majority of strokes are caused by either cerebral infarction or cerebral haemorrhage. In this patient's case there is a necrotic lesion in the left hemisphere and, although the CT appearances are not pathognomonic, a cerebral infarct is the most likely underlying pathology here.

5. G – Hypertrophy

As described in the answer to the first scenario in this group, hypertrophy is an increase in size of cells without an increase in number and usually occurs in response to an increased workload. In patients with chronic lung disease the right ventricle has to pump against increased vascular resistance and its workload is therefore increased. The consequent increase in the size of the cardiac myocytes leads to right ventricular hypertrophy and eventually to right-sided heart failure. Right ventricular hypertrophy as a consequence of chronic lung disease is termed known as 'cor pulmonale'.

13. CHEST RADIOGRAPHS – CLINICAL SCENARIOS

1. **(P1–P2) H – Globular heart**
   This patient has developed a significant pericardial effusion secondary to a probable viral pericarditis. The radiograph shows a large, globular heart. Significant pericardial effusions can cause a cardiac tamponade which in turn can lead to 'pulsus parodoxus'. Originally described by Kussmaul, the paradox is said to be that the patient is seen to be alive despite having no palpable peripheral pulses or audible heart sounds.

2. **(P1–P2) D – Mitralised left heart border**
   This patient has signs of significant mitral stenosis, including the 'ruby cheeks' (mitral facies) and a low rumbling mid-diastolic murmur. Other signs include atrial fibrillation (due to the enlarged left atrium), a low-volume pulse, an undisplaced, 'tapping' apex beat and an early-diastolic opening snap. Severe mitral stenosis leads to biventricular failure and is commonly associated with tricuspid regurgitation due to stretching of the tricuspid valve ring as the right ventricle enlarges.

3. **(P1–P2) A – Left ventricular failure**
   This patient has developed acute pulmonary oedema after suffering an acute anterior ST-elevation myocardial infarction (STEMI). A large anterior STEMI can severely compromise the left ventricle (particularly without thrombolytic or angiography-led intervention) and in turn can lead to acute severe left ventricular failure. The incidence of such severe acute (and later chronic) complications, such as arrhythmias and heart failure, have been significantly reduced by thrombolysis and angiography-led interventions.

4. **(P1–P2) B – Bronchiectasis**
   This gentleman has developed bronchiectasis, which is caused by dilation and destruction of the distal airways. Common causes include cystic fibrosis, proximal obstruction due to plugging (eg in tuberculosis) and large obstructing tumours.

5. **(P1–P2) J – Thoracic aortic aneurysm**
   This woman has the symptoms and signs of a dissecting thoracic aortic aneurysm. Classically, dissection involving the ascending thoracic aorta can cause angina-like chest pain, but radiation of the pain between the scapulae should always raise the possibility of a dissection. Other signs include asymmetrical radial pulses and blood pressures in the upper limb (as in this case).

IMAGES: pages 345–347

14. INNERVATION OF THE MUSCLES OF THE UPPER LIMB

1. **C – Long thoracic nerve**
    The nerve arises from the fifth, sixth and seventh roots of the brachial plexus and passes downwards behind the trunks and vessels to reach the medial wall of the axilla and supply the muscle.

2. **G – Musculocutaneous nerve**
    The nerve is a terminal branch of the lateral cord of the brachial plexus. It passes laterally to supply coracobrachialis, biceps and brachialis, and emerges lateral to these muscles to pierce the deep fascia in front of the elbow and become the lateral cutaneous nerve of the forearm.

3. **I – Radial nerve**
    This nerve is the continuation of the posterior cord of the brachial plexus. It passes obliquely over the spiral groove of the humerus in the posterior compartment of the arm. It supplies triceps, brachioradialis and extensor carpi radialis longus. Its posterior interosseous branch supplies the muscles arising from the common extensor origin and from the extensor aspect of the forearm.

4. **F – Median nerve**
    The median nerve passes between the heads of the pronator teres and deep to the flexor digitorum superficialis in the forearm. It supplies both these muscles, together with the flexor carpi radialis, palmaris longus, the thenar muscles (except adductor longus), the lateral two lumbricals and, through its anterior interosseous branch, the flexor pollicis longus, pronator quadratus and the lateral half of the flexor digitorum profundus.

5. **J – Ulnar nerve**
    The ulnar nerve enters the forearm between the heads of the flexor carpi ulnaris and supplies it and the medial half of the flexor digitorum profundus, the hypothenar and interosseous muscles, the medial two lumbricals and the adductor pollicis muscle.

PAPER 3

Paper 3 Questions

1. THEME: CARDIAC THERAPIES

A   Abciximab
B   Aspirin
C   Atenolol
D   Bisoprolol
E   Clopidogrel
F   Insulin
G   Isosorbide mononitrate
H   Nicorandil
I   Streptokinase
J   tPA

The following patients have all presented with cardiac disease. Please choose the NEXT most appropriate therapeutic intervention from the above list. The options may be used once, more than once or not at all.

1. A 61-year-old man with long-standing ischaemic heart disease is re-referred to the Cardiology Out-patient Clinic with a 3-month history of worsening shortness of breath on exertion and occasional episodes of angina lasting no longer than 2–3 minutes and always relieved with glyceryl trinitrate (GTN) spray. His ECG shows mild to moderate left ventricular dysfunction. He is on clopidogrel (he could not tolerate aspirin) and also takes GTN spray as required.

2. A 79-year-old woman presents in the Emergency Department with a 3-hour history of angina-like chest pain, which is now resolving. She is haemodynamically stable but her ECG shows ST depression in leads V_1–V_4. She is admitted and placed on aspirin and metoprolol. Her subsequent troponin I is negative.

3. A 44-year-old man who is awaiting transfer for coronary stenting develops further angina pain that persists despite low-molecular-weight heparin, a nitrate infusion and maximal oral anti-anginal therapy.

4. A 38-year-old man with a strong family history of ischaemic heart disease (IHD) presents in the Emergency Department with a 90-minute history of severe central chest pain. On examination in the resuscitation area, he is tachycardic, hypotensive and looks distressed and unwell. His ECG confirms ST elevation in leads V_1–V_4. He was given aspirin by the paramedics and has received some diamorphine and antiemetic for the pain.

5. A 64-year-old man presents to his GP with a 3-month history of worsening angina. He is placed on a β-blocker and aspirin and is told to use a GTN spray if and when he gets any further pain. Six months later he returns complaining of worsening pains. He is referred to the Cardiology Clinic for further assessment.

2. THEME: BACK PAIN

A Acute disc prolapse
B Ankylosing spondylitis
C Lytic metastases
D Multiple myeloma
E Osteoarthritis
F Osteoporotic collapse
G Paget's disease of bone
H Pott's disease of the spine
I Retroperitoneal haematoma
J Sclerotic metastases

The following patients have all presented with back pain. Please choose the most appropriate cause from the above list. The options may be used once, more than once or not at all.

1. A 25-year-old man presents to his GP with a 4-month history of increasing pain in his lumbar spine radiating into his buttocks and down the backs of his lower limbs. He has also had painful red eyes over the last few weeks. Radiographs of his lumbar spine and pelvis reveal erosions of his sacroiliac joints.

2. A 67-year-old man presents to his GP with increasing pain in his lower back, malaise and lethargy. On examination, he is clinically anaemic and has marked purpura over his forearms. He has hepatosplenomegaly but no associated lymphadenopathy and is tender over L3/L4. Routine investigations show: haemoglobin 6.1 g/dl, MCV 89 fl, WCC 3.2×10^9/l, platelets 21×10^9/l; ESR 117 mm/h.

3. A 39-year-old homeless man is admitted to hospital with severe mid-thoracic back pain. On examination, he is unwell, pyrexial and is very tender over T8/T9. The radiograph of his thoracic spine shows loss of the intervertebral space between T8 and T9 and erosion of the two vertebral bodies.

4. A 47-year-old woman presents to her GP with a 5-month history of change in bowel habit and weight loss. Colonoscopy reveals a large polypoid tumour 37 cm from the anal margin, which is surgically excised. Four months later she returns to the GP with severe lumbar back pain.

5. A 74-year-old man presents to his GP with severe lower back, hip and pelvic pain. Radiographs of his pelvis show: 'increased trabecular pattern with cortical thickening'.

3. THEME: LIVER TESTS

	Total bilirubin (μmol/l)	Unconjugated /conjugated bilirubin (μmol/l)	AST (IU/L)	ALT (IU/l)	Alkaline phosphatase (IU/l)	γGT (IU/l)	Albumin (g/l)
A	32	28/4	12	16	143	23	40
B	69	4/65	1453	1619	250	45	38
C	71	5/66	52	73	1323	258	37
D	10	3/7	21	32	212	34	16
E	7	1/6	23	17	204	13	40
F	8	2/6	13	14	1089	16	39
G	9	1/8	17	20	1089	434	40
H	6	1/5	479	13	188	18	40

The following patients have all presented with conditions leading to derangement of their liver tests. Please choose the most appropriate set of liver tests from the above list. You may use the options once, more than once or not at all.

1. A 23-year-old medical student returns from her elective in Thailand with a 10-day history of a flu-like illness, which is now associated with 48 hours of jaundice. Of note, she had been staying in a very poor fishing community where they ate lots of shellfish. The diagnosis is confirmed when a specific IgM is found to be raised in her serum.

2. A 54-year-old man is admitted to hospital for a routine left total knee replacement. Two days postoperatively he is found to have deranged liver tests but the consultant on-call is 'unimpressed' and diagnoses the patient as simply having Gilbert's syndrome.

3. An 83-year-old woman is admitted to hospital with severe hip and pelvic pain, leading her inability to manage at home. Her liver tests and radiological investigations confirm that she has Paget's disease of bone.

4. A 97-year-old woman is admitted to her local hospital after being found on the floor by her neighbour. On examination, she has multiple carpet burns and is pyrexial and delirious. Investigations show that her serum creatin kinase is 21,000 IU/l and she has myoglobinuria.

5. A 67-year-old man is admitted to hospital with a 5-day history of painless jaundice on a background of several months of weight loss and anorexia. An ultrasound scan of the abdomen reveals a large mass in the head of his pancreas.

4. THEME: CAUSES OF ABDOMINAL PAIN

A   Acute intermittent porphyria
B   Acute pancreatitis
C   Diabetes mellitus
D   Diverticulitis
E   Gallstones
F   Incarcerated femoral hernia
G   Mesenteric ischaemia
H   Peptic ulcer
I   Splenic infarct
J   Spontaneous bacterial peritonitis

The following patients have all presented with abdominal pain. Please choose the most appropriate cause from the above list. Each cause may be used once, more than once or not at all.

1. A 29-year-old man presents in the Emergency Department with severe, generalised abdominal pain and vomiting after a night out celebrating his birthday. On examination, he is tachycardic, hypertensive and is obviously inebriated. Investigations show: haemoglobin 13.9 g/dl, MCV 86 fl, WCC 11.9 × 10^9/l, platelets 299 × 10^9/l; Na$^+$ 134 mmol/l, K$^+$ 3.9 mmol/l, urea 6.6 mmol/l, creatinine 84 μmol/l, amylase 67 IU/l; total bilirubin 29 μmol/l, AST 54 IU/l, alkaline phosphatase 127 IU/l, albumin 39 g/l.

2. An overweight, 34-year-old woman presents to her GP with severe upper abdominal pain and vomiting. On examination she is unwell, jaundiced and pyrexial. She has a positive Murphy's sign. She is admitted to hospital and improves with intravenous cefuroxime and metronidazole. Investigations show: haemoglobin 13.9 g/dl, WCC 23.5 × 10^9/l, platelets 322 × 10^9/l; total bilirubin 41 μmol/l, AST 39 IU/l, alkaline phosphatase 347 IU/l, albumin 37 g/l, γGT 184 IU/l; amylase 210 IU/l.

3. A 91-year-old woman is admitted to hospital with severe left lower quadrant pain. On examination, she is unwell and distressed and has obvious left lower quadrant rebound and tenderness. The admitting doctor documents that there is no hernia but the abdominal radiograph reveals dilated loops of small bowel consistent with obstruction.

4. A 42-year-old man with a long history of alcohol excess presents with severe general abdominal pain. He is encephalopathic, jaundiced and has clinical ascites. He has severe general abdominal tenderness. An ascitic tap reveals > 250 white cells/mm^3.

5. A 47-year-old smoker presents to his GP with recurrent upper abdominal pain associated with meals. Of note, he has had two previous myocardial infarctions and experiences intermittent claudication in the calves (on the right more than the left). Routine blood tests, including FBC, U&Es, LFTs and amylase are normal and an oesophagogastroduodenoscopy shows mild gastritis, with a negative *Campylobacter*-like organism (CLO) test.

5. THEME: DELIRIUM

A   Atypical pneumonia
B   Encephalopathy
C   Hypercalcaemia
D   Hypercapnia
E   Hypoglycaemia
F   Hyponatraemia
G   Meningitis
H   Opiate narcosis
I   Subdural haemorrhage
J   Uraemia

The following patients have all presented with delirium. Please choose the most appropriate cause from the above list. The options may be used once, more than once or not at all.

1. An 83-year-old woman is visited at home by her son. She is very confused and is dragging her left leg. He takes her to the local hospital and tells the admitting doctor that she has been deteriorating over the past 10 days since she fell down a flight of steps while out on a coach trip with her friends.

2. A previously fit and well 92-year-old woman is admitted to hospital with diarrhoea, faecal incontinence and increasing confusion. Routine investigations reveal: haemoglobin 12.2 g/dl, MCV 85 fl, WCC 7.8 × 10^9/l (with a relative lymphopenia), platelets 377 × 10^9/l; Na$^+$ 127 mmol/l, K$^+$ 4.3 mmol/l, urea 9.7 mmol/l, creatinine 107 μmol/l. She is noted to have type-I respiratory failure despite a relatively normal chest radiograph.

3. A 78-year-old woman is started on paroxetine by her GP following the death of her son in a motorbike accident. Three weeks later the GP is called out by the patient's youngest son who is concerned that she has become increasingly confused. The GP can find no abnormalities on examination, urinalysis or capillary blood glucose. The son does not want her admitted to hospital, so the GP stops the paroxetine and sends some routine blood tests. She improves over the next week, as do her abnormal tests.

4. A 79-year-old woman with known hypertension and ischaemic heart disease is started on ramipril. Her other medications include bendroflumethiazide and spironolactone. Six weeks later she is admitted to hospital with increasing confusion and is noted to have hiccups and 'twitches'.

5. A 79-year-old woman is started on chlorpropamide in Pakistan after being admitted to hospital with chest pains and a high blood glucose. Several months after her return to the UK she is found at home by her daughter very clammy and confused. She improves with some glucagon administered by paramedics.

6. THEME: SKIN RASHES

A   Contact dermatitis
B   Discoid lupus
C   Erythema multiforme
D   Erythema nodosum
E   Lupus vulgaris
F   Pemphigoid
G   Pemphigus
H   Psoriasis
I   Pyoderma gangrenosum
J   Rosacea

The following patients have all presented with a skin rash. Please choose the most appropriate cause from the above list. Each condition may be used once, more than once or not at all.

1. A 17-year-old girl who has recently been started on the oral contraceptive pill presents to her GP with a painful rash over her shins. On examination, the GP notes that the lesions have coalesced and are tender to palpation.

2. A previously fit and well, 27-year-old man is referred to the 'leg ulcer' clinic with an ulcerating lesion on the left shin. He describes the lesion as starting several weeks ago as an area of pustules, which 'joined up' to form the bigger ulcer.

3. A 69-year-old woman is admitted to hospital with delirium secondary to a urinary tract infection. She is started on trimethoprim but 2 days later she develops a severe blistering rash over her limbs, back, chest and abdomen. The ST4 Registrar comments on the presence of 'target lesions'.

4. A 77-year-old man presents in the Emergency Department with a severe blistering rash involving 'most areas of his skin'. The FY1 doctor notes the blisters are 'completely popped and raw' and involve his face and oral mucosa. He improves slowly with oral prednisolone.

5. A 21-year-old Asian man is admitted to hospital with a severe pneumonia, haemoptysis and fever. The ST1 doctor notes a scaling plaque-like lesion over his shin. A biopsy confirms 'granulomatous infiltration with positive staining for AAFBs'.

7. THEME: RECTAL BLEEDING

A   Anal carcinoma
B   Anal fissure
C   Angiodysplasia
D   Colonic carcinoma
E   Colonic polyp
F   Crohn's disease
G   Diverticular disease
H   Haemorrhoids
I   Infective colitis
J   Ischaemic colitis
K   Ulcerative colitis

The following patients have all presented with rectal bleeding. Please select the most appropriate diagnosis from the above list. The options may be used once, more than once or not at all.

1. An 18-year-old mother presents with a 1-week history of bright-red rectal bleeding and severe anal pain on defecation. Her symptoms started post-partum. On examination, rectal examination is impossible because of discomfort but no obvious abnormality is seen.

2. A 32-year-old man presents with a 3-week history of lower abdominal colicky pain, diarrhoea (bowels opening 6–10 per day) and the passage of blood mixed with the stool. Investigations show: haemoglobin 9.8 g/dl, MCV 78.6 fl; WCC 12.1 × 10^9/l ESR 62 mm/h.

3. A 76-year-old woman with a 10–year history of intermittent constipation and left-sided abdominal pain presents in the Emergency Department with a 48-hour history of dark-red rectal bleeding. Rectal examination is unremarkable and sigmoidoscopy only demonstrates blood in the lumen. She had a similar episode investigated 1 year previously with no site of bleeding found.

4. A 37-year-old homosexual man presents with a 3-month history of episodes of bright-red rectal bleeding associated with soreness and pruritis ani. On examination, he has widespread excoriations perianally, and an area of ulceration at the anal verge with an everted irregular edge.

5. A 92-year-old woman presents with painless, bright-red rectal bleeding with no other associated symptoms. She has a normal barium enema and is sent back to the nursing home where she lives. One week later she rebleeds and returns to the Emergency Department. Again, the bleeding settles and after another transfusion she undergoes a gastroscopy and colonoscopy. No abnormality is found and she is referred for mesenteric angiography.

8. THEME: COMMON FRACTURE EPONYMS

A Barton's fracture
B Bennett's fracture
C Colles' fracture
D Galeazzi fracture
E Garden II fracture
F Garden IV fracture
G Monteggia fracture–dislocation
H Pott's fracture
I Salter–Harris fracture
J Smith's fracture

The following are descriptions of fractures. Please select the most appropriate fracture from the above list. These are all commonly used in current clinical practice (and so remain important). The options may be used once, more than once or not at all.

1. An injury in which the upper half of the ulna is fractured and the radial head is dislocated.

2. An injury in a child involving the growth plate (physis).

3. An injury in which the fibula and tibia are fractured at the ankle.

4. A complete but undisplaced fracture of the neck of femur.

5. A fracture–subluxation of the first metacarpal.

9. THEME: SALIVARY GLAND DISEASE

A Adenoid cystic carcinoma
B Bacterial sialadenitis
C HIV-associated sialadenitis
D Lymphoma
E Pleomorphic adenoma
F Sjögren's syndrome
G Sialolithiasis
H Viral parotitis
I Warthin's tumour

The following are descriptions of patients with salivary gland disorders. Please select the most appropriate descriptive term from the above list. The options may be used once, more than once or not at all.

1. A 67-year-old man with progressive dysphagia and cachexia is nil by mouth in preparation for an endoscopy. You are called to see him on the ward where you find him to be dehydrated and pyrexial, with a left parotid swelling which is hot and tender.

2. A 21-year-old man presents in Ophthalmology Out-patients with dry eyes and recurrent conjunctivitis. On direct questioning, he admits to having a dry mouth. On examination, there is swelling of his salivary glands and cervical lymphadenopathy. There is no history of polyarthritis and a full autoantibody screen is negative.

3. A 32-year-old man presents with a short history of acute left submandibular pain and swelling immediately (1 minute) after eating.

4. A 44-year-old woman is referred to Surgical Out-patients by her GP with a 3-cm swelling in the region of the right parotid gland. The swelling is smooth and non-tender. There is no lymphadenopathy. Facial nerve function is intact.

5. An 80-year-old man has a long-standing swelling of the left parotid gland, which he declined to have removed because of ill health. Recently, the mass has grown markedly and is causing pain. Of note, he has a lower motor neurone facial nerve palsy.

10. THEME: INTRAPARTUM COMPLICATIONS

A   Cephalopelvic disproportion (CPD)
B   Chorioamnionitis
C   Cord prolapse
D   Malposition of the occiput
E   Meconium-stained liquor
F   Placental abruption
G   Ruptured uterus
H   Shoulder dystocia
I   Uterine hyperstimulation
J   Uterine inertia

From the above list please choose the condition most likely to have caused the clinical picture described. Each option may be used once, more than once or not at all.

1.   A 30-year-old primiparous woman is being induced at 42 weeks' gestation for prolonged pregnancy. Her antenatal period has been complicated by idiopathic polyhydramnios. The presenting part (cephalic) is five-fifths palpable. Immediately after a controlled artificial rupture of membranes (ARM) there is a fetal bradycardia to 60 bpm. There is no vaginal bleeding and the uterus is soft and non-tender. After a vaginal examination, the Registrar positions the woman on all-fours with elbows to knees and head down before taking her straight for emergency Caesarean section.

2.   A 30-year-old primiparous woman is in spontaneous labour at term. Her antenatal period has been uneventful. She is 5-cm dilated at 6 am. At her next vaginal examination at 10 am she is still 5-cm dilated.

3.   A 30-year-old, primiparous, low-risk woman is in spontaneous labour at term. Her antenatal period has been uneventful. She is 5-cm dilated at 6 am and is being monitored by intermittent auscultation. After spontaneous rupture of membranes (SROM), however, the Registrar now recommends continuous cardiotocography (CTG) monitoring with a quick recourse to fetal blood sampling in the presence of CTG abnormalities.

4.   A 30-year-old, primiparous, low-risk woman is in spontaneous labour at term. Her antenatal period has been uneventful. She is on a Syntocinon® infusion for slow progress and is now contracting 5–6× in 10 minutes, strongly. The CTG shows repeated late decelerations. The Registrar attends and stops the Syntocinon® infusion and awaits events over the next few minutes.

5.   A 30-year-old, multiparous, low-risk woman is in spontaneous labour at term. Her antenatal period has been uneventful. Her labour has progressed well to 8-cm dilatation but after a further 2 hours she is still 8-cm dilated. She is contracting 3× in 10 minutes, strongly. The Registrar examines her vaginally and is unwilling to use Syntocinon®, preferring to reassess her in 1 hour.

11. THEME: BACTERIAL INFECTIONS

A   *Campylobacter jejuni*
B   *Clostridium difficile*
C   *Clostridium perfringens*
D   *Escherichia coli*
E   *Helicobacter pylori*
F   *Neisseria meningitidis*
G   *Salmonella typhi*
H   *Staphylococcus aureus*
I   *Streptococcus pneumoniae*
J   *Streptococcus pyogenes*

From the above list, please select the bacterium that each of the following descriptions applies to. You may use each organism once, more than once or not at all.

1. A Gram-negative, lactose-fermenting bacillus that is a common cause of urinary tract infection.

2. A Gram-negative coccus that is a common cause of meningitis in adults.

3. A Gram-positive, α-haemolytic diplococcus that causes lobar pneumonia.

4. A Gram-positive, cytotoxin-producing bacillus that causes pseudomembranous colitis.

5. An S-shaped, urease-positive bacillus that is the major cause of chronic gastritis and peptic ulcer disease. The organism stains poorly with Gram stain.

12. THEME: CHEST RADIOGRAPHS – ASSOCIATED DISORDERS

*Using the radiographic images **A-J on pages (348 – 350)**, please match the associated disorders shown described below to the correct image. You may use each image once, more than once or not at all. There may be more than one image appropriate for each disorder.*

1. Rheumatic fever. ☐

2. Hypertension. ☐

3. Myasthenia gravis. ☐

4. Dressler's syndrome. ☐

5. Childhood measles infection. ☐

6. Iodine deficiency. ☐

13. THEME: CRANIAL NERVES

A Abducent nerve
B Accessory nerve
C Facial nerve
D Glossopharyngeal nerve
E Hypoglossal nerve
F Oculomotor nerve
G Trigeminal nerve
H Trochlear nerve
I Vagus nerve
J Vestibular nerve

For each of the following descriptions, please choose the most appropriate nerve from the above list. Each nerve may be used once, more than once or not at all.

1. Has a branch passing through the foramen rotundum.

2. Provides secretomotor fibres to the parotid gland.

3. Innervates lateral gaze.

4. Innervates the cricothyroid muscle.

5. Transmits the taste fibres from the anterior two-thirds of the tongue to the tractus solitarius.

14. THEME: MUSCLES CONCERNED WITH MASTICATION

A   Anterior belly of digastric
B   Buccinator
C   Genioglossus
D   Hyoglossus
E   Lateral pterygoid
F   Masseter
G   Medial pterygoid
H   Mylohyoid
I   Palatoglossus
J   Temporalis

For each of the following descriptions, please choose the most appropriate muscle from the above list. Each muscle may be used once, more than once or not at all.

1. Supplied by the facial nerve.

2. Attached to the body of the hyoid bone.

3. Has the submandibular duct as a lateral relation.

4. Is attached to the lower border of the anterior two-thirds of the zygomatic arch.

5. Is attached to the intra-articular disc of the temporomandibular joint.

Paper 3 Answers

1. CARDIAC THERAPIES

1. D – Bisoprolol
This patient has unstable angina and symptoms suggestive of the mild to moderate heart failure seen on the ECG. Recent cardiology studies have contradicted previous thinking on the use of β-blockers in cardiac failure and have shown improvements in both morbidity and mortality, particularly with the use of the cardioselective β-blockers such as bisoprolol, carvedilol and metoprolol. In this case the β-blocker effects will also improve his anginal symptoms.

2. E – Clopidogrel
This woman has developed an acute coronary syndrome. Her subsequent troponin I suggests that no significant myocardial damage has been sustained. She has been placed on aspirin and metoprolol and results of the recent CURE (Clopidogrel in Unstable angina to prevent Recurrent Events) study have suggested that such patients should also be placed on clopidogrel. The benefits of this combination of antiplatelet therapy must be balanced against the increased risk of upper gastrointestinal bleeding, particularly in the elderly.

3. A – Abciximab
This patient has unstable angina and is awaiting a definitive procedure. He is on maximal anti-anginal therapy and low-molecular-weight heparin and until he can be transferred for his stenting he should be placed on abciximab, the GIIb/IIIa-receptor antagonist. This class of drugs has been licensed for use in non-ST-elevation myocardial infarctions (non-STEMIs) but they are principally used in patients waiting for coronary investigations and procedures. The glycoprotein GIIb/IIIa receptor is a platelet receptor and blocking it stops platelet and fibrinogen binding and so clot formation.

4. J – tPA
This young man presents with hypotension, tachycardia and ECG changes suggestive of an acute anterior myocardial infarction. He has received analgesia and aspirin and should now have thrombolytic therapy. He has presented with the four criteria for administering tissue plasminogen activator (tPA) rather than streptokinase – he is young, male, has presented early (within 4 hours) and has an acute anterior myocardial infarction. However, the principal reason for administering tPA rather than streptokinase is his hypotension. Streptokinase can cause hypotension and so is contraindicated in this case.

5. H – Nicorandil
This man has ongoing unstable angina despite the β-blocker and aspirin he is taking. He should have his anti-anginal therapy increased and secondary risk factors addressed (eg smoking, hyperlipidaemia and hyperglycaemia), and he may require coronary angiography. The recent IONA study has suggested the potassium-gate agonist, nicorandil, should be considered as the second-line therapy after β-blockade, rather than calcium-channel blockers or nitrates. Side-effects are similar to those for nitrates and include headaches, flushing and hypotension.

2. BACK PAIN

1. **B – Ankylosing spondylitis**
   This patient has developed ankylosing spondylitis with associated iritis. It principally affects young men and presents with low back pain and stiffness. It has a genetic association with HLA-B27. The classic pain of sacroiliitis is felt in the buttocks and radiates down the back of the legs. The diagnosis is confirmed by radiographic evidence of sacroiliac erosion. Later in the disease the sacroiliac joints fuse and the lumbar vertebrae develop outgrowths known as 'syndesmophytes', which cause the classic appearance of 'bamboo spine'.

2. **D – Multiple myeloma**
   This man has developed signs and symptoms of a pancytopenia secondary to multiple myeloma. He has myelomatous lytic lesions in the spine causing the back pain. He has a grossly elevated ESR and might also have renal impairment, a monoclonal gammopathy and urinary Bence Jones proteins. Myeloma and metastatic disease should always be excluded in any older patient presenting with anaemia and back pain.

3. **H – Pott's disease of the spine**
   This man has developed tuberculosis, which has caused osteomyelitis of the thoracic vertebrae and subsequent tuberculous abscess, eponymously called 'Pott's disease of the spine'. Patients can present with severe local back pain and fever, as well as pulmonary and other systemic features of tuberculosis. If the abscess is left unchecked it can also cause 'long tract' signs in the limbs, with paraplegia asociated with absolute constipation and urinary retention. Treatment includes decompression and drainage if there are cord symptoms and antituberculous therapy, including rifampicin, isoniazid, (pyridoxine) and pyrazinamide for at least 2 months, with rifampicin and isoniazid continued for a further 4 months.

4. **C – Lytic metastases**
   This patient has developed bony metastases from her colonic carcinoma. Breast, lung, thyroid and kidney usually cause lytic lesions while prostate can cause both lytic and osteosclerotic lesions.

5. **G – Paget's disease of bone**
   This man has developed Paget's disease of bone, as evidenced by the radiographic findings and the raised alkaline phosphatase in the presence of normal liver function tests and serum calcium. Complications of Paget's disease of bone include local pain, pathological fractures and, rarely, osteosarcoma. It can also cause deafness due to otosclerosis and nerve compression, and brainstem and high cervical cord signs due to invagination at the skull base, which is known as 'platybasia'.

3. LIVER TESTS

The 'liver functions tests' (LFTs) are in fact a mixture of tests for enzymes and other molecules. True liver function or synthesis ability is reflected by the albumin level and the clotting factors, reflected by the INR and the activated partial thromboplastin time (APTT) and prothrombin time (PT). In practice, only the total bilirubin is provided and you have to request a breakdown of the conjugated and unconjugated components to differentiate pre-hepatic from hepatic causes of abnormality. The transaminases (aspartate transaminase or AST and alanine transaminase or ALT) reflect hepatocyte function and so when they rise significantly with respect to the alkaline phosphatase this is classified as 'hepatitic' jaundice. When the reverse is true, the predominant rise being in the alkaline phosphatase, the jaundice is said to be 'obstructive' (both alkaline phosphatae and gamma-glutamyltransferase [γGT] are produced within the smooth muscle of the biliary tree and rise in parallel). However, though this classification has been taught to undergraduates since the discovery of these different enzymes, in everyday practice there is often a mixed picture, where both sets of enzymes rising almost in unison and this division therefore becomes slightly academic.

1. **B – Bilirubin 69 μmol/l (unconjugated/conjugated 4/65), AST 1453 IU/l, ALT 1619 IU/l, alkaline phosphatase 250 IU/l, γGT 45 IU/l, albumin 38 g/l**
   This student has acquired hepatitis A, which causes a transient hepatitic jaundice, reflected by the raised transaminases. In the patients who do become frankly jaundiced, this is often short-lived, and is paradoxically ofen the time when they start to feel better. Hepatitis A is diagnosed by a rise in a specific IgM against the virus. The spread of hepatitis S is via the faecal–oral route and is the infection is prevalent in any areas of poor sanitation. It is also commonly associated with shellfish growing in infected waters.

2. **A – Bilirubin 32 μmol/l (unconjucated/conjugated 28/4), AST 12 IU/l, ALT 16 IU/l, alkaline phosphatase 143 IU/l, γGT 23 IU/l, albumin 40 g/l**
   Gilbert's syndrome (first described by French gastroenterologist Augustin Nicolas Gilbert, 1858–1927) is a hereditary liver disorder caused by a defect of the enzyme glucuronyl transferase. This leads to defective conjugation of bilirubin, causing an unconjugated hyperbilirubinaemia. Unlike haemolytic causes of unconjugated hyperbilirubinaemia, the reticulocyte count will be normal and the other markers of haemolysis (eg reduced haptoglobins) are also normal. Gilbert's syndrome is a common, benign finding in acutely unwell or stressed patients (eg postoperatively) but rarely if ever causes levels of hyperbilirubinaemia high enough to cause frank jaundice.

3. **F – Bilirubin 8 μmol/l (unconjugated/conjugated 2/6), AST 13 IU/l, ALT 14 IU/l, alkaline phosphatase 1089 IU/l, γGT 16 IU/l, albumin 39 g/l**
   Alkaline phosphatase is included in most liver test profiles. This enzyme is found throughout the body's cells but is concentrated in the liver, bile duct, kidney and bone cells, and so when the alkaline phosphatase is raised with no other derangement of the routine liver tests, a gamma-glutamyltransferase (γGT) should be requested. If this is raised, the alkaline phosphatase can be presumed to be hepatic in origin; if it is normal, the alkaline phosphatase is most likely to be derived from a pathological condition of the bone. In this case, radiology, a bone profile (calcium and phosphate) and urinary hydroxyl-proline will confirm the diagnosis of Pagets' bone disease.

4. **H – Bilirubin 6 μmol/l (unconjugated/conjugated 1/5), AST 479 IU/l, ALT 13 IU/l, alkaline phosphatase 188 IU/l, γGT 18 IU/l, albumin 40 g/l**

    This patient has been lying on the floor for a prolonged period of time and has suffered a 'crush injury', leading to rhabdomyolysis. The insult to the large muscles causes release of muscle enzymes, including creatine kinase and AST. Although common in most tissues in the body, AST is found in high concentrations in skeletal and cardiac muscle and in the liver. It is included as one of the transaminases in a liver profile but when the other components are normal, other sources should be considered.

5. **C – Bilirubin 71 μmol/l (unconjugated/conjugated 5/66), AST 52 IU/l, ALT 73 IU/l, alkaline phosphatase 1323 IU/l, γGT 258 IU/l, albumin 37 g/l**

    Painless jaundice in older patients is a sinister sign and implies that they probably have a malignant obstruction of the biliary tree. This is usually caused by a large mass in the head of the pancreas but it also can be caused by a cholangiocarcinoma or the relatively rare carcinoma at the ampulla of Vater (in the duodenum). Obstruction associated with pain signifies cholangitis, associated with gallstones and other less malignant (but no less dangerous) causes of jaundice.

4. CAUSES OF ABDOMINAL PAIN

1. **A – Acute intermittent porphyria**
   This man has acute intermittent porphyria (AIP) precipitated by his 'alcoholic' celebrations. Patients present with severe abdominal pain but their initial investigations, including FBC, U&Es, glucose and amylase are often unremarkable other than a slight leucocytosis. Other common acute precipitants include drugs.

2. **E – Gallstones**
   This woman has developed acute cholecystitis secondary to her gallstones. These can also cause acute pancreatitis. The diagnosis should be confirmed by an ultrasound scan of the liver and biliary tree. If this shows dilatation of the biliary tract, an endoscopic retrograde cholangiopancreatography (ERCP) should be undertaken.

3. **F – Incarcerated femoral hernia**
   Older women often present with incarcerated femoral rather than inguinal herniae and these are often be missed by the inexperienced clinician. If otherwise well, the patient requires urgent operative intervention or the incarcerated bowel will become ischaemic and perforate.

4. **J – Spontaneous bacterial peritonitis**
   This patient with alcohol-related chronic liver disease has developed spontaneous bacterial peritonitis, which in turn has led to encephalopathy and acute hepatic decompensation. The peritonitis is thought to be due to bacteria crossing the bowel mucosa into the previously established ascites, leading to an acute infection. This is confirmed by the high WCC in the ascites. Treatment includes intravenous cefuroxime and metronidazole, intravenous fluids and good nursing care while the patient remains encephalopathic.

5. **G – Mesenteric ischaemia**
   This man has mesenteric ischaemia or 'abdominal angina'. The patient classically experiences ischaemic-type pain with or after meals. Invariably, as with this man, they have arterial disease. The diagnosis can be confirmed by mesenteric angiography and it might be possible to perform bypass or revascularisation procedures. The classic presentation is 'food fear' (due to the pain), diarrhoea and weight loss. There is often a delay in making this diagnosis as the presentation can mimic many other abdominal conditions. The patient can often be subjected to numerous other investigations before a definitive diagnosis is made.

5. DELIRIUM

1. **I – Subdural haemorrhage**
   This patient's fall down some stairs has led to a subdural haemorrhage and subsequent right-sided space-occupying effects, including a left monoparesis and confusion suggestive of raised intracranial pressure. The diagnosis should be confirmed on a CT head scan, which will show a hyperdense concave rim around the right cortex. Early subdural haematomas appear as white (fresh blood) or hypodense areas. Subdural haemorrhages that are around 10 days old can be difficult to define as they are of the same density as underlying brain tissue. This patient needs urgent neurosurgical evacuation of the haemorrhage, which should reverse her monoparesis and confusion.

2. **A – Atypical pneumonia**
   This previously fit and well elderly patient has presented with atypical symptoms (confusion and diarrhoea) and atypical investigation findings (a normal WCC with relative lymphopenia and hyponatraemia) and improves rapidly with cefuroxime and clarithromycin. These are the features of an atypical pneumonia, possibly due to *Legionella pneumophila*. The diagnosis can be confirmed by rising antibody titres and detection of urinary *Legionella* antigen.

3. **F – Hyponatraemia**
   This scenario implies that this older patient has developed significant hyponatraemia secondary to her selective serotonin re-uptake inhibitor (SSRI) treatment. Examination is unremarkable and she rapidly improves with withdrawal of the paroxetine. The diagnosis is confirmed by a set of U&Es but a second set must be sent, even with rapid clinical resolution of the symptoms, to exclude ongoing hyponatraemia. If this is the case, SIADH should be excluded with paired urinary and serum osmolalities.

4. **J – Uraemia**
   This woman has developed signs of uraemia, as evidenced by the confusion, hiccups and 'twitches'. The combination of ramipril (an ACE inhibitor), spironolactone and bendroflumethiazide has caused progressive renal impairment and has led to frank uraemia. The combination of spironolactone and an ACE inhibitor can also lead to hyperkalaemia and careful monitoring of such patients is advisable.

5. **E – Hypoglycaemia**
   This older woman has been placed on chlorpropamide, which is relatively contraindicated in the older patient. This sulphonylurea has a relatively long half-life and will cause hypoglycaemia due to the overlapping effect of two consecutive doses. The patient should be changed either to a shorter-acting sulphonylurea such as gliclazide or to the biguanide metformin. All diabetics need expert multidisciplinary care and follow-up in dedicated specialist clinics.

6. SKIN RASHES

1. **D – Erythema nodosum**

   This girl has developed erythema nodosum secondary to her oral contraceptive pill. Erythema nodosum is a tender, red, plaque-like or nodular rash that classically occurs over the shins. Rarely, it can also affect the upper limbs. Common causes in the UK include inflammatory bowel disease, sarcoid, TB, streptococcal infection and drugs such as the oral contraceptive pill and antibiotics. Around 50% of cases are idiopathic.

2. **I – Pyoderma gangrenosum**

   This man has developed pyoderma gangrenosum, a violaceous, ulcerating lesion that also commonly occurs over the shins. The lesion often begins as pustules and these coalesce to form a large necrotic ulcerating lesion. Around 50% of cases are idiopathic but common associations include inflammatory bowel disease, rheumatoid and the seronegative arthropathies and the haematological malignancies, particularly the paraproteinaemias and acute leukaemias.

3. **C – Erythema multiforme**

   This patient has developed a severe blistering rash secondary to her trimethoprim treatment. This rash is characterised by the presence of annular 'target lesions'. Erythema multiforme is a relatively common side-effect of several classes of drugs (particularly antibiotics), infections such as herpes simplex virus, *Mycoplasma pneumoniae*, *Streptococcus* and TB infections and, more rarely, the systemic arthritides and malignancy. A more malignant form of the condition that involves the mucous membranes, genitalia and eyes, known as 'Stevens–Johnson syndrome', causes a severe systemic illness and can be fatal, particularly in the elderly.

4. **G – Pemphigus**

   Pemphigus and pemphigoid are severe, autoimmune, blistering conditions which occur in late middle age and in the elderly. PemphiguS forms Superficial blisters that typically Sheer and leave large raw areas, commonly in a generalised distribution and involving the mucous membranes. Nikolsky's sign is positive in apparent normal areas of skin. The antibody is found in the epidermiS and is typically an IgG. PemphigoiD, in contrast, is a Deeper lesion that forms large tense blisters over localised areas of the skin such as a limb or the back; the antibody is an IgG and attaches to at the level of the basement membrane in the Dermis. Both conditions require steroid treatment for a prolonged period and this should be accompanied by a bone-sparing agent.

5. **E – Lupus vulgaris**

   Lupus vulgaris is a TB-associated skin condition caused by direct infiltration of the skin by the acid-fast bacilli, usually through haematogenous spread. The chronic lesion can take on a bitten, gnarled appearance (hence its name, lupus meaning 'wolf-like'). The patient often has evidence of pulmonary or systemic TB infection and should be treated with antituberculous therapy for at least 6 months. TB can also be associated with erythema nodosum and erythema multiforme.

7. RECTAL BLEEDING

1. B – Anal fissure

The presentation (acute pain and bleeding) is typical of this condition, which can be precipitated by constipation, acute diarrhoea, pregnancy or childbirth. The condition can be acute (as in this case) or chronic. Treatment is medical (GTN 0.2% ointment heals 50–75% in 8 weeks) or surgical (with lateral sphincterotomy) although this carries a risk of incontinence.

2. K – Ulcerative colitis

This is the commonest diagnosis in a young patient with a long history of bloody diarrhoea. The microcytic anaemia reflects chronic blood loss, and the WCC and ESR reflect the underlying inflammatory condition.

3. G – Diverticular disease

The long history of characteristic symptoms in a woman of this age indicates this as the most likely diagnosis. A carcinoma could present similarly but she has presumably had negative investigations for this the year before.

4. A – Anal carcinoma

While this condition is relatively rare, it has an increased incidence in homosexual men due to anal infection with HPV. Lesions are of epithelial origin and are most commonly squamous. Historically, treatment was by radical surgery (abdominoperineal excision of the rectum) but a long course of chemoradiotherapy is now the preferred first-line treatment in most specialist centres.

5. C – Angiodysplasia

This is a type of arteriovenous malformation and is one of the common causes of significant lower gastrointestinal bleeding in the elderly. As in this case, it is notoriously difficult to pinpoint the offending vessel. Where direct vision fails to do this, mesenteric angiography or radionuclide scans can sometimes be helpful in finding the source but these also often yield negative results if the vessel is not actively bleeding at the time of investigation. Patients therefore sometimes have to undergo a total colectomy as a life-saving measure.

8. COMMON FRACTURE EPONYMS

1. **G – Monteggia fracture–dislocation**
   There are two common fracture–dislocations of the forearm, best known by their Italian eponyms. The other (also in the list) is the Galeazzi fracture and this is an injury in which the lower half of the radius is fractured and the inferior radioulnar joint is dislocated.

2. **I – Salter–Harris fracture**
   Injuries involving the growth plate ('physeal' injuries) are common in children and are a special problem because of the risk of abnormal subsequent bone growth. Salter and Harris' classification of such injuries is useful and defines five types depending on the exact morphology of the injury: types 1 and 2 are milder forms with a good prognosis, but types 3–5 can often result in arrested, slowed or asymmetric growth.

3. **H – Pott's fracture**
   Fractures and fracture–dislocations of the ankle were first described by Percival Pott in 1768. The modern classification is the Danis–Weber classification, which defines three types of injury (A, B and C), depending on level of the fibula fracture and resultant instability. These are, however, still grouped together for convenience as 'Pott's fractures'. The student should note that Pott was not a man whose discoveries were limited to one body region – his name is given to Pott's disease of the spine (TB of the vertebrae) and to Pott's puffy tumour (osteomyelitis of the frontal bone of the skull). He is perhaps best remembered, however, for his description in 1775 of the first occupational cancer, scrotal carcinoma in chimney sweeps.

4. **E – Garden II fracture**
   Garden's classification is perhaps the best known and most commonly used of all fracture classifications. It defines four types, with stage I = incomplete, impacted; stage II = complete, undisplaced; stage III = complete with moderate displacement; and stage IV = severely displaced.

5. **B – Bennett's fracture**
   Bennett described a special case of metacarpal fracture involving the base of the thumb in which an oblique fracture extends into the first metacarpal joint, producing an unstable fracture–subluxation.

9. SALIVARY GLAND DISEASE

1. **B – Bacterial sialadenitis**
This is a typical description of this uncommon condition, which used to occur classically in cases such as that described when salivary flow is reduced. With better attention to in-patient oral hygiene and nutrition, it is now seen equally commonly in patients without any obvious predisposition. Pain is made worse on eating and pus can occasionally be expressed from the duct. Treatment is with antibacterial therapy against the causative staphylococcal and streptococcal organisms.

2. **C – HIV-associated sialadenitis**
The presentation is one of keratoconjunctivitis sicca (dry eyes) and xerostomia (dry mouth). The differential diagnosis is between primary or secondary (ie in association with connective tissue disease) Sjögren's syndrome or HIV infection. The latter is indistinguishable in presentation from Sjögren's syndrome but the autoantibody screen is negative. In addition, Sjögren's syndrome is much less common in males (the female to male ratio is 10 : 1).

3. **G – Sialolithiasis (salivary duct stones)**
The typical history provides the diagnosis. The submandibular gland is most commonly affected (80%) and 80% are radio-opaque. The diagnosis can be confirmed by a contrast sialogram and treatment is largely surgical (stone extraction from Wharton's duct).

4. **E – Pleomorphic adenoma**
This is the most common benign salivary gland tumour (75% of parotid tumours). They can occur at any age (mean age 42) and occur equally in both sexes. Although they are histologically benign, they require complete excision (usually superficial, conservative parotidectomy) to prevent recurrence and the long-term risk of malignant change.

5. **A – Adenoid cystic carcinoma**
There are a number of variants of epidermoid tumours in the salivary gland (squamous, adenosquamous, adenoid cystic, adenocarcinoma) of which this is the most common. In this case, the tumour has arisen from a long-standing pleomorphic adenoma in the parotid (the most common site of malignant as well as benign tumours). Invasion is direct, with a propensity to perineural spread, leading to palsies and eventually CNS destruction and by metastasis to the lung. The prognosis is usually poor. Treatment can involve surgery (radical total parotidectomy) and sometimes radiotherapy.

10. INTRAPARTUM COMPLICATIONS

1. C – Cord prolapse

Polyhydramnios and a high head are risk factors for cord prolapse at the time of artificial rupture of membranes (ARM). If the cord prolapses into the vagina, the change in temperature can cause vasospasm in the umbilical vessels, leading to a fetal bradycardia and fetal death if the baby is not delivered urgently. The manoeuvre described aims to take pressure off the cord by the presenting part. In this context, a placental abruption, which is also more common at the time of ARM with polyhydramnios, is much less likely as there is no evident bleeding and no abdominal signs.

2. J – Uterine inertia

From the list there are only three possible choices for slow progress in labour: uterine inertia ('powers'), malposition of the occiput ('passenger') and cephalopelvic disproportion ('passages and passenger'). True cephalopelvic disproportion is very rare and is usually due to an abnormal pelvis (eg a previous pelvic fracture). In primiparous women, up to 50% (higher in some series) need augmentation due to uterine inertia (inadequate or inco-ordinate contractions). Multiparous women who have laboured before rarely have this problem as their uterine action is more efficient. It is in the multiparous group where malpositions of the occiput are most common.

3. E – Meconium-stained liquor

Intermittent auscultation is recommended for all low-risk women in labour, as cardiotocograph (CTG) monitoring doubles the Caesarian section rate with no reduction in perinatal morbidity or mortality. The risk status can, however, change to high-risk due to the dynamic nature of labour, for example the appearance of meconium-stained liquor, which is only recognised after spontaneous rupture of membranes (SROM). In the presence of meconium-stained liquor, CTG monitoring is recommended and this should be backed up with fetal blood sampling in the presence of CTG abnormalities.

4. I – Uterine hyperstimulation

Syntocinon® is a synthetic oxytocin used to augment or induce labour. It should be titrated against the strength and frequency of uterine contractions, aiming for not more than four in 10 minutes: more frequent contractions represent uterine hyperstimulation. If there is insufficient time for relaxation between contractions, fetal hypoxia can occur relatively rapidly, manifesting as an abnormal CTG. The timing of the contractions and the fact that the infusion was switched off to see if the situation improved indicates that this is the most likely cause. Cord prolapse and abruption are possible, but much less likely.

5. **D – Malposition of the occiput**

From the list there are only three possible choices for slow progress in labour – uterine inertia ('powers'), malposition of the occiput ('passenger') and cephalopelvic disproportion ('passages and passenger'). True cephalopelvic disproportion is rare (usually due to a previous pelvic injury) and multiparous women who have laboured before rarely have a problem with uterine action as it is more efficient than in primiparous women. Her contractions are also described as '3 in 10, strong'. It is in the multiparous group that malpositions of the occiput, especially occipito-posterior (OP) presentation, are the most common cause of slow progress in labour. Syntocinon® should never be used in multiparous women if there is any clinical suspicion of obstructed labour.

11. BACTERIAL INFECTIONS

1. **D –** *Escherichia coli*
    Escherichia coli is the cause of 60–90% of urinary tract infections. It is a Gram-negative, lactose-fermenting bacillus that is a normal commensal of the large intestine. Transfer to the urinary tract can be via the bloodstream, via lymphatics or by direct extension (eg from a vesico-colic fistula) but is most frequently via the ascending transurethral route, particularly in women.

2. **F –** *Neisseria meningitidis*
    The two most likely causes of meningitis from the list are *Neisseria meningitidis* (meningococcus) and *Streptococcus pneumoniae* (pneumococcus). Both organisms are cocci but the former is Gram-negative while the latter is Gram-positive. Diagnosis depends on identifying the organism in CSF or blood culture.

3. **I –** *Streptococcus pneumoniae*
    In about 90% of cases of lobar pneumonia the causative organism is *Streptococcus pneumoniae*. This organism is a Gram-positive diplococcus that shows α-haemolysis on blood agar. The colonies are typically described as 'draughtsman-shaped' on account of their sunken centre. Vagrants and alcoholics who have poor social and medical care are particularly prone to lobar pneumonia.

4. **B –** *Clostridium difficile*
    The organism that causes pseudomembranous colitis is a toxigenic strain of *Clostridium difficile*, an anaerobic Gram-positive bacillus. *C. difficile* produces two toxins: toxin A is an enterotoxin responsible for the gut symptoms; toxin B is a cytotoxin that has a cytopathic effect in cell cultures.

5. **E –** *Helicobacter pylori*
    Helicobacter pylori is an S-shaped, urease-producing, flagellate bacillus that colonises the gastric antrum. In some parts of the third world the prevalence of infection exceeds 80%, and even in industrialised countries the prevalence has been estimated to be 40–50%. Up to 85% of cases of chronic gastritis and 90% of cases of duodenal ulcer are caused by *H. pylori*. The organism has also been implicated in the development of gastric adenocarcinoma and primary gastric lymphoma. *H. pylori* infection can be diagnosed by non-invasive methods such as serology for IgG antibodies or the ^{13}C or ^{14}C urea breath tests. Invasive diagnostic methods require endoscopy and include the rapid urease test, microbiological culture of the organism and histological identification in gastric biopsies. *H. pylori* is found in greatest numbers in the mucus layer on the surface epithelium or in gastric pits. The organism stains poorly with Gram stain and is best visualised using a modified Giemsa stain.

12. CHEST RADIOGRAPHS – ASSOCIATED DISORDERS

1. **(P3–P4) D, H – Mitralised left heart border and globular heart**
   Rheumatic fever can cause a pancarditis, including significant pericarditis and subsequent effusion. Rheumatic fever is still the commonest cause of mitral valve disease worldwide.

2. **(P3–P4) A, J – Left ventricular failure and thoracic aortic aneurysm**
   Hypertension can cause cardiomyopathy, leading to cardiomegaly and biventricular failure. It can also contribute to the formation and subsequent dissection of a thoracic aortic aneurysm.

3. **(P3–P4) E – Sail sign**
   Myasthenia gravis is associated with the development of a thymoma. Myasthenia is an autoimmune disorder characterised by the formation of autoantibodies against the post-synaptic part of the acetylcholine receptor at the neuromuscular junction. The antibodies are positive in about 85–90% of patients. Myasthenia characteristically presents with skeletal muscle weakness and fatiguability. The diagnosis is normally confirmed by an edrophonium or Tensilon® test, which leads to rapid improvement in symptoms and signs. The mainstays of treatment are acetylcholine esterase inhibitors but thymectomy and plasma exchange are also sometimes performed.

4. **(P3–P4) H – Globular heart**
   Dressler's syndrome is an autoimmune pericarditis associated with an acute myocardial infarction. It classically occurs within 2 weeks but can present up to 6 months after a myocardial infarction. This differentiates it from non-immune pericarditis, which occurs within a few days of the myocardial infarction. Treatment includes non-steroidal anti-inflammatory drug (NSAID) analgesia and/or steroids and bedrest.

5. **(P3–P4) B – Bronchiectasis**
   Childhood measles can be associated with the later development of bronchiectasis. Other associations include childhood whooping cough and respiratory syncytial virus (RSV) infection, tuberculosis and other cavitating pneumonias, aspergillosis, proximal, obstructing malignant tumours and cystic fibrosis.

6. **(P3–P4) I – Goitre causing tracheal deviation**
   Iodine deficiency, previously common in mountainous regions of the world and still prevalent in regions of the Indian subcontinent and in central Africa, predisposes to the development of large goitres. In eighteenth-century Britain, this association (iodine deficiency and goitre) was common in the Midlands (hence 'Derbyshire neck'). However, iodine is now routinely added to table salt and so deficiency is rare in the developed world.

IMAGES: pages 348–350

13. CRANIAL NERVES

1. **G – Trigeminal nerve**
    The maxillary division of the trigeminal nerve passes through the foramen rotundum into the pterygopalatine fossa. Here it gives off sensory fibres to the pterygopalatine ganglion that pass, without synapsing, to the nose, palate and nasopharynx.

2. **D – Glossopharyngeal nerve**
    These parasympathetic secretomotor fibres synapse in the otic ganglion before passing in the auriculotemporal nerve to the parotid gland. The glossopharyngeal nerve also supplies taste fibres to the posterior third of the tongue and innervates the carotid baro- and chemoreceptors.

3. **A – Abducent nerve**
    The lateral rectus is supplied by the abducent nerve; the superior oblique is supplied by the trochlear nerve (LR_6SO_4) and the other extraocular muscles are supplied by the oculomotor nerve.

4. **I – Vagus nerve**
    All the laryngeal muscles are supplied by the vagus nerve, the cricothyroid by the external laryngeal nerve and the remainder through the recurrent laryngeal nerve.

5. **C – Facial nerve**
    Taste fibres from the tongue, mouth and pharynx are carried in the facial, glossopharyngeal and vagus nerves to the nucleus of the tractus solitarius in the floor of the fourth ventricle. Fibres from the anterior two-thirds of the tongue pass via the chorda tympani to the seventh nerve.

14. MUSCLES CONCERNED WITH MASTICATION

1. **B – Buccinator**
   Food is retained between the teeth for chewing by the buccinator from the outside and by the muscles of the tongue and the floor of the mouth from the inside.

2. **H – Mylohyoid**
   The two mylohyoid muscles meet as a midline raphé, and are attached laterally to the mylohyoid line on the medial aspect of the body of the mandible. The mylohyoid and the anterior belly of the digastric are supplied by the inferior alveolar branch of the mandibular nerve.

3. **D – Hyoglossus**
   Other lateral relationships are the styloglossus, lingual nerve, submandibular ganglion, submandibular gland and hypoglossal nerve. The last supplies this muscle, genioglossus, styloglossus and all the intrinsic muscles of the tongue.

4. **F – Masseter**
   The mandibular attachment is to the lateral surface of the ramus and angle of the mandible. A similar area gives attachment to the medial pterygoid muscle on the medial surface of the mandible. Both the pterygoids and the masseter and temporalis muscles are supplied by the mandibular branch of the fifth nerve.

5. **E – Lateral pterygoid**
   This attachment is also to the neck of the mandible and the joint capsule. The two heads of the lateral pterygoid are attached to the inferior temporal surface of the greater wing of the sphenoid and the lateral surface of the pterygoid plate. The latter is embraced by the two heads of the medial pterygoid.

PAPER 4

Paper 4 Questions

1. THEME: CARDIAC CHEST PAIN

A   Acute anterior ST-elevation myocardial infarction
B   Acute inferior ST-elevation myocardial infarction
C   Decubitus angina
D   Dissecting thoracic aortic aneurysm
E   Myocarditis
F   Non-ST-elevation myocardial infarction
G   Pericarditis
H   Prinzmetal's angina
I   Syndrome X
J   True posterior myocardial infarction

The following patients have all presented with cardiac chest pains. Please choose the most appropriate cause from the above list. Each option may be used once, more than once or not at all.

1.   A 39-year-old woman with a strong family history of ischaemic heart disease presents in the Emergency Department with a 4-hour history of severe central chest pain radiating to the left shoulder and the neck associated with nausea, sweating and shortness of breath. Examination is unremarkable, as are her initial blood tests, including the creatine kinase. Her subsequent troponin I is normal. Her ECG shows sinus tachycardia with a normal axis and flattening of the T-waves in leads II, III and aVF. Her exercise stress test shows 'pseudonormalisation' of the T-waves but her coronary angiogram is totally unremarkable.

2.   A 48-year-old man who has smoked since the age of 8 presents in the Emergency Department with a 2-hour history of severe angina-like chest pain associated with sweating and feeling faint and dizzy. His pain is poorly relieved with GTN and oxygen. His ECG shows deep ST depression in leads V_1–V_3 associated with dominant R-waves in leads V_1 and V_2. His creatine kinase is 567 IU/l.

3.   A 27-year-old smoker presents in the Emergency Department with central chest pain which he says is worse when he moves around on the trolley but seems to be eased a little if he leans forward over the trolley bars. His ECG shows saddle-shaped ST elevation in leads V_1, V_5, V_6, aVL, I and II. His creatine kinase is 567 IU/l and troponin 6.9 ng/ml.

4. A 61-year-old diabetic woman is admitted to hospital with an 8–10-hour history of dull central chest pain and shortness of breath. Her ECG shows T-wave inversion in leads V_4–V_6, I and aVL; a subsequent troponin I is 7.6 ng/ml and the creatine kinase is 1099 IU/l.

5. A 76-year-old woman with known hypertension and diabetes mellitus presents in the Emergency Department with severe epigastric and low chest pains radiating to her shoulders. Her ECG shows ST elevation in leads II, III and aVF. Her creatine kinase is 397 IU/l and her troponin is 4.9 ng/ml.

2. THEME: MONOARTHRITIS

A   Brucellosis
B   Charcot's joint
C   Gonococcal arthritis
D   Haemophilia A-induced haemarthrosis
E   Haemophilia B-induced haemarthrosis
F   Osteoarthritis
G   Reiter's syndrome
H   Pyrophosphate arthropathy
I   Syphilitic arthropathy
J   Tuberculous arthritis

The following patients have all presented with a monoarthritis. Please choose the most appropriate cause from the above list. Each diagnosis may be used once, more than once or not at all.

1. A 26-year-old, HIV-positive man attends his GP with a 3-day history of increasing pain and swelling in his left knee, 2 weeks after a febrile illness and dysuria. Aspiration of the joint shows no organisms or crystals but a urethral swab shows Gram-negative intracellular diplococci.

2. A 29-year-old alcohol abuser is admitted to hospital acutely unwell with fever and rigors. On examination, he has signs of a left apical pneumonia and a hot, swollen right knee.

3. A 31-year-old, HIV-positive man is seen in the Genitourinary Medicine Clinic with a swollen, hot left ankle associated with dysuria and conjunctivitis. This is similar to a previous episode he had 3 months ago secondary to a *Chlamydia* infection.

4. A 79-year-old man presents in the Emergency Department with a 3-day history of pain and swelling in the left knee, despite having been placed on allopurinol 2 months earlier by his GP for a similar event. Microscopy of the joint aspirate confirms the presence of weakly positive birefringent crystals under polarised light. No organisms are seen.

5. A 17-year-old boy presents to his GP with a badly swollen left knee 2 days after a rugby match. Subsequent investigation reveals a normal INR, bleeding time and prothrombin time, with reduced factor VIII:C levels at 85% of normal.

3. THEME: GASTROINTESTINAL BLOOD LOSS

A   Barrett's oesophagus
B   Colonic carcinoma
C   Crohn's disease
D   Diverticular disease
E   Duodenal ulcer
F   Gastric ulcer
G   Gastro-oesophageal reflux disease
H   Meckel's diverticulum
I   Oesophageal varices
J   Ulcerative colitis

The following patients have all presented with occult or frank gastrointestinal blood loss. Please choose the most appropriate cause from the above list. Each diagnosis may be used once, more than once or not at all.

1. A 41-year-old man presents to his GP with upper abdominal pain, which is worse before meals and occasionally radiates through to his back. The pain comes and goes and is associated with 'burping' and dyspepsia. Routine investigations reveal: haemoglobin 8.2 g/dl, MCV 74 fl, WCC 9.2 × 10^9/l, platelets 412 × 10^9/l. He declines an oesophagogastroduodenoscopy but a ^{14}C breath test is positive.

2. A 64-year-old woman presents to her GP with weight loss and constipation. Investigations reveal: haemoglobin 7.9 g/dl, MCV 69 fl, WCC5.9 × 10^9/l, platelets 513 × 10^9/l; ESR 78 mm/h; corrected Ca^{2+} 2.27 mmol/l; total bilirubin 32 μmol/l, AST 44 IU/l, ALT 51 IU/l, alkaline phosphatase 449 IU/l, albumin 32 g/l. An ultrasound scan of her abdomen confirms 'multiple hypoechogenic lesions in the liver'.

3. A 39-year-old-man presents to his GP with lethargy and jaundice. Routine investigations reveal: haemoglobin 9.2 g/dl, MCV 104 fl, WCC 4.4 × 10^9/l, platelets 61 × 10^9/l; total bilirubin 42 μmol/l, AST 314 IU/l, ALT 211 IU/l, alkaline phosphatase 565 IU/l, albumin 26 g/l, γGT 207 IU/l; INR 1.8. He is referred to Gastroenterology Out-patients but before this appointment he is admitted with a large, fresh haemetemesis.

4. A 67-year-old woman presents in the Emergency Department with severe left iliac fossa pain. On examination, she is obviously distressed, is vomiting and is pyrexial (temperature 39.5 °C). She is very tender in the left iliac fossa with guarding but with no signs of peritonism. Investigations show: haemoglobin 7.4 g/dl, MCV 71 fl, WCC 29.2 × 10^9/l, platelets 445 × 10^9/l; Na^+ 156 mmol/l, K^+ 4.9 mmol/l, urea 29.7 mmol/l, creatinine 288 μmol/l. Blood cultures confirm an *Escherichia coli* bacteraemia.

5. A 54-year-old man is referred to Gastroenterology Out-patients with a microcytic anaemia. He denies having any upper or lower gastroenterological symptoms. Subsequent upper and lower gastrointestinal endoscopy are unremarkable, but a 'special scan' confirms the diagnosis, showing an ileal lesion 50–60 cm from the ileocaecal valve.

4. THEME: TUMOUR MARKERS

A α-FP
B β-hCG
C CA-15.3
D CA-19.9
E CA-27.29
F CA-125
G CEA
H HER-2
I Philadelphia chromosome
J PSA
K Thyroglobulin
L Tyrosinase

The following patients have all presented with malignant tumours or have been treated in the past for a malignancy. Please choose the most appropriate tumour marker for their condition from the above list. You may use the markers once, more than once, in combination or not at all.

1. A 79-year-old man presents to his GP with increasing lower back and left femur pain, associated with recent significant weight loss and haematuria.

2. A 34-year-old Australian man who came to the UK 7 years ago is seen by his GP with a large pigmented naevus on his left calf. There are satellite lesions surrounding the main lesion and the GP feels several large hard lymph nodes in his left inguinal region.

3. A 41-year-old man who is HIV- and hepatitis C-positive presents in Out-patients with jaundice and hepatomegaly. An ultrasound scan shows a large solitary mass in the left lobe of his liver.

4. A 58-year-old man with a history of a Whipple's procedure performed for carcinoma of the head of the pancreas presents in Surgical Out-patients 18 months after his surgery with lumbar back pain and weight loss.

5. A 51-year-old woman with a history of a left mastectomy and radiotherapy presents in Oncology Out-patients with a mass in her right breast and several hard, fixed lymph nodes in her axillae and supraclavicular fossae.

5. THEME: STROKE

A   Cerebellar
B   Cervical
C   Frontal
D   Medullary
E   Midbrain
F   Occipital
G   Parietal
H   Pontine
I   Temporal
J   Thalamic

The following patients have all presented with signs of a stroke. Please choose the most appropriate site of their lesion from the above list. The sites may be used once, more than once or not at all.

1. A 64-year-old, left-handed man with known hypertension presents in the Emergency Department with an episode of collapse. On examination he is well but his BP is 210/135 mmHg. He is noted by the admitting doctor to have marked nystagmus to the right, right-sided dysdiadochokinesia and past-pointing.

2. A 67-year-old, right-handed woman calls her GP out because of sudden difficulty with her speech. On arrival, she finds the patient has no obvious limb weakness but has marked dysarthria. Her pupils and eye movements are normal but her palate deviates to the left when asked to say 'aagh' and her tongue deviates to the right on protrusion.

3. An 84-year-old, right-handed woman with a previous history of stroke presents in the Emergency Department with a collapse. On examination, she has signs of her old right hemiparesis but has a new right homonymous hemianopia.

4. A 59-year-old man is brought to the Emergency Department with a GCS of 3. He has bilateral pupillary constriction which does not improve with several doses of naloxone. A CT head scan fails to demonstrate any abnormalities and, remarkably, he shows some improvement. The diagnosis is confirmed on magnetic resonance imaging (MRI).

5. A 78-year-old, right-handed woman is admitted to hospital with a right hemisphere stroke. On the stroke rehabilitation ward she complains of shooting pains down her left arm and leg, which improve somewhat with gabapentin.

6. THEME: GENITAL ULCERATION

A Behçet's syndrome
B Chancroid
C Donovanosis
D Herpes simplex
E Herpes zoster
F Lymphogranuloma venereum
G Pemphigus
H Stevens–Johnson syndrome
I Syphilitic chancre
J Syphilitic gumma

The following patients have all presented with genital ulceration. Please choose the most appropriate cause from the above list. Each diagnosis may be used once, more than once or not at all.

1. A 29-year-old Asian man presents in Genitourinary Medicine Clinic 10 days after having unprotected sexual intercourse on holiday in India. On examination, he has a painless, ulcerating, papular rash over the glans penis. He has had no urethral discharge. Diagnosis is confirmed on cell culture which shows an obligate intracellular organism. Both gonococcal and Venereal Disease Research Laboratory (VDRL) tests are negative. He improves with doxycycline.

2. A 24-year-old, HIV-positive African woman presents in the Genitourinary Medicine Clinic with a 2-week history of an ulcerating lesion extending over her labia and perineum. The ulcerated area is friable and bleeds on contact. It is very painful. The Gram stain taken from swabs shows a characteristic coccobacillus.

3. A 37-year-old Afro-Caribbean man presents in the Genitourinary Medicine Clinic 2 weeks after having unprotected sexual intercourse at a party in Jamaica. On examination, he has a 'heaped', ulcerated lesion on his glans but no discharge. Gonococcal and *Chlamydia* investigations are negative, as are tests for herpes simplex virus and the VDRL. A short, encapsulated, Gram-negative bacillus is grown on culture.

4. A 18-year-old woman presents to her GP with multiple, painful, ulcerating lesions over her vulva. She has a fever and feels 'achey' all over. The VDRL is negative, as are gonococcal and bacterial screens. Culture confirms the presence of an icosahedral virus.

5. A 24-year-old homosexual man is seen by his GP with a 4-week history of a painless ulcerating lesion over the glans penis, 6 weeks after unprotected sex. Subsequent investigations identify a motile spirochaete under dark-ground microscopy.

7. THEME: COMPLICATIONS OF GALLSTONE DISEASE

A   Acute cholecystitis
B   Acute pancreatitis
C   Ascending cholangitis
D   Biliary colic
E   Bilioenteric fistula
F   Chronic cholecystitis
G   Empyema of the gallbladder
H   Gallstone ileus
I   Mucocele
J   Perforated gallbladder
K   Obstructive jaundice

The following are descriptions of patients with complications of gallstone disease. Please select the most appropriate diagnosis from the above list. Each diagnosis may be used once, more than once or not at all.

1. A 58-year-old man presents in the Emergency Department with sudden onset of severe upper abdominal pain with exacerbations and associated nausea. On examination, there is tenderness and guarding, maximal in the right upper quadrant. Investigations show: total bilirubin 35 µmol/l, AST 18 IU/l, ALT 22 IU/l, alkaline phosphatase 180 IU/l, albumin 41 g/l.

2. A 45-year-old woman attends her GP with a 6-month history of episodic indigestion. Attacks commonly occur after eating. On direct questioning, she also admits to having post-prandial belching. She is not jaundiced and the abdominal examination is unremarkable other than mild obesity and a previous hysterectomy scar. Her LFTs are normal.

3. A 75-year-old woman presents in the Emergency Department with a 1-day history of colicky central and right-sided abdominal pain, bilious vomiting and distension. On examination, she is dehydrated but not jaundiced. The abdomen is distended and tympanic, with obstructed bowel sounds. Her LFTs are normal.

4. A 68-year-old man presents in the Emergency Department with a 12-hour history of severe upper abdominal pain radiating to the back, associated with nausea and vomiting. On examination, he is dehydrated and tachycardic, with tenderness and guarding in the epigastrium and left hypochondrium. Investigations show: total bilirubin 32 µmol/l, AST 40 IU/l, ALT 27 IU/l, alkaline phosphatase 155 IU/l, albumin 39 g/l, lactate dehydrogenase (LDH) 610 IU/l, amylase 2150 U/l.

5. A 72-year-old woman presents in the Emergency Department with a 2-day history of severe right hypochondrial pain, nausea and vomiting and fever. On examination, she is distressed and dehydrated but not jaundiced. There is guarding and rebound in the right upper quadrant, with a suspicion of an underlying mass extending from beneath the costal margin. Tests show: WCC 27.6 × 10⁹/l; total bilirubin 32 µmol/l, AST 85 IU/l, ALT 95 IU/l, alkaline phosphatase 175 IU/l, albumin 38 g/l.

8. THEME: CHEST TRAUMA

A   Cardiac tamponade
B   Diaphragmatic rupture
C   Flail chest
D   Haemothorax
E   Massive haemothorax
F   Myocardial contusion
G   Open pneumothorax
H   Pulmonary contusion
I   Simple pneumothorax
J   Tension pneumothorax
K   Tracheobronchial disruption
L   Traumatic aortic disruption

The following patients have all had thoracic injuries. Please select the most appropriate diagnosis from the above list. Each option may be used once, more than once or not at all.

1. A 19-year-old man is brought to the Emergency Department following a stab wound to the right side of the chest. He is shocked (pulse 115 bpm, BP 90/50 mmHg) and slightly dyspnoeic. Examination of the chest shows some decreased breath sounds and dullness to percussion on the left side. A chest radiograph demonstrates a moderate pleural effusion on the right side and a chest drain is inserted which drains 500 ml of blood.

2. A 26-year-old pedestrian is brought to the Emergency Department after being hit by a car travelling at approximately 50 mph. He has serious lower extremity injuries and a minor head injury. Shortly after arrival he becomes acutely dyspnoeic, cyanotic, tachycardic and hypotensive. Examination of the chest reveals reduced breath sounds and increased resonance to percussion on the left side. The neck veins are distended.

3. A 45-year-old man is brought to the Emergency Department having been hit by a train. Although he was thrown clear of the track, he has serious chest and abdominal injuries. He is dyspnoeic and in considerable distress. Examination reveals evidence of blunt injury to both sides of the chest. On the right side there is paradoxical movement of the chest wall with inspiration and expiration.

4. A 21-year-old man is brought to hospital after sustaining an isolated stab wound to the left side of the chest. There is little external haemorrhage and a chest radiograph demonstrates a simple small pneumothorax, which is treated by insertion of a chest drain. In the Emergency Department he rapidly becomes severely hypotensive (BP 70/30 mmHg). Re-examination of the chest shows bilateral, equal breath sounds and expansion, and the chest drain is swinging but not draining any significant blood (100 ml total). His neck veins are distended.

5. A 52-year-old, unrestrained driver hits a tree at 50 mph. She has some bruising over the sternum and tenderness on palpation. There is no evidence of shock. A chest radiograph demonstrates widening of the mediastinum.

9. THEME: SURGICAL INCISIONS

A Gridiron/McBurney's
B Kocher's
C Lanz
D Long midline
E Lower midline
F Paramedian
G Pfannenstiel
H Rooftop/gable
I Rutherford-Morrison
J Upper midline

The following are descriptions of patients requiring operations. Please select the most appropriate/commonly-used surgical incision from the above list. Each incision may be used once, more than once or not at all.

1. A 24-year-old man is brought to the Emergency Department following a major road traffic accident. He is cardiovascularly shocked despite fluid resuscitation and has a blunt abdominal injury. He is taken for emergency laparotomy.

2. A 65-year-old woman with symptomatic gallstone disease has had two previous laparotomies for adhesional small-bowel obstruction following a hysterectomy 15 years ago. She requires a cholecystectomy.

3. A 34-year-old woman has a complicated second stage of labour. She requires an emergency Caesarean section.

4. A 65-year-old man with cirrhosis and hepatic failure is to undergo a cadaveric liver transplantation.

5. A 72-year-old woman requires a sigmoid colectomy for colorectal carcinoma.

10. THEME: GYNAECOLOGICAL THERAPEUTIC AGENTS

A   Combined oral contraceptive pill (COCP)
B   Cyproterone acetate
C   Danazol
D   Goserelin (GnRH analogue)
E   Medroxyprogesterone acetate
F   Mefenamic acid
G   Oestrogen-only hormone-replacement therapy (HRT)
H   Oestrogen–progesterone HRT
I   Tamoxifen
J   Tranexamic acid

From the above list please choose the agent that is being described in the statements below. The options may be used once, more than once or not at all.

1. This agent is used to downregulate the hypothalamic-pituitary axis, prior to in-vitro fertilisation (IVF) cycles. It is taken non-orally and commonly has the side-effects of hot flushes and night sweats. ☐

2. This agent is commonly used for the treatment of menorrhagia and dysmenorrhoea. It is taken orally and is relatively contraindicated in patients with asthma. ☐

3. This oral agent has some beneficial side-effects, including a reduction in ovarian and endometrial cancer with long-term use. ☐

4. This oral agent is known to reduce hirsutism and acne with long-term use. It needs to be given with oestrogen to prevent feminisation of a male fetus if the patient becomes pregnant. ☐

5. This agent is commonly be used in women after hysterectomy, to prevent or treat hot flushes and night sweats. ☐

11. THEME: CHEST RADIOGRAPHS – CLINICAL SIGNS

*Using the radiographic images **A–J on pages 348 – 350** please match the clinical signs shown below with the correct image. You may use each images once, more than once or not at all.*

1. The patient is slightly distressed and tachypnoeic but is otherwise well, with normal oxygen saturations. The trachea is central, there is reduced expansion on the right, a resonant percussion note, reduced tactile vocal fremitus and vocal fremitus, and absent breath sounds.

2. The patient is in extremis, the trachea is deviated to the left, with poor chest expansion (R<L), and absent vocal fremitus and breath sounds on the right.

3. The patient looks cachectic and chronically unwell. The trachea is deviated to the right, with reduced expansion on the right and dullness to percussion in the upper zone with associated reduced breath sounds.

4. The patient looks 'septic' and unwell. The trachea is central, expansion is reduced due to pleuritic chest pain and there is dullness to percussion with associated coarse crackles and bronchial breathing in the right axilla.

5. The patient looks thin but well. Their trachea is central and there is bronchial breathing and fine inspiratory crepitations in the apices.

12. THEME: PATHOGENIC VIRUSES

A   Coronavirus
B   Cytomegalovirus
C   Epstein–Barr virus
D   Hepatitis C virus
E   Herpes simplex virus type 2
F   Human papillomavirus
G   Measles virus
H   Rhinovirus
I   Rotavirus
J   Varicella zoster virus

From the above list, please select the virus that is the most likely cause of each of the following diseases. Each virus may be used once, more than once or not at all.

1. Cirrhosis of the liver. ☐

2. Severe acute respiratory syndrome (SARS). ☐

3. Shingles. ☐

4. Verruca vulgaris. ☐

5. Infectious mononucleosis. ☐

13. THEME: PHARYNGEAL MUSCLES

A   Inferior constrictor
B   Levator palatini
C   Middle constrictor
D   Palatoglossus
E   Palatopharyngeus
F   Pharyngobasilar fascia
G   Salpingopharyngeus
H   Stylopharyngeus
I   Superior constrictor
J   Tensor palatini

For each of the following descriptions, please choose the most appropriate structure from the above list. Each option may be used once, more than once or not at all.

1. Attached to the lateral aspect of the cricoid cartilage.

2. Underlies the anterior pillar of the fauces.

3. Attached to the upper border of the greater horn of the hyoid bone.

4. Encircles the opening of the eustachian tube.

5. Innervated by the trigeminal nerve.

14. THEME: MUSCLE ATTACHMENTS IN THE UPPER LIMB

A   Biceps
B   Brachialis
C   Deltoid
D   Extensor carpi radialis longus
E   Flexor carpi ulnaris
F   Flexor digitorum profundus
G   Flexor digitorum superficialis
H   Flexor pollicis longus
I   Pronator teres
J   Triceps

For each of the following attachments please choose the most appropriate muscle from the above list. Each muscle may be used once, more than once or not at all.

1.   Along the upper border of the radial groove of the humerus.

2.   Anterior aspect of the lower humerus.

3.   Lateral supracondylar ridge on the humerus.

4.   Lateral aspect of the mid-radius.

5.   Anterior aspect of the base of the distal phalanx of the middle finger.

Paper 4 Answers

1. CARDIAC CHEST PAIN

1. I – Syndrome X

This patient has a strong family history of ischaemic heart disease, a history highly suggestive of angina, and an abnormal ECG. She has no rise in her cardiac enzymes but her exercise tolerance test shows 'pseudonormalisation' of her inverted T-waves. This change occurs when the ECG shows permanent T-wave inversion and 'right' themselves on exertion. However, despite these changes her subsequent coronary arteriogram is normal. This suggests she either has another cause for her pain (eg oesophageal spasm) or has cardiac syndrome X, or microvascular angina. This diagnosis of exclusion is more common in females. They can present with angina-like chest pain, ECG changes and a positive exercise stress test, but coronary angiography is normal. Such patients should still have their macrovascular risk factors addressed and receive symptomatic treatment with calcium-channel blockers. There is no proof that the addition of antiplatelet therapy is of benefit.

2. J – True posterior myocardial infarction

This middle-aged man has a history consistent with an acute coronary syndrome and his ECG confirms a true posterior myocardial infarction, as evidenced by the deep ST depression in the anterior leads associated with the dominant R-waves in leads V_1 and V_2. He should be treated as if he was having an ST-elevation myocardial infarction (STEMI) – with aspirin, thrombolysis and other prognosis-changing drugs such as insulin, β-blockers, statins and ACE inhibitors. Symptomatic relievers such as nitrates, diuretics, calcium-channel blockers and nicorandil might also be required.

3. G – Pericarditis

This young man has the historical features and ECG changes of acute pericarditis. He has sharp chest pain that is eased on leaning forwards and 'saddle' ST elevation in a non-anatomical distribution. He should be treated symptomatically with non-steroidal anti-inflammatory drugs (NSAIDs) and rest. The most likely cause in an otherwise well individual is a viral infection. Other causes, such as ischaemic heart disease, uraemia, malignant invasion and sepsis (TB) should be excluded.

4. F – Non-ST-elevation myocardial infarction (non-STEMI)

Recently, patients presenting with unstable chest pain (increasing in frequency, severity and/or duration) have been classified as having an 'acute coronary syndrome'. Patients are then subdivided on the basis of their ECG changes and cardiac enzyme results into: (1) patients with ST-elevation myocardial infarction (STEMI); and (2) patients with non-ST-elevation myocardial infarction and unstable angina. Both groups of patients should have macrovascular risk factors addressed and receive aspirin, β-blockers and other prognosis-changing drugs (see above). Patients with an STEMI should receive thrombolysis and patients with non-STEMI and unstable angina should receive low-molecular-weight heparin and/or abciximab. Non-STEMI and unstable angina patients should have an early exercise stress test, whereas STEMI patients might require early coronary angiography and intervention.

5. B – Acute inferior ST-elevation myocardial infarction (inferior STEMI)

This patient has presented with an acute coronary syndrome with ECG changes suggestive of an acute inferior STEMI (leads II, III and aVF). She requires thrombolysis, her secondary risk factors need to be addressed and she also needs prognosis-changing drugs.

2. MONOARTHRITIS

1. **C – Gonococcal arthritis**
    This patient has developed a gonococcal arthritis. This condition is usually manifest as a flitting polyarthritis or arthralgia primarily affecting the large joints of the upper and lower limbs. There can be associated effusions and tenosynovitis but it does not cause progressive joint destruction. The diagnosis can be confirmed from synovial fluid or blood cultures but it is usually made from anal or genital swabs. The treatment, as with all gonococcal infections, is penicillin, co-trimoxazole or, in resistant cases, ciprofloxacin.

2. **J – Tuberculous arthritis**
    This patient has a left lower lobe pneumonia and an associated acute arthritis of the right knee. As with most systemic involvement of TB, this is due to direct haematogenous spread from the primary pulmonary infection. The diagnosis can be confirmed on microscopy of joint aspirate, sputum and blood cultures. Treatment is with standard antituberculous therapy for at least 6 months.

3. **G – Reiter's syndrome**
    This patient has developed Reiter's syndrome secondary to his *Chlamydia* infection. He has the classic triad of arthritis, urethritis and conjunctivitis. Other features include keratoderma blennorrhagica, plantar fasciitis, Achilles tendonitis, circinate balanitis (in males) and sacroiliitis.

4. **H – Pyrophosphate arthropathy**
    This older man has developed a monoarthritis of the knee associated with weakly positive birefringent crystals. Pyrophosphate arthropathy or 'pseudogout' is commoner in older people, presenting as a 'new' arthritis, compared with gout, which starts in late middle age. Aspiration of the joint and microscopy is important to confirm or exclude one or both of these diagnoses. Analgesia without long-term gout prophylaxis (allopurinol) is given to patients with pyrophosphate arthropathy.

5. **D – Haemophilia A-induced haemarthrosis**
    This young man has a haemarthrosis secondary to haemophilia A. This is an autosomal recessive disorder characterised by a low factor VIII:C. The severity of presentation depends on the residual levels of the factor. Levels of more than 5% of normal lead to a mild disorder (as in this case), with later onset of symptoms and often discovered only on excessive bleeding after trauma. Levels between 1% and 5% of normal lead to occasional spontaneous bleeds (eg haemarthrosis), but patients with levels at 3–4% are often diagnosed after trauma. Patients with levels at less than 1% of normal present in the neonatal period or early childhood with spontaneous bleeding into joints and muscles or even intracranial bleeds. The treatment is with factor VIII:C replacement.

3. GASTROINTESTINAL BLOOD LOSS

1. **E – Duodenal ulcer**
   This man has developed a peptic ulcer that is most likely to be duodenal. He has 'hunger' pains, associated with dyspepsia and upper gastrointestinal flatulence, which are suggestive of duodenal rather than gastric ulceration. His ^{14}C breath test confirms the presence of *Helicobacter pylori*, which is found in 90–95% of patients with duodenal ulcer but in only 60% patients with gastric ulcer. He should be treated with a 1-week course of eradication therapy using a proton-pump inhibitor (eg lansoprazole, esomeprazole or pantoprazole) combined with two antibiotics (eg amoxicillin, clarithromycin or metronidazole).

2. **B – Colonic carcinoma**
   This woman has a colonic carcinoma with hepatic metastases. Her investigations show a microcytic anaemia and deranged liver function tests and her ultrasound scan confirms the presence of multiple metastases. She might need surgical resection and adjuvant chemotherapy and radiotherapy.

3. **I – Oesophageal varices**
   This man's investigations confirm that he has a hepatitic jaundice and a macrocytic anaemia associated with a raised INR and thrombocytopenia. This combination of results is highly suggestive of alcohol excess. His subsequent presentation with a large upper gastrointestinal bleed is most likely to be due to oesophageal varices. He will need urgent blood transfusion and, once he is haemodynamically stable (if possible), urgent upper gastrointestinal endoscopy. If varices are confirmed these should be injected with a sclerosant agent or banded.

4. **D – Diverticular disease**
   This woman has presented with the classic picture of acute diverticulitis. She has left iliac fossa pain (diverticulitis is commonly called 'left-sided appendicitis'), vomiting, pyrexia and severe left iliac fossa tenderness. She should be treated with intravenous fluids, antibiotics (cefuroxime and metronidazole) and she should be 'nil by mouth'. She should have an erect chest radiograph and an abdominal radiograph to exclude perforation or obstruction. Diverticular disease is a common complication of the low-fibre diet seen in the Western world and patients must be encouraged to increase roughage in their diet and avoid prolonged episodes of constipation.

5. **H – Meckel's diverticulum**
   This man has a Meckel's diverticulum, which is usually an asymptomatic lesion found in the ileum, classically 60 cm from the ileocaecal valve. In adults it is a 'diagnosis of exclusion', made when more common causes of upper and lower gastrointestinal blood loss have been excluded. It is demonstrated radiologically using a radionuclide scan using technetium-99, which concentrates in the gastric mucosa. The ectopic mucosa within the diverticulum shows up using a gamma camera.

4. TUMOUR MARKERS

The identification and utilisation of tumour markers has become increasingly sophisticated over the past 5 years. This is a rapidly developing and changing area and, as with similar areas such as monoclonal antibody therapies and autoimmune markers of disease, we all need to watch their development and use them very carefully. However, it should be noted that despite increasing recognition of specific tumour markers (the carbohydrate antigens or CAs), their use is still principally limited to prediction of relapse and management success, and few are used at present as screening or diagnostic aids.

1. **J – Prostatic-specific antigen (PSA)**
    This patient has a history suggestive of metastatic cancer of the prostate. Prostatic-specific antigen (PSA) is one of the only tumour markers currently used as a screening test, a diagnostic test, a measure of management success and a marker of recurrence. It should be noted that a normal PSA does not exclude carcinoma in situ and a moderately raised PSA does not necessarily imply carcinoma. A prostatic biopsy is the only true method of discriminating between the two at levels of PSA at the upper end of normal or only mildly elevated.

2. **L – Tyrosinase**
    Metastatic malignant disease is accompanied by the presence of circulating malignant cells in the blood. One of the common methods of screening for early metastatic disease is to look for these cells using the techniques of reverse transcriptase polymerase chain reaction (RT-PCR) and resulting amplification. This method has been used to look for tyrosinase, an enzyme involved in melanin synthesis, which is overexpressed in malignant melanoma. At present this technique is still unproved in clinical trials but it is used in large centres to try to pick up early metastatic melanoma.

3. **A – α-FP**
    This patient has developed primary hepatocellular carcinoma (HCC), which rarely occurs without a background of chronic liver disease. It is therefore a common tumour associated with chronic viral hepatitis and alcoholic liver disease. The tumour marker, α-fetoprotein (α-FP) is one of the most specific tumour markers and in this context gross elevation is almost pathognomonic of malignant HCC. It is also a useful screening and monitoring tool in patents with non-seminomatous germ-cell tumours and in patients presenting with ascites or disseminated malignancy with an unknown primary tumour. Other causes of elevated α-FP levels include pancreatic, bronchogenic, gastric and colonic carcinoma (but it is not used in the management of these diseases), cirrhosis and hepatitis.

4. **D – CA-19.9**
    CA-19.9 is used in oncology to confirm the diagnosis of malignant pancreatic tumours, differentiating them from chronic pancreatic disease (pancreatitis) where the diagnosis may be more complex than normal. It is also used for monitoring the response to therapy and for confirming metastatic or recurrent disease. Levels can also be elevated in hepatobiliary disease, but it is not used clinically in this setting.

5.   C, E – CA-15.3 and CA-27.29

Even in the relatively new world of tumour markers, specificity, and thus the utilisation of these proteins, continues to change. As acid phosphatase was superseded by PSA as the marker for prostatic disease, so our understanding of the newer markers has led to changes in their use. CA-15.3 was used as a marker of treatment success, recurrence and metastatic disease in breast malignancy until relatively recently. However this has now been superseded by CA-27.29 which is more specific in this role. CA-27.29 is a mucin-1-associated antigenic component expressed by tumour cells, including breast, pancreatic, ovarian and bronchogenic malignancies. Levels are raised in a third of patients with stage I and stage II disease and in two-thirds of patients with stage III and stage IV disease. It was hoped that this would be a linear relationship but, as yet, differentiating the various stages (I from II and III from IV) using this marker has not been successful.

NB: For a very understandable and comprehensive overview of this subject please see: www.aafp.org/afp/20030915/1075.pdf

5. STROKE

1. **A – Cerebellar**

   This man has suffered a right-sided cerebellar stroke, as evidenced by the nystagmus to the right, right-sided dysdiadochokinesia and past-pointing. Posterior fossa strokes might not be visualised on a CT head scan because of the artefact effect of the closely surrounding bone. However, a CT head scan is still the radiological investigation of choice in most hospitals because it will exclude large cerebellar bleeds or space-occupying lesions which are neurosurgical emergencies and require urgent intervention.

2. **D – Medullary**

   This woman has a right vagus nerve palsy, causing the palate to deviate to the left on asking the patient to say 'aagh' and a right-sided hypoglossal nerve palsy, which is causing the tongue to deviate to the right on protrusion. These lesions lead to a dysarthria and are consistent with a medullary or bulbar stroke (the medulla is known as the 'bulb'). She will invariably have swallowing difficulties and will need speech and language therapy.

3. **F – Occipital**

   This patient has developed a new right homonymous hemianopia, which localises the lesion to the left optic tract, radiation or occipital cortex, ie the left optic pathways distal to the optic chiasma.

4. **H – Pontine**

   This man presents with pupillary constriction and a GCS of 3/15. As with all unconscious patients, your should follow the simple rules of **A**irway, **B**reathing, **C**irculation (ABC) and in the patient with bilaterally constricted pupils you should try intravenous naloxone to exclude opiate toxicity. Pontine strokes will cause constricted pupils, whereas mid-brain strokes will often affect both sympathetic innervation (dilation) and parasympathetic innervation (constriction), leading to an unresponsive mid-dilated pupil.

5. **J – Thalamic**

   It is not uncommon for patients to complain of burning or shooting pains down their affected hemiparetic limbs following a stroke. This is considered to be thalamic in origin and should be treated as with other causes of neuropathic pain with gabapentin or carbamazepine.

6. GENITAL ULCERATION

1. **F – Lymphogranuloma venereum**
   This patient has developed lymphogranuloma venereum, which is caused by *Chlamydia trachomatis*. The primary lesion is a painless ulcerating lesion over the genitalia. This heals and is followed by painful lymphadenopathy (local), which can turn into buboes and rupture. In a rectal infection, a proctitis occurs with associated abscess formation.

2. **B – Chancroid**
   This patient has developed chancroid sexually transmitted disease caused by *Haemophilus ducreyi*. This ulcerating condition can be difficult to differentiate clinically from other sexually transmitted diseases such as lymphogranuloma venereum and herpes simplex virus infection and the diagnosis should be confirmed by testing swabs of the ulcerated areas or pus from the resulting abscesses. The lesion initially starts as a small papule, which ulcerates to form a painful necrotic lesion. Multiple ulcers often coalesce to form a single, painful ulcer with associated local lymphadenopathy.

3. **C – Donovanosis**
   This patient has developed donovanosis or granuloma inguinale. This is an endemic infection in the Caribbean, in South-East Asia and in Southern India and is caused by the Gram-negative bacillus, Calymmatobacterium *granulomatis*. This infection causes a characteristic 'heaped', ulcerating lesion on skin contact areas. The primary infection then spreads to the local lymph nodes, leading to the formation of the characteristic 'pseudo-buboes'.

4. **D – Herpes simplex**
   This patient has developed a genital herpes infection caused predominantly by herpes simplex virus 2 (HSV2). In women, the infection can be asymptomatic if it is intravaginal but classically there is painful genital ulceration with associated dysuria and regional lymphadenopathy. The virus invades the sacral ganglia where it lies dormant until episodically it causes secondary infections, with associated genital ulceration and pain in the buttocks, thighs and inguinal regions.

5. **I – Syphilitic chancre**
   This patient has developed a syphilitic chancre, a painless, ulcerating lesion which is associated with primary syphilis infection. The chancre which develops at the primary site of contact (ie the penis, labia, anus or even the mouth) is associated with painless lymphadenopathy (local) and heals within a few weeks. Syphilitic gummas are ulcerating lesions that occur in tertiary syphilis.

7. COMPLICATIONS OF GALLSTONE DISEASE

1. **D – Biliary colic**
   The characteristic history, especially the sudden onset of severe pain, gives the diagnosis in this case. While described as a colic, patients typically have pain even in-between exacerbations. The pain is caused by impaction of a stone in the cystic duct and the resultant spasm of the gallbladder, which occurs in an attempt to force the stone distally. Approximately 20% of patients will develop clinical jaundice, although a larger proportion of patients will have subclinically deranged LFTs, as in this case.

2. **F – Chronic cholecystitis**
   This woman has the characteristic symptoms of 'flatulent dyspepsia'. Classically, pain is said to start some 15–30 minutes after eating and usually lasts 30–90 minutes. It is often worse after fatty foods. The diagnosis is usually based on the history and the finding of gallstones on ultrasound (and the exclusion of other causes). Treatment is by elective surgery, with a laparoscopic cholecystectomy (provided there are no contraindications).

3. **H – Gallstone ileus**
   These symptoms are those of small-bowel obstruction. Gallstones are a relatively rare cause of intestinal obstruction (well down the list compared with adhesions and hernias) and gallstone ileus is a rare complication of gallstone disease (2%). A large gallstone enters the duodenum, usually by means of a bilioenteric fistula, and typically impacts in the narrower terminal ileum where it causes acute obstruction. This rarely resolves spontaneously, and emergency laparotomy is required.

4. **B – Acute pancreatitis**
   The patient has the classic clinical presentation of this disorder, which is further suggested by the raised lactate dehydrogenase (LDH) and confirmed by the raised amylase. In Western populations, gallstones and alcohol are the two commonest causes. Gallstone pancreatitis typically occurs in patients over the age of 60 and can be severe and lead to serious complications. Initial management is the same as for pancreatitis (starting with resuscitation and fluid management), with subsequent treatment of the cause.

5. **G – Empyema of the gallbladder**
   The presentation is that of acute cholecystitis, but the finding of a palpable, distended gallbladder, especially with the severity of the symptoms and the marked leucocytosis, suggests empyema of the gallbladder. The mildly deranged LFTs (a mixed picture) reflect local inflammation. This is a relatively uncommon complication of acute cholecystitis in which obstructed bile in the gallbladder becomes infected and replaced eventually by pus. Treatment is by resuscitation and prompt surgery (drainage or cholecystectomy). The other two complications of severe acute cholecystitis are perforation and gangrene.

8. CHEST TRAUMA

1. **D – Haemothorax**
This is caused by a laceration of the lung or of an intercostal vessel. It is best treated using a large-calibre chest drain and is usually self-limiting unless bleeding continues, in which case thoracotomy might be required. It is distinguished from 'massive haemothorax', which is defined as a rapid accumulation of more than 1.5 litres of blood in the chest cavity with subsequent respiratory compromise.

2. **J – Tension pneumothorax**
This develops when a 'one-way valve' air leak occurs, either from the lung or the chest wall. Air is forced into the thoracic cavity without any means of escape, completely collapsing the affected lung. The mediastinum is displaced to the opposite side, decreasing venous return and compressing the opposite lung. The commonest cause of tension pneumothorax is mechanical (positive-pressure) ventilation in the patient with a visceral pleural injury. Rapid decompression is required (with a needle, then a chest drain) to prevent rapid death.

3. **C – Flail chest**
This occurs when a segment of chest wall has no bony continuity with the rest of the thoracic cage. There will be multiple rib fractures, with fractures in two places (usually front and back) resulting from a significant force, usually a crush injury. While the flail segment moves paradoxically and compromises respiration slightly, it is the underlying severe pulmonary contusion that is the main cause of morbidity and mortality. Treatment is by positive-pressure ventilation/oxygen therapy; surgical fixation is not usually required.

4. **A – Cardiac tamponade**
The pericardium can fill with blood from the heart, especially after penetrating injuries. Only a small amount of pericardial blood is required to restrict cardiac activity and prevent filling. The diagnosis of cardiac tamponade can be difficult. The classic diagnostic Beck's triad consists of increased central venous pressure, decreased BP and muffled heart sounds, but muffled heart sounds are difficult to assess in a trauma-care scenario and distended neck veins are difficult to assess with a hard collar in place. In general, marked hypotension or cardiac arrest with pulseless electrical activity (PEA) in the absence of hypovolaemia or tension pneumothorax should prompt consideration of this diagnosis. Treatment is with needle pericardiocentesis and/or thoracotomy.

5. **L – Traumatic aortic disruption**
This is usually a cause of sudden death at the scene after a road traffic accident or a fall from a height. However, a proportion of patients have a small laceration that becomes contained by a mediastinal haematoma (at least for a while). The diagnosis is suggested by the mechanism of injury (blunt force to the sternum) and should be strongly suspected after the findings of a sternal fracture. The chest radiographic findings of a widened mediastinum in this context are almost confirmatory and should prompt urgent arteriography and surgery.

9. SURGICAL INCISIONS

1. **D – Long midline**
    In such cases there might be multiple visceral injuries requiring attention. This incision allows adequate exposure of all the abdominal contents. It can extend from xiphisternum to the symphysis pubis.

2. **B – Kocher's**
    Before the advent of laparoscopic cholecystectomy, this was the most commonly used incision for open gallbladder surgery. It is an oblique right subcostal incision, extending for approximately 15 cm, parallel to the costal margin. In this patient, a laparoscopic cholecystectomy would probably be contraindicated because of adhesions and the risk of small-bowel injury.

3. **G – Pfannenstiel**
    This is a suprapubic transverse incision, separating the rectus abdominal muscles. The lower-segment uterine incision is almost universally employed. This can be performed via a lower midline incision, but is best and most commonly performed by a Pfannenstiel incision.

4. **H – Rooftop/gable**
    This incision is formed by making bilateral oblique subcostal incisions that meet in the middle, giving an inverted 'V' appearance. It provides excellent exposure for major, especially hepatobiliary, surgery in the upper abdomen. To gain even greater exposure, a vertical extension can be added from the midpoint to the xiphisternum (often called a 'mercedes incision' because of its similarity to the car emblem).

5. **E – Lower midline**
    This is the commonly used incision for surgical operations involving the sigmoid colon and rectum, including sigmoid colectomy, anterior resection and abdominoperineal resection. It consistes of a midline incision extending from just above the umbilicus to the symphysis pubis. If difficulty is encountered, and especially if the splenic flexure requires mobilisation, this incision can be extended upwards into a longer midline incision.

10. GYNAECOLOGICAL THERAPEUTIC AGENTS

1. **D – Goserelin (GnRH analogue)**

    Gonadotrophin-releasing hormone (GnRH) analogues cannot be given orally because they are small peptides that are broken down quickly if swallowed. They act by initial stimulation of the hypothalamus and pituitary GnRH receptors, followed quickly by competitive blockade of the receptor sites. They effectively switch off the hypothalamic–pituitary–ovarian axis (leading to a temporary medical menopause, hence the side-effects due to hypo-oestrogenism) so that stimulated cycles in in-vitro fertilisation (IVF) start from a basal level. Tamoxifen can cause similar side-effects but is taken orally and acts as an ovulation-induction agent, not a downregulator.

2. **F – Mefenamic acid**

    The combined oral contraceptive pill (COCP), mefenamic acid, tranexamic acid, medroxyprogesterone acetate, GnRH analogues (non-oral) and even danazol (rarely nowadays) are all used for the treatment of menorrhagia. The COCP and mefenamic acid are also used extensively for dysmenorrhoea. Mefenamic acid is a NSAID that alters prostaglandin balance and therefore menstrual flow and pain. It can induce bronchospasm in asthmatics via its action on prostaglandins so is relatively contraindicated in these patients. The COCP has no such effects and is therefore safe in asthmatic patients.

3. **A – Combined oral contraceptive pill (COCP)**

    The COCP stops ovulation and endometrial proliferation and significantly reduces the user's risk of both endometrial and ovarian cancer with long-term use (5–10 years). However, there is a slightly increased incidence of breast and cervical cancers. Tamoxifen increases the risk of endometrial cancer. Hormone-replacement therapy (HRT, either oestrogen-only or combined) is not associated with a reduction in endometrial cancer (but possibly with a slight, non-significant increase). The evidence about long-term progestagens is confusing but these should be considered to have no effect on the incidence of these cancers. GnRH analogues are not given alone long term due to a deleterious effect on bone mineral density.

4. **B – Cyproterone acetate**

    The COCP, GnRH analogues and cyproterone acetate are the only agents that have an anti-androgenic effect, reducing hirsutism and acne. GnRH analogues are not given alone long term due to a deleterious effect on bone mineral density. Cyproterone acetate is a competitive blocker of androgen action. It is usually given as part of Dianette®, a form of COCP. The COCP already contains oestrogen by definition and does not cause feminisation of male fetuses if pregnancy occurs while taking it.

5. **G – Oestrogen-only HRT**

    Oestrogen-only HRT is all that is required after hysterectomy and is highly effective at preventing or treating vasomotor symptoms of the menopause. If the patient still has a uterus, then combined oestrogen-progesterone HRT is required to prevent endometrial stimulation. The COCP already contains oestrogen and progesterone by definition and is therefore not appropriate. Medroxyprogesterone acetate (as Depo-Provera®) can be effective in the management of vasomotor symptoms but is only given to patients in whom oestrogen is contraindicated or best avoided (so is not commonly used).

11. CHEST RADIOGRAPHS – CLINICAL SIGNS

1. **(P3–P4) D – Right-sided pneumothorax**
   These are the signs of a significant right-sided pneumothorax. The management will include analgesia and insertion of a chest drain connected to an underwater system.

2. **(P3–P4) J – Right-sided tension pneumothorax**
   These are the signs of a right-sided tension pneumothorax and the patient requires urgent treatment to relieve the increasing intrathoracic pressure. Without relief this will cause cardiac compression and cardiorespiratory arrest will follow. Under the controlled conditions of a hospital environment, a chest drain should be inserted immediately. Under more challenging conditions (eg at the scene of a road traffic accident) a large-bore intravenous cannula or a similar implement should be inserted.

3. **(P3–P4) H – Right upper lobe collapse**
   These are the signs of right upper lobe collapse. Lobar collapse can produce similar signs to a pleural effusion, with reduced percussion note, vocal and tactile vocal fremitus and reduced or absent breath sounds.

4. **(P3–P4) C – Right middle lobe pneumonia**
   The signs of a right middle lobe pneumonia are commonly missed as students and junior doctors alike commonly miss out (ie forget) to examine the patient's right axillary region. The radiographic findings might of course prompt you to re-examine the patient fully!

5. **(P3–P4) A – Apical fibrosis**
   Localised fibrosis (as in apical fibrosis) is one of the causes of bronchial breathing. Others include consolidation and the air–fluid interface above a pleural effusion.

IMAGES: pages 348–350

12. PATHOGENIC VIRUSES

1. **D – Hepatitis C virus**

   Hepatitis C is an RNA virus belonging to the flavivirus family. The major routes of infection are through blood transfusion and intravenous inoculation, but the incidence of transmission by both these routes is falling. At least 75% of patients infected with hepatitis C eventually develop chronic liver disease. Cirrhosis is seen in up to 20% of patients and of these, 7–15% will go on to develop hepatocellular carcinoma. Fulminant hepatitis is rare. Patients who are infected after the age of 40, particularly men, and patients infected with genotypes 1 and 4 show more rapid progression of fibrosis.

2. **A – Coronavirus**

   Severe acute respiratory syndrome (SARS) is a condition that was first described in the Far East and Canada in early 2003. It is characterised by a prodromal fever followed by dry cough, dyspnoea and hypoxia. In 10–20% of cases, the disease is severe enough that the patient requires mechanical ventilation. The mortality is in the region of 5%. The responsible virus is a novel coronavirus, an RNA virus named after its halo-(corona-)like appearance on electron microscopy. Before it came to prominence as the cause of SARS, coronavirus was better known as one of the viruses causing the common cold.

3. **J – Varicella zoster virus**

   Varicella zoster virus is a DNA virus of the α herpesvirus family. It causes two distinct diseases, varicella (chickenpox) and herpes zoster (shingles). Varicella is the primary infection and usually occurs in children. Shingles can occur at any age but is most common in the elderly. It produces vesicular skin lesions similar to chickenpox, usually in the distribution of a single dermatome. The lesions are often preceded by severe dermatomal pain, indicating the involvement of sensory nerves. Shingles never occurs as a primary infection but results from reactivation of latent virus from dorsal root and/or cranial nerve ganglia.

4. **F – Human papillomavirus**

   Verrucas or warts are benign tumours of squamous epithelium known as 'squamous-cell papillomas'. They arise not only in keratinised squamous epithelium, such as the skin, but also in non-keratinised squamous epithelium such as that lining the ectocervix. All warts are caused by human papillomavirus (HPV), a DNA virus belonging to the papovavirus family. There are almost 50 different serotypes of HPV. Genital warts are usually caused by HPV types 6 and 11. Other serotypes, notably types 16, 18 and 31, have been implicated in the development of high-grade cervical intraepithelial neoplasia (CIN) and invasive cervical carcinoma.

5. **C – Epstein–Barr virus**

   Infectious mononucleosis is a multisystem disorder caused by Epstein–Barr virus (EBV). This is a DNA virus belonging to the herpesvirus family. Diagnosis of infectious mononucleosis is made by finding heterophil antibodies to sheep erythrocytes in the patient's serum. As well as causing infectious mononucleosis, EBV has a strong association with certain human malignancies, particularly Burkitt's lymphoma and nasopharyngeal carcinoma.

13. PHARYNGEAL MUSCLES

1. **A – Inferior constrictor**
   A further component of the muscle is attached to the oblique line on the thyroid cartilage. Between the crico- and thyro-pharyngeal components, there is a potential weakness (the dehiscence of Killian), this being the site of protrusion of a pharyngeal pouch.

2. **D – Palatoglossus**
   The posterior pillar is underlaid by the palatopharyngeus. The palatine tonsil lies between the anterior and posterior pillars on the superior constrictor, which separates it from the facial artery and the carotid sheath.

3. **C – Middle constrictor**
   The anterior attachment is also from the stylohyoid ligament. Posteriorly, the three constrictors meet in the midline raphé, the superior being within the middle, which is within the inferior constrictor muscle.

4. **F – Pharyngobasilar fascia**
   The fascia completes the pharyngeal wall superolaterally, being continuous with the superior constrictor and attached to the skull base. The eustachian (auditory) tube passes from the lateral wall of the pharynx to the anterior wall of the middle ear. Its medial two-thirds is cartilaginous but it passes laterally into the petrous temporal bone.

5. **J – Tensor palatini**
   The stylopharyngeus is supplied by the glossopharyngeal nerve. The remainder of the muscles in the option list are supplied by the vagus nerve through the pharyngeal plexus.

14. MUSCLE ATTACHMENTS IN THE UPPER LIMB

1. **J – Triceps**
    The description is that of the attachment of the lateral head of the triceps. The medial head comes from the posterior aspect to the humerus below the radial groove; the long head is attached proximally to the infraglenoid aspect of the scapula. The three heads are attached distally to the olecranon process of the ulna. The muscle is a powerful extensor of the forearm.

2. **B – Brachialis**
    From its extensive humeral attachment the tendon is attached to the coronoid process of the ulna. The muscle is a powerful flexor of the forearm.

3. **D – Extensor carpi radialis longus**
    The ridge also gives rise to the brachioradialis muscle. Extensor carpi radialis brevis arises from the common extensor origin on the lateral epicondyle of the humerus; distally the tendons are attached to the base of the second and third metacarpal bones. They extend the wrist and have a weak action across the elbow.

4. **I – Pronator teres**
    Proximally the muscle has two heads, one just above the common flexor origin on the humerus and the second from the medial side of the coronoid process on the ulna. The muscle is a pronator of the forearm and forms the medial border of the cubital fossa.

5. **F – Flexor digitorum profundus**
    These are long flexor tendons passing deep to the flexor retinaculum, deep to the flexor digitorum superficialis. They gain attachment to the palmar surface of the base of the terminal phalanx of the fingers, and they also give attachment to the lumbrical muscles in the palm. The tendons of the flexor digitorum superficialis split over the proximal phalanx, each half encircling the corresponding tendon of the flexor digitorum profundus; after partial decussation, the tendon is attached to the sides of the middle phalanx. These two muscles flex the wrist and phalanges.

PAPER 5

Paper 5 questions

1. THEME: HEART FAILURE

A Alcoholic cardiomyopathy
B Aortic regurgitation
C Aortic stenosis
D Beriberi
E Cardiac tamponade
F Chronic obstructive pulmonary disease (COPD)
G Ischaemic cardiomyopathy
H Mitral regurgitation
I Mitral stenosis
J Pulmonary fibrosis

The following patients have all presented with heart failure. Please choose the most appropriate cause from the above list. The options may be used once, more than once or not at all.

1. A 59-year-old diabetic man presents in the Emergency Department with a 4-day history of increasing shortness of breath and ankle oedema. On examination, he is unwell and has signs of biventricular failure. Cardiac enzymes are within normal limits. The ECG shows sinus tachycardia, 120 bpm, left axis deviation and poor anterior 'R-wave' progression with a partial left bundle branch block.

2. A 29-year-old man is recovering in hospital after a severe pneumonia for which he has been on intravenous antibiotics for 1 week. He becomes acutely unwell with pyrexia and shortness of breath. On examination, he has several splinter haemorrhages and signs of left ventricular failure. There is a loud early diastolic murmur heard primarily at the left sternal edge. An old intravenous cannula is noted in the left antecubital fossa.

3. A 71-year-old woman is seen in Medical Out-patients for her 6-monthly check-up. She has been increasingly unwell, with shortness of breath on exercise, paroxysmal nocturnal dyspnoea (PND), orthopnoea and leg oedema. On examination, she has signs of biventricular failure and a low-volume pulse in atrial fibrillation. Auscultation reveals a soft, mid-diastolic murmur at the apex with a loud pansystolic murmur at the left sternal edge.

4. A 19-year-old Somalian man is admitted to hospital with suspected pulmonary tuberculosis. He has a positive Kussmaul's sign and his heart sounds are difficult to hear. His ECG confirms low-voltage complexes.

5. A 72-year-old man is admitted to hospital with worsening oedema and
shortness of breath. On examination, he is short of breath at rest and his
oxygen saturation is 84% on air. He has marked clubbing of the fingernails and
fixed inspiratory bibasal crepitations, as well as signs of biventricular failure.

2. THEME: DEFINITIVE UROLOGICAL INVESTIGATIONS

A   Anti-dsDNA antibody
B   Anti-GBM antibody
C   Blood glucose
D   c-ANCA
E   Plasma electrophoresis
F   Prostate-specific antigen (PSA)
G   Renal angiogram
H   Renal biopsy
I   Urine cytology
J   Ultrasound scan of the renal tract

The following patients have all presented with urological problems. Please choose the most definitive investigation to confirm the diagnosis in each case from the above list. Each investigation may be used once, more than once or not at all.

1. A 61-year-old man presents to his GP with increasing problems with passing urine. He has hesitancy, poor stream and terminal dribbling. Examination is unremarkable, other than the per rectal examination, which reveals a smoothly enlarged prostate gland. Subsequent investigations, including FBC, U&Es, corrected Ca^{2+} and chest radiograph are all within normal limits.

2. A 27-year-old woman presents in the Emergency Department with increasing peripheral and facial oedema. On examination, she is noted to have a malar rash as well as marked ascites and facial and ankle oedema. Urinalysis confirms protein+++ and microscopy shows the presence of renal casts. Blood tests show: haemoglobin 9.2 g/dl, MCV 88 fl, WCC 4.2 × 10^9/l, platelets 191 × 10^9/l; Na^+ 132 mmol/l, K^+ 6.9 mmol/l, urea 34.7 mmol/l, creatinine 553 μmol/l.

3. A 59-year-old man presents in the Emergency Department with a 10–day history of a flu-like illness associated with myalgia, arthralgia and shortness of breath, episodic haemoptysis and a 2-day history of oliguria and ankle oedema. Investigations show: Na^+ 133 mmol/l, K^+ 5.8 mmol/l, urea 17.1 mmol/l, creatinine 303 μmol/l. His chest radiograph shows hazy shadowing throughout both lung fields.

4. A 24-year-old woman presents in the Emergency Department with vague abdominal pains and haematuria. Of note, she has a strong family history of 'kidney problems' and her grandmother and aunt both died suddenly of 'brain haemorrhages'. Urinalysis shows: blood +++, protein++, nitrites negative and microscopy shows no organisms or renal casts. Other investigations show: haemoglobin 16.7 g/dl, haematocrit 54.8, WCC 14.2 × 10^9/l, platelets 553 × 10^9/l; Na^+ 129 mmol/l, K^+ 5.7 mmol/l, urea 25.8 mmol/l, creatinine 401 μmol/l.

5. An 87-year-old woman presents with severe back pain and general malaise. Routine investigations reveal: haemoglobin 5.9 g/dl, MCV 93 fl, WCC 2.8 × 10^9/l, platelets 33 × 10^9/l; Na^+ 131 mmol/l, K^+ 6.2 mmol/l, urea 18.0 mmol/l, creatinine 322 μmol/l; corrected Ca^{2+} 3.43 mmol/l; ESR 110 mm/h.

3. THEME: DYSPHAGIA

A   Achalasia
B   External oesophageal compression
C   Motor neurone disease
D   Oesophageal candidiasis
E   Oesophageal carcinoma
F   Oesophageal diverticulum
G   Oesophageal peptic stricture
H   Pharyngeal pouch
I   Presbyoesophagus
J   Systemic sclerosis

The following patients have all presented with difficulty in swallowing (dysphagia). Please choose the most appropriate cause from the above list. Each cause may be used once, more than once or not at all.

1. A 62-year-old woman presents in Medical Out-patients with a 3-month history of worsening 'high-level' dysphagia associated with nasal regurgitation. She has now developed speech problems and increasing limb weakness.

2. A 49-year-old man who has been in hospital for several weeks with a severe infective exacerbation of COPD and who has required several courses of antibiotics and steroids complains to the FY1 of worsening retrosternal pain and dysphagia to solids. Oesophagogastroduodenoscopy shows circumferential erosions and ulceration with linear white plaques.

3. A 91-year-old woman presents in the Health Care of the Older Person Out-patient Department with a 6-month history of worsening dysphagia to solids and liquids. A barium swallow reveals no intrinsic lesion but shows severe 'corkscrew' dysmotility.

4. A 54-year-old Hong Kong Chinese man presents with dysphagia to solids and liquids. A barium swallow confirms a long, irregular stricture extending over several centimetres.

5. A 31-year-old man presents to his GP with an 8-month history of worsening dysphagia to solids, with occasional regurgitation of unaltered food. The dysphagia is not as bad if he eats small amounts and washes everything down with lots of fluids. The diagnosis is confirmed on a barium swallow, which shows a 'bird's beak' deformity in the lower oesophagus.

4. THEME: WEAKNESS

A   Alcoholic myopathy
B   Amyotrophy
C   Cervical myelopathy
D   Demyelination
E   Duchenne muscular dystrophy
F   Guillain–Barré syndrome
G   Hypokalaemia
H   Motor neurone disease
I   Paraneoplastic motor neuropathy
J   Thyrotoxic proximal myopathy

The following patients have all presented with muscle weakness. Please choose the most appropriate cause from the above list. Each cause may be used once, more than once or not at all.

1. A 73-year-old man presents to his GP with increasing weakness in all four limbs, associated with nasal regurgitation of fluids and speech difficulties. Initial investigations, including FBC, U&Es, random blood glucose, LFTs, corrected Ca^{2+}, chest radiography, ECG and CT head scan, are all normal.

2. A 64-year-old woman presents to the Emergency Department with severe generalised weakness. She was recently started on metolazone and furosemide for peripheral oedema which had begun after she was put on nifedipine for hypertension.

3. A 19-year-old woman is seen by her GP with increasing difficulty water ski-ing. On examination, she is thin, peripherally vasodilated, tachycardic and tremulous.

4. A 34-year-old man is admitted to hospital with a 10-day history of an upper respiratory tract infection, which was followed by increasing difficulty with walking and the development of pins and needles and numbness in his feet. Two days after admission he has to be electively ventilated because of decreasing FEV_1 (forced expiratory volume in 1 second) and FVC (forced vital capacity).

5. A 63-year-old man on gliclazide for type 2 diabetes sees his GP with increasing pain and weakness in his thighs. His symptoms improve with insulin.

5. THEME: LESS COMMON INVESTIGATIONS

A   Bubble-contrast transoesophageal echocardiogram
B ^{13}C urea breath test
C   Electromyography (EMG)
D   Hydrogen breath test
E   PET scan
F   Rectal biopsy
G   Technetium-99-labelled red cell scan
H   Schirmer's test
I   Tensilon® test
J   Visual-evoked responses

The following patients have all presented with conditions requiring less common diagnostic tests to confirm the diagnosis. Please choose the most appropriate investigation for each of the patients from the above list. You may use each items once, more than once or not at all.

1. A 36-year-old man presents to the Emergency Department with sudden onset of right-sided weakness and slurred speech 24 hours after returning from the Far East by plane. Examination confirms that he has grade 2/5 right hemiparesis and dysarthria but the consultant in the stroke unit also thinks that he can hear a soft systolic murmur over the upper left sternal edge.

2. A 41-year-old man with a 'phobia' about hospitals and needles, presents to his GP with a 3–month history of worsening dyspepsia and reflux. The GP arranges for him to have a special test to detect possible *Helicobacter* infection.

3. A 29-year-old woman presents to her GP with pins and needles in her hands and episodic visual blurring, on one occasion leading to transient blindness in her left eye. Her GP refers her to Neurology Out-patients where an MRI scan of the brain and another diagnostic test are arranged.

4. A 39-year-old man presents to Out-patients with a second episode of melaena in 2 months. His first episode led to an upper gastrointestinal endoscopy, which was entirely normal, as was a subsequent colonoscopy.

5. A 49-year-old woman with long-standing rheumatoid arthritis presents to her GP with increasing exertional dyspnoea, ankle oedema and 'frothy' urine. On examination, she has a large left pleural effusion and moderate ascites. Her urinalysis shows protein ++++. Amyloidosis is confirmed on further testing.

6. THEME: NEW THERAPEUTIC INTERVENTIONS

A Abciximab
B Aldesleukin
C Alemtuzumab
D α-Interferon
E Basiliximab
F β-Interferon
G Granulocyte colony-stimulating factor (GCSF)
H Infliximab
I Rituximab
J Trastuzumab

The following patients have all presented with disorders requiring one of the newer therapeutic interventions. Please choose the most appropriate intervention from the above list. Each option may be used once, more than once or not at all.

1. A 39-year-old woman is admitted to her local hospital under the consultant neurologist with a third relapse of her multiple sclerosis in the past 18 months. He has discussed starting a new therapy that might help prevent these frequent relapses.

2. A 29-year-old man with severe Crohn's disease is re-admitted to hospital with another acute flare-up of his colitis. He is noted to have an infected anal fistula which has been resistant to treatment in the past.

3. A 63-year-old man with known ischaemic heart disease is re-admitted to hospital with a prolonged episode of angina-like chest pain. His troponin I is significantly raised but his ECG shows only T-wave inversion through the anterolateral leads. He continues to experience angina pains on minimal exertion and is referred for in-patient angiography at the local cardiology centre.

4. A 25-year-old previous intravenous drug user is seen in the Hepatology Clinic to be told that his recent blood tests have confirmed he has active hepatitis C virus infection. The consultant discusses the possibility of starting him on a relatively new treatment but after reviewing his notes he tells him that he is unfortunately not eligible because of a recent episode of severe depression and attempted suicide.

5. A 31-year-old woman who is undergoing her third course of chemotherapy for metastatic breast cancer is given a new drug which she is told might stop her getting infections related to her very low WCC.

7. THEME: JAUNDICE

A   Acute viral hepatitis
B   Ascending cholangitis
C   Carcinoma of the gallbladder
D   Cholangiocarcinoma
E   Cirrhosis
F   Gallstones
G   Hepatocellular carcinoma
H   Multiple hepatic metastases
I   Pancreatic carcinoma
J   Sclerosing cholangitis

The following are descriptions of patients with jaundice. Please select the most appropriate diagnosis from the above list. Each diagnosis may be used once, more than once or not at all.

1. A 78-year-old woman is seen in the Emergency Department with a 2-week history of progressive jaundice and pruritis. On direct questioning, she has a 3-month history of anorexia and weight loss. On examination, she is cachectic and deeply icteric, with a palpable gallbladder but no hepatomegaly. The LFTs show: total bilirubin 262 μmol/l, AST 62 IU/l, ALT 56 IU/l, alkaline phosphatase 695 IU/l, albumin 31 g/l.

2. A 65-year-old woman attends her GP with a 3-day history of increasing jaundice, nausea and upper abdominal pain. She has had several previous bouts of acute abdominal pain and a long history of dyspeptic symptoms. Examination reveals jaundice and slight tenderness in the right hypochondrium but no masses. The LFTs show: total bilirubin 90 μmol/l, AST 37 IU/l, ALT 23 IU/l, alkaline phosphatase 312 IU/l, albumin 39 g/l.

3. A 39-year-old man with known ulcerative colitis presents to his GP with a 2-week history of increasingly severe but painless jaundice. He is admitted to hospital, where an abdominal ultrasound scan demonstrates dilated intrahepatic ducts but a normal-diameter common bile duct.

4. A 43-year-old man presents in the Emergency Department with acute jaundice, nausea, vomiting and upper abdominal pain. On examination, he is unwell and pyrexial and there is tender hepatomegaly. The LFTs show: total bilirubin 96 μmol/l, AST 435 IU/l, ALT 570 IU/l, alkaline phosphatase 212 IU/l, albumin 42 g/l.

5. A 49-year-old woman presents with recent onset of jaundice. On further questioning, she says that she has noticed bouts of pruritis and dark urine for several months. The LFTs show: total bilirubin 63 μmol/l, AST 40 IU/l, ALT 27 IU/l, alkaline phosphatase 509 IU/l, albumin 36 g/l. An autoantibody screen shows a positive titre (> 1/80) for antimitochondrial antibodies.

8. THEME: INTESTINAL OBSTRUCTION

A   Adhesions
B   Bezoar
C   Colonic carcinoma
D   Crohn's stricture
E   Diverticular stricture
F   Gallstones
G   Hernia
H   Intussusception
I   Small-bowel lymphoma
J   Tuberculous stricture
K   Volvulus

The following patients have all presented with intestinal (large- or small-bowel) obstruction. Please select the most appropriate diagnosis from the above list. Each diagnosis may be used once, more than once or not at all.

1. A 90-year-old woman presents in the Emergency Department with a 3-day history of vomiting and colicky central and right-sided abdominal pain. She has had no previous surgery. On examination, she is dehydrated and her abdomen is distended and tympanic, with obstructed bowel sounds. There is a 2-cm tender swelling in the right groin with overlying erythema.

2. A 46-year-old woman is referred by her GP to the Emergency Department with a 48-hour history of abdominal pain, distension and vomiting. She has had several previous admissions for similar symptoms. On examination, she has scars from previous operations which include a hysterectomy and a laparotomy.

3. A 6-month-old baby is referred to the paediatric on-call team because of attacks of screaming associated with drawing up of the legs. The baby has vomited and is clinically dehydrated and unwell. On examination there is blood and mucus per rectum.

4. A 67-year-old man presents in the Emergency Department with a 4-day history of severe lower abdominal cramps and vomiting. He has not opened his bowels for 3 days and has not passed flatus today. On direct questioning, he admits to having had vague lower abdominal pains and some diarrhoea for some months and might have lost some weight. The abdomen is distended on examination and bowel sounds are obstructed. The rectum is empty.

5. An 80-year-old man with severe Parkinson's disease is a long-term resident in a nursing home. The nurses have called the GP out because he has been distressed for some days and has not been eating or drinking. The patient has a reduced level of consciousness and is dehydrated. The abdomen is very distended and a plain abdominal radiograph demonstrates a single, hugely dilated loop of colon.

9. THEME: POSTOPERATIVE PYREXIA

A   Anaesthetic drugs
B   Anastomotic dehiscence
C   Basal atelectasis
D   Deep vein thrombosis
E   Pelvic abscess
F   Phlebitis
G   Respiratory tract infection
H   Subphrenic abscess
I   Transfusion reaction
J   Urinary tract infection
K   Wound infection

The following are descriptions of patients with postoperative pyrexia, with or without associated pain. Please select the most appropriate diagnosis from the above list. Each diagnosis may be used once, more than once or not at all.

1. A 62-year-old woman undergoes a right hemicolectomy for caecal carcinoma. She is given an epidural for pain relief but this falls out on leaving theatre recovery. Patient-controlled analgesia is started but only after some delay, during which she has significant pain. On the first postoperative day she has a temperature of 37.9 °C.

2. A 92-year-old woman undergoes a laparotomy for small-bowel obstruction. She has a protracted recovery and is still catheterised at day 14 after the operation because of problems with mobilisation. You are called because she develops a temperature of 38.7 °C. She has no cough or gastrointestinal symptoms and is eating and drinking normally.

3. A 12-year-old boy undergoes a difficult appendicectomy for gangrenous appendicitis. He makes a rapid recovery initially and goes home on the third post-operative day. Four days later, however, his mother brings him back to the Emergency Department with further lower abdominal pain and a swinging pyrexia of 39 °C. The wound is clean but there is tenderness and guarding in the right iliac fossa.

4. A 66-year-old woman undergoes a laparotomy with oversewing of a perforated duodenal ulcer. Five days post-operatively, she develops a swinging pyrexia of 38.6 °C with rigors. On examination, there is some right upper quadrant tenderness. She has right basal crackles and a small right pleural effusion on a chest radiograph.

5. A 76-year-old man undergoes an anterior resection for rectal cancer. On the third post-operative day he develops severe lower abdominal pain. On examination, he is septic with a high temperature, has a reduced conscious level and has abdominal distension with peritonism in the lower abdomen.

10. THEME: UROGENITAL RADIOLOGY – RADIOLOGICAL DIAGNOSIS

*Using the radiographic images **A–J on pages 351–353**, please match the radiological diagnoses with the correct image. You may use the images once, more than once or not at all. There may be more than one image appropriate for each of the diagnoses.*

1. Downward displacement of the kidney.

2. Renal enlargement.

3. Dilated, obstructed pelvicalyceal system.

4. Congenital abnormality of the renal tract.

5. Abnormal calcification within the renal tract.

11. THEME: UROGYNAECOLOGICAL DISORDERS

A   Congenital abnormality of the genitourinary tract
B   Cystocoele
C   Detrusor overactivity
D   Enterocoele
E   Genuine stress incontinence (GSI)
F   Interstitial cystitis
G   Rectocoele
H   Urinary tract infection (UTI)
I   Uterovaginal prolapse
J   Vesicovaginal fistula

From the above list please choose the condition most likely to cause the clinical picture described. Each option may be used once, more than once or not at all.

1. A 38-year-old woman describes urinary frequency, urgency and stress incontinence on coughing and laughing for the last 6 months. Examination of the urogenital tract reveals no abnormality. Her symptoms improve markedly on tolterodine, an anticholinergic agent.

2. A 45-year-old woman describes having urinary incontinence almost continuously. It started shortly after a 'difficult' hysterectomy for fibroids. Examination reveals a moist vagina and vulva but no demonstrable stress incontinence on coughing.

3. A 60-year-old woman describes a feeling of 'something coming down' in the vagina. She also describes frequency and difficulty passing urine, having to insert a finger into the vagina to aid voiding.

4. A 28-year-old woman describes urinary frequency, urgency and dysuria. She had a diagnostic laparoscopy 1 week ago for pelvic pain (with no cause found for the pain). Examination reveals no abnormality.

5. A 58-year-old woman describes urinary frequency and stress incontinence on coughing and laughing for the last 6 months. Examination of the urogenital tract reveals moderate urogenital atrophy but no other abnormalities. Urodynamic investigation shows no increase in detrusor pressure during witnessed episodes of stress incontinence.

12. THEME: DISEASES OF THE LARGE INTESTINE

A Adenocarcinoma
B Adenoma
C Amoebiasis
D Angiodysplasia
E Crohn's disease
F Diverticular disease
G Hirschsprung's disease
H Ischaemic colitis
I Pseudomembranous colitis
J Ulcerative colitis

From the above list, please select the disease that each of the following patients is most likely to have. Each diagnosis may be used once, more than once or not at all.

1. A 50-year-old man presents with recent onset of bright-red rectal bleeding. Flexible sigmoidoscopy shows a pedunculated polyp in the rectum. The polyp has a red, lobulated surface and is 1 cm in diameter.

2. A 75-year-old woman who had a total hip replacement 5 days ago develops diarrhoea on the orthopaedic ward. She was treated with prophylactic antibiotics around the time of surgery. Stool culture grows *Clostridium difficile*.

3. A 35-year-old man presents with abdominal pain and bloody diarrhoea 1 month after returning from holiday in India. Colonoscopy shows multiple flask-shaped ulcers throughout the colon. Biopsies of the ulcerated areas shows periodic acid–Schiff (PAS-)positive trophozoites with ingested red cells in the ulcer slough.

4. A 75-year-old man presents with a 2-month history of left-sided abdominal pain and altered bowel habit. On examination, he has a pyrexia of 37.8 °C and is tender in the left iliac fossa. Barium enema shows narrowing of the sigmoid colon and multiple outpouchings that communicate with the lumen. No evidence of a mass lesion is seen.

5. A 23-year-old woman presents with a 4-week history of profuse bloody diarrhoea and abdominal pain. Colonoscopy reveals diffuse mucosal erythema starting in the rectum and extending continuously to the splenic flexure. Stool cultures on three consecutive occasions are negative. Colonic biopsies show diffuse chronic inflammation in the lamina propria with crypt abscesses and crypt distortion. No granulomas are seen.

13. THEME: THE LARYNX

A   Arytenoid cartilage
B   Cricoid cartilage
C   Epiglottis
D   External laryngeal nerve
E   Inferior thyroid artery
F   Internal laryngeal nerve
G   Recurrent laryngeal nerve
H   Superior laryngeal nerve
I   Thyrohyoid membrane
J   Thyroid cartilage

For each of the following descriptions, please choose the most appropriate structure from the above list. Each structure may be used once, more than once or not at all.

1. Innervates the lateral cricoarytenoid muscle.   ☐

2. Gives attachment to both sides of the conus elasticus.   ☐

3. Gives anterior attachment to the vocal fold.   ☐

4. Gives posterior attachment to the quadrangular membrane.   ☐

5. Is a posterior relation of the tongue.   ☐

14. THEME: NERVE SUPPLY OF THE MUSCLES OF THE LOWER LIMB

A   Common peroneal (lateral popliteal) nerve
B   Deep peroneal (anterior tibial) nerve
C   Femoral nerve
D   Medial plantar nerve
E   Obturator nerve
F   Sciatic nerve
G   Superficial peroneal (musculocutaneous) nerve
H   Superior gluteal nerve
I   Sural nerve
J   Tibial (posterior tibial) nerve

For each of the following muscles please choose the nerve that innervates it from the above list. Each nerve may be used once, more than once or not at all.

1.   Gluteus medius.   ☐

2.   Semimembranosus.   ☐

3.   Tibialis anterior.   ☐

4.   Peroneus longus.   ☐

5.   Soleus.   ☐

Paper 5 answers

1. HEART FAILURE

1. **G – Ischaemic cardiomyopathy**
   This man has signs of biventricular failure. He has peripheral oedema and dyspnoea, which could be due to pulmonary oedema, a pleural effusion or, indeed, low-output failure. His ECG confirms signs of old (ie non-acute) ischaemic heart disease with left axis deviation, poor anterior R-wave progression and a partial left bundle branch block. He will need treatment with diuretics and, if possible, with an ACE inhibitor and/or cardioselective β-blocker.

2. **B – Aortic regurgitation**
   This young man has developed acute infective endocarditis, probably caused by a staphylococcal infection. He has had an intravenous cannula, which is probably the source of the infection, and shows the importance of the aseptic insertion and removal of these as soon as they are no longer required. He will require intravenous flucloxacillin and probably aortic valve replacement.

3. **I – Mitral stenosis**
   This woman has signs consistent with mitral stenosis and secondary tricuspid regurgitation. She has a soft mid-diastolic murmur (mitral stenosis) and a loud pansystolic murmur (tricuspid regurgitation) with a low-volume pulse in atrial fibrillation. She has now developed cardiac failure and will need treatment with diuretics, digoxin and prophylactic warfarin or aspirin. If she is agreeable she should be considered for mitral valve replacement.

4. **E – Cardiac tamponade**
   This young man probably has a TB pericardial effusion with signs of a potential tamponade. Kussmaul's sign (the paradoxical rise in the jugulovenous pressure with inspiration), the poorly heard heart sounds and the low-voltage complexes on his ECG are all consistent with a tamponade and he requires urgent pericardiocentesis. He will also need antituberculous treatment for at least 6 months.

5. **J – Pulmonary fibrosis**
   This man has developed cor pulmonale, ie cardiac failure secondary to his chronic lung condition. He has signs of pulmonary fibrosis, as evidenced by the fixed bibasal crepitations and finger clubbing with associated hypoxia and desaturation. This chronic condition has led to pulmonary hypertension and secondary right, and then left heart failure.

2. DEFINITIVE UROLOGICAL INVESTIGATIONS

1. **F – Prostate-specific antigen (PSA)**

   This man has developed symptoms of bladder outflow tract obstruction. In a middle-aged man this is most likely to be due to prostatic enlargement, which can be confirmed on per rectal examination. He has no associated systemic symptoms, normal FBC, U&Es, corrected Ca^{2+} and chest radiograph. The most likely diagnosis is benign prostatic hypertrophy, although carcinoma must still be excluded. The differentiating investigation is a serum prostatic-specific antigen (PSA). If the PSA is within the normal range the patient should be started on an α-blocker or considered for surgical resection.

2. **A – Anti-dsDNA antibody**

   This patient has developed systemic lupus erythematosus (SLE) as evidenced by her malar rash and renal failure. The renal impairment is secondary to a glomerulonephritis, which maybe membranous, focal segmental, diffuse or even minimal change disease. However it may be that even lupus patients with apparently normal renal function have some immune-mediated changes within the kidney visible only on microscopy. SLE is characterised by the presence of dsDNA antibodies, particularly in the presence of active nephritis. This may be associated with low C3 and C4 levels and a raised ESR in the presence of relatively normal CRP levels.

3. **B – Anti-glomerular basement membrane (-GMB) antibody**

   This patient has developed renal impairment and pulmonary changes consistent with haemorrhage. This combination can be associated with Goodpasture's syndrome, more recently renamed 'anti-glomerular basement membrane disease' (anti-GBM disease) or, in a chronic setting, Wegner's granulomatosis can present in a similar manner but would usually involve the upper respiratory tract as well. The common antigen in anti-GBM disease is a component of type-IV collagen, which forms a major structural component of the basement membrane found within both the alveolus and the glomerulus.

4. **J – Ultrasound scan of the renal tract**

   This patient has a strong family history of renal disease and two relatives have died suddenly of intracranial haemorrhage. She now presents with renal failure, haematuria and polycythaemia. This clinical picture is highly suggestive of adult polycystic kidney disease (APCKD). The diagnosis can be easily confirmed on renal ultrasound scan. APCKD is the commonest congenital abnormality of the renal tract leading to renal failure and should be screened for in all first-degree relatives. It is an autosomal dominant disorder, unlike the childhood form, which is inherited in an autosomal recessive manner.

5. **E – Plasma electrophoresis**

This elderly woman has presented with back pain. Subsequent routine investigations have confirmed a pancytopenia, an ESR > 100 mm/h, hypercalcaemia and acute renal failure, suggesting probable multiple myeloma. The diagnosis is confirmed by the presence of a monclonal gammopathy with associated immunoparesis on plasma electrophoresis, Bence Jones proteins in the urine and plasma cells on a blood film or in the bone marrow. Renal failure occurs as a result of four or five processes in myeloma, collectively called 'myeloma kidney':

- Dehydration – due to being unwell
- Glomerulonephritis
- Increased incidence of urinary tract infections – due to the immunoparesis
- Hypercalcaemia – leading to nephrocalcinosis and renal stones
- Obstruction of the tubules by the light chains.

3. DYSPHAGIA

1. **C – Motor neurone disease**
This woman has symptoms of 'bulbar problems'. She has high-level dysphagia and nasal regurgitation, which are suggestive of an oropharyngeal neuromuscular problem. She has also developed speech problems and limb weakness. This clinical picture is highly suggestive of motor neurone disease, although the diagnosis is one of exclusion and other pathologies should be excluded using magnetic resonance imaging (MRI) of the cervical spine and brain, electroencephalography (EEG) and electromyography (EMG).

2. **D – Oesophageal candidiasis**
This patient has had multiple courses of antibiotics and steroids, implying he has been seriously ill, and this will lead to opportunistic infections such as candidiasis, *Clostridium difficile* and methicillin-resistant *Staphylococcus aureus* (MRSA) infections. Patients often complain of hoarseness of the voice if the candidiasis has affected their pharynx or has caused dysphagia, as in this case. Patients should be treated with a single dose of fluconazole 150 mg, nystatin or amphotericin.

3 **I – Presbyoesophagus**
Presbyoesophagus or 'corkscrew' oesophagus is another diagnosis of exclusion and is due to dysfunctional peristalsis. This can occur throughout the gastrointestinal tract in older patients and leads to dysphagia in the upper gastrointestinal tract and constipation in the colon. Benign and malignant lesions are both common in the older patient and dysphagia should be investigated with a barium swallow and/or upper gastrointestinal endoscopy, constipation with colonoscopy or CT abdomen with contrast.

4. **E – Oesophageal carcinoma**
Carcinoma of the oesophagus is more common in Chinese people and presents with increasing dysphagia, initially to solids and then progressively to liquids. Risk factors include underlying oesophageal disorders such as achalasia and Barrett's oesophagus, cigarette smoking and spicy foods.

5. **A – Achalasia**
Achalasia of the oesophagus is an idiopathic disorder caused by an atonic segment in the lower oesophagus, similar to Hirschsprung's disease in the rectum. It leads to low-level dysphagia to solids and patients often complain of vomiting of undigested food. It is improved symptomatically if the patient takes smaller mouthfuls and washes the food down with large volumes of liquid. Definitive treatment involves forceful dilation of the lower oesophageal sphincter or, in poorly responsive cases, surgical division of the segmental muscle wall.

4. WEAKNESS

1. **H – Motor neurone disease**
   This patient has signs and symptoms of limb weakness and bulbar problems, ie speech and swallowing difficulties, consistent with motor neurone disease. Motor neurone disease is a diagnosis of exclusion and must be differentiated from other pathological conditions. such as multi-infarct disease and late-onset myasthenic syndrome.

2. **G – Hypokalaemia**
   Hypokalaemia can make patients feel very weak and lethargic and is common in patients on several diuretics. The hypokalaemia can be avoided by the addition of spironolactone, amiloride and/or an ACE inhibitor.

3. **J – Thyrotoxic proximal myopathy**
   This young woman has developed a proximal myopathy secondary to thyrotoxicosis. The major endocrine disorders associated with 'excess', ie acromegaly, Cushing's and diabetes (hyperglycaemia), can all cause a proximal myopathy.

4. **F – Guillain–Barré syndrome**
   This patient has developed a mixed motor-sensory neuropathy 10 days after a respiratory tract infection. This is consistent with Guillain–Barré syndrome. Patients with *Campylobacter* antibodies or evidence of HIV infection suffer a more rapidly progressive, malignant form of this disorder and often require ventilatory support. The patient's respiratory function should be monitored using serial spirometry measurements (not the peak expiratory flow rate, PEFR).

5. **B – Amyotrophy**
   This man has developed a proximal motor neuropathy associated with his diabetes. This is known as 'diabetic amyotrophy'. The patient should improve with insulin therapy. Other causes of proximal myopathy need to be excluded in patients who do not respond to this therapy.

5. LESS COMMON INVESTIGATIONS

1. **A – Bubble-contrast transoesophageal echocardiogram**
   This man has presented with a 'paradoxical embolism', which is an embolism that has travelled from the right-sided circulation to the left, ie from venous to arterial. His long-distance flight has caused a deep vein thrombosis (DVT), which would normally lead to a pulmonary embolism. The only way that the DVT can travel into the left side of the circulation, and thus cause a stroke, is if there is a arteriovenous connection, in this case an atrial septal defect. The method of confirming this diagnosis is to inject the patient with contrast medium, which has been shaken (but not stirred) to create tiny bubbles within it. The flow of contrast is then viewed using transoesophageal echocardiography, the diagnosis confirmed when bubbles are seen to cross the atrial septum into the left atrium.

2. **B – ^{13}C urea breath test**
   Helicobacter pylori is a urease-producing, Gram-negative organism that is has been closely linked to upper gastrointestinal inflammation, peptic ulcer disease and, more recently, upper gastrointestinal malignancy. The easiest method to confirm infection is by a CLO (*Campylobacter*-like organism) test on biopsy materials recovered at endoscopy or by direct visualisation on microscopy. If the patent is unwilling to have upper endoscopy, however, a blood antibody or stool antigen test can be undertaken. Alternatively, a labelled carbon breath test can be done. Both the CLO test and the ^{13}C urea breath test rely on the ability of *H. pylori* to produce urease, which splits urea: in the CLO test this causes a rise in pH (through the release of ammonia) and a colour change; in the ^{13}C urea test this leads to the release of ^{13}C, which is then expired in carbon dioxide and quantified using mass spectrometry.

3. **J – Visual-evoked responses**
   This young woman has symptoms suggestive of demyelination secondary to multiple sclerosis. The main diagnostic test in this condition is MRI of the brain and cervical cord, looking for plaques of demyelination. These are most commonly found in the periventricular areas, the cerebellum, the brainstem and the cervical spine. The other mainstay of diagnosis is visual-evoked responses (VERs) and examination of the CSF (obtained by lumbar puncture) for oligoclonal bands. VERs are measured by shining lights into the eyes of the patient and recording when they are registered in the visual cortices using scalp electrodes. The presence of demyelination causes prolongation of the visual pathways and thus delayed responses.

4. **G – Technetium-99-labelled red cell scan**
   Most patients presenting with upper or lower gastrointestinal bleeding have a diagnosis confirmed at endoscopy. If this fails, further imaging might be performed using arteriography or, in some cases, a labelled red cell scan. Both arteriography and the labelled red cell scan rely on continued bleeding and their use is limited to patients who are bleeding enough to cause haemodynamic instability or an acute drop in haemoglobin. These two procedures are principally used when trying to localise a bleeding source prior to radical surgical intervention in very sick patients with life-threatening haemorrhage or, as in this case, in patients with recurrent occult bleeds.

5. **F – Rectal biopsy**

    This patient has symptoms suggestive of fluid overload and heavy proteinuria (as evidenced by the frothy urine). The unifying diagnosis in this case is amyloidosis, which is diagnosed on biopsy of affected organs, but often less invasively by its presence on rectal biopsy. Amyloid appears apple-green under polarised light when stained with Congo red.

6. NEW THERAPEUTIC INTERVENTIONS

This set of questions is difficult for the undergraduate (and probably for most postgraduates too), but we have included them because they illustrate that medicine is an ever-changing field and that keeping up with innovation and change requires the doctor of today to commit to lifelong learning. The alternative is that they will find themselves very quickly 'behind the times'. Immunomodulators and monoclonal antibody therapies will become increasingly common, particularly in autoimmune disease, chronic inflammatory conditions and malignancies.

1. **F – β-Interferon**
    This patient has relapsing-remitting multiple sclerosis. Several new agents have been licensed recently that have been shown to reduce the frequency of the relapses. Beta-interferon and glatiramer are given to patients who have had at least one relapse in the past 18 months (both should only be given in specialist centres). Beta-interferon commonly causes a flu-like illness but can also cause personality changes, severe depression and even suicidal ideation. Glatiramer is an 'immunomodulator' made up of synthetic peptides. Like β-interferon, it can cause local irritation at the injection site but its main side-effects are tachycardia, palpitations and shortness of breath.

2. **H – Infliximab**
    This patient should be given the monoclonal antibody therapy, infliximab, which is used in specialist centres for severe, relapsing Crohn's disease and, in particular, for treatment-resistant fistulae. It works against the pro-inflammatory cytokine, tumour necrosis factor-α (TNF-α). It can cause worsening of heart failure and reactivate tuberculosis infection. Infliximab is also used in the treatment of rheumatoid arthritis.

3. **A – Abciximab**
    This man has unstable angina following a prolonged episode of chest pain. Despite being in hospital and on maximal therapy, he continues to get exertional chest pain and should be started on the glycoprotein-receptor antagonist, abciximab. This monoclonal agent is directed against the GIIb/IIIa receptor on the platelet, stopping it binding to fibrinogen and thus blocking clot formation.

4. **D – α-Interferon**
    This patient has active hepatitis C virus infection and would be eligible for α-interferon therapy but its use is contraindicated because of his history of depression and parasuicide. In approximately 40% of treated patients, α-interferon causes seroconversion from HBe antigen to antibody (showing viral replication has been inhibited). This in turn can cause reversal of some of the liver damage sustained during the active infection. Paradoxically, patients with more severe disease are more likely to respond than those with minimal changes in the liver. Alpha-interferon can also be given for its anti-tumour effects in the treatment of lymphoma and some solid tumours.

5. **G – Granulocyte colony-stimulating factor**

Granulocyte colony-stimulating factor (GCSF) is used prophylactically in patients undergoing chemotherapy to try to avoid neutropenia and severe sepsis, particularly in patients who have already had one such episode. Others (and there will be more in the near future) include:

- Aldesleukin – recombinant IL2, used in metastatic renal carcinoma with limited success. It is very toxic and has several severe side-effects.
- Alemtuzumab – monoclonal therapy directed against B-cell lymphocytes. It is principally used in chemotherapy-resistant chronic lymphocytic leukaemia (CLL). Both alemtuzumab and rituximab can cause severe acute dyspnoea 1–2 hours after infusion, due to the sudden release of cytokines (cytokine release syndrome).
- Basiliximab – monoclonal therapy directed against T-cell lymphocyte proliferation. It is used with ciclosporin and steroid immunosuppression to avoid acute rejection in allogenic renal transplantation.
- Rituximab –like alemtuzumab, this is a monoclonal therapy directed against B-cell lymphocytes. It is used in chemotherapy-resistant follicular and large-B-cell non-Hodgkin's lymphoma.
- Trastuzumab – this is a monoclonal therapy directed against the human epidermal growth factor receptor 2 (HER2), which is overexpressed by some breast cancers.

7. JAUNDICE

1. **I – Pancreatic carcinoma**
   The patient has an obstructive jaundice picture with progressive symptoms, suggestive of underlying pancreatic carcinoma. Cholangiocarcinoma and multiple liver metastases can present similarly, but the former is much less common than pancreatic cancer (this is therefore the more likely diagnosis) and the latter is associated with a palpable liver, not a palpable gallbladder. Other characteristic symptoms of pancreatic cancer include severe abdominal and back pain. Investigations include ultrasound, CT, ERCP and cytology.

2. **F – Gallstones**
   This woman has previous characteristic symptoms of gallstones and now presents with obstructive jaundice due to impaction of gallstone in the common bile duct. The gallbladder is not palpable because, despite the obstruction, the gallbladder will not expand due to previous inflammation and scarring. This forms the essence of Courvoisier's law, which roughly states that 'when the gallbladder is palpable and the patient is jaundiced, the cause is not gallstones' (as in patient 1). In practice there are a few exceptions, but this is at least a useful guide, especially during your student years.

3. **J – Sclerosing cholangitis**
   Benign stricturing of the bile ducts can occur in response to localised inflammation (chronic pancreatitis, chronic duodenal ulceration, parasitic infection) or trauma (usually operative) or can be due to sclerosing cholangitis. This is an obscure disorder of uncertain aetiology that results in fibrous obliteration of the biliary tract. It is a relatively uncommon complication of ulcerative colitis and is more common in males with the disease.

4. **A – Acute viral hepatitis**
   The patient has an acute presentation with jaundice and systemic upset. While this could also be typical of ascending cholangitis, the patient's young age and tender hepatomegaly make acute viral hepatitis the most likely diagnosis. The diagnosis can be confirmed by viral serological testing.

5. **E – Cirrhosis (in this case primary biliary cirrhosis)**
   The presentation is typical for this disorder in terms of sex and age. This autoimmune disorder is confirmed by the finding of antimitochondrial antibodies and proven by characteristic histology from liver biopsy. Cirrhosis is one of the principal causes of jaundice and itself has many causes of which primary biliary cirrhosis is a less frequent cause than alcohol and chronic active (viral) hepatitis.

8. INTESTINAL OBSTRUCTION

1. G – Hernia, in this case a femoral hernia

Hernia is the second most common cause of small-intestinal obstruction in the West after adhesions. The presence of a hernia should always be sought by careful examination. Femoral hernias, while less common than inguinal hernias, are particular offenders for causing obstruction. Surgical treatment is indicated.

2. A – Adhesions

This is the most common cause of small-intestinal obstruction in the West. Why some patients develop adhesions and others do not is a cause for much speculation. Treatment should be conservative for about 48 hours (nil by mouth, intravenous fluids, nasogastric tube, correction of any U&Es abnormalities), provided there are no signs of strangulation. Thereafter, the decision regarding surgery depends on individual case findings.

3. H – Intussusception

Intussusception is telescoping of a segment of intestine into an adjacent one. The condition is encountered most commonly in infancy but can occur in adults, when a precipitating factor (ie a 'lead point') is usually present, such as a polyp. Treatment can be hydrostatic (barium enema) or surgical.

4. C – Colonic carcinoma

The presentation is of large-bowel obstruction, the common causes of which in this age group include carcinoma, diverticular disease and volvulus. Carcinoma is suggested by the preceding history. Treatment is by resuscitation and then surgical resection.

5. K – Volvulus

This occurs when a segment of bowel twists on its mesentery, causing obstruction, often leading later to strangulation. The common sites are the sigmoid colon and the caecum but the condition can also affect the small intestine. The patient is commonly very elderly and infirm, as in this case. Treatment consists of resuscitation and surgical resection, often with end-stoma formation, for example a Hartmann's procedure (although endoscopic attempts at reduction can be made initially).

9. POSTOPERATIVE PYREXIA

The postoperative patient with pyrexia is a common source of difficulty during your surgical house post. This requires an organised approach and the diagnosis is usually evident if you are aware of the common causes listed in the question.

1. **C – Basal atelectasis**
   This is the commonest cause of early pyrexia postoperatively (the other being anaesthetic drugs). It classically occurs in a patient in whom inadequate analgesia leads to reduced respiratory excursion and coughing. The resultant hypoventilation of the lung bases leads to localised small-airway collapse and is usually accompanied by low-grade pyrexia.

2. **J – Urinary tract infection**
   This should always be near the top of the list in any patient who is catheterised, especially the elderly convalescent patient.

3. **E – Pelvic abscess**
   This is the only common significant complication of appendicectomy. Wound infections are more common but less serious. The patient (or parent) should be warned about these two complications when they are giving consent for surgery.

4. **H – Subphrenic abscess**
   This can occur after any inflammatory/infective process in the upper abdomen but also commonly results from secondary infection of a haematoma in the region (eg post-splenectomy. The swinging nature of the pyrexia again suggests a collection of pus and the chest radiograph findings are supportive – these caused by transdiaphragmatic irritation of the pleura.

5. **B – Anastomotic dehiscence**
   The nature of the surgery (anterior resection, ie a left-sided anastomosis) and the clinical findings suggest this diagnosis. This is a serious complication that carries a significant mortality. Treatment is urgent resuscitation and surgery and (usually) postoperative care in an intensive care unit.

10. UROGENITAL RADIOLOGY – RADIOLOGICAL DIAGNOSIS

1. **(P5–P7) F – Displaced left-sided kidney**
   This intravenous urogram (IVU) shows a downwardly displaced, abnormal, left-sided pelvicalyceal system. This displacement is due to a large renal mass which could be either benign (eg renal cyst) or malignant. In this case it was due to a large renal-cell carcinoma.

2. **(P5–P7) A – Polycystic kidneys**
   This plain radiograph shows bilaterally enlarged renal shadows. In this case it is due to adult polycystic kidney disease, but large kidneys can be caused by multiple bilateral 'simple' cysts, by bilateral malignant tumours, or by any cause of hydronephrosis.

3. **(P5–P7) E, G, H – Obstructed right kidney, duplex kidneys and obstructed left kidney**
   These three IVU images show an obstructed and dilated right pelvicalyceal system (**E**), an obstructed and dilated left pelvicalyceal system (**H**) and a dilated pelvicalyceal system in a duplex system on the left (**G**). Obstruction at the ureteric–pelvic junction can be functional due to an inelastic ring of tissue at the junction, or can occur as a result of calculi or benign or malignant strictures.

4. **(P5–P7) C, H – Horseshoe kidney and obstructed left kidney**
   The IVU in radiograph **C** demonstrates the characteristic appearances of a 'horseshoe' kidney, with both pelvicalyceal systems rotated through 90° degrees, so seen 'end on'. The IVU in radiograph **H** shows a duplex system of both renal tracts. Bilaterally there are two kidneys and ureters with a dilated, abnormal pelvicalyceal system of the lower kidney on the left. Such abnormalities predispose patients to urinary tract infections and subsequent chronic renal problems, such as reflux nephropathy.

5. **(P5–P7) D, I, J – Vesical calculus, right-sided nephrocalcinosis and right staghorn calculus**
   Radiographs **D** and **J** show large, calcified calculi within the bladder and the right kidney respectively. Radiograph **I** shows nephrocalcinosis of the right kidney, particularly in the upper pole. Nephrocalcinosis is commonly associated with chronic hypercalcaemia (hyperparathyroidism, sarcoidosis), medullary sponge kidney and renal tubular acidosis. Localised areas of calcification can occur after trauma (iatrogenic or non-iatrogenic), with tuberculous infection or within cysts or malignant tumours.

IMAGES: pages 351–353

11. UROGYNAECOLOGICAL DISORDERS

1. **C – Detrusor overactivity**
    The two most common causes of stress incontinence are 'genuine stress incontinence' (GSI) and detrusor overactivity. GSI is most common in the peri- and post-menopausal period due to pelvic floor and sphincter deficiencies, exacerbated by the hypo-oestrogenic state. GSI is a not particularly likely in a 38-year-old but is still possible. The symptoms described can occur in most of the listed conditions but the irritative symptom of urgency is more common with detrusor overactivity than it is in GSI. The fact that the symptoms improve with tolterodine (an anticholinergic) makes detrusor overactivity most likely diagnosis because this would be unlikely to improve the symptoms of a urinary tract infection, interstitial cystitis or GSI.

2. **J – Vesicovaginal fistula**
    Continuous urinary incontinence suggests either bypass of the normal sphincter mechanism (vesicovaginal fistula or a congenital abnormality such as an aberrant ureter) or very severe sphincter deficiency (ie GSI). The timing of the symptoms (immediately after a difficult surgical procedure) is again highly suggestive of a vesicovaginal fistula as unrecognised bladder trauma (more likely during a difficult operation) can lead to subsequent fistula formation in the postoperative period. An aberrant ureter usually presents in childhood or adolescence. Intrinsic sphincter deficiency severe enough for continuous leakage is rare.

3. **B – Cystocoele**
    'Something coming down' is a common pressure symptom of prolapse, depending on whether there is laxity of the anterior vaginal wall (cystocoele) or the posterior vaginal wall (rectocoele) or direct utero–vaginal prolapse. An enterocoele is commonly seen when bowel contents prolapse into the top of the vaginal vault after hysterectomy. The fact that the symptoms are urinary tends to suggest prolapse of the anterior compartment. Difficulty in voiding is rare in women and is likely to be due to a significant cystocoele which is allowing the bladder to move from its normal anatomical position and kink the urethra, causing obstruction to outflow and hence frequency and voiding difficulty. Manual replacement of the cystocoele corrects this and aids micturition.

4. **H – Urinary tract infection (UTI)**
    Sudden onset of frequency, urgency and dysuria in a young, fit woman suggests urinary tract infection as the most likely cause. The fact that she has had a laparoscopy the previous week means she was likely to have been catheterised, further increasing the risk of infection. Interstitial cystitis and detrusor overactivity are possible but the former is rare and the latter does not usually cause dysuria.

5. **E – Genuine stress incontinence (GSI)**
    Genuine stress incontinence is most common in the peri- and post-menopausal period, due to pelvic floor and sphincter deficiencies, exacerbated by the hypo-oestrogenic state. Frequency tends to become a habit in order to try and reduce the number of episodes of incontinence. The main indication for urodynamic investigations is to make a firm diagnosis when there are mixed urinary symptoms and also before any bladder neck surgery. Detrusor pressure is calculated by subtracting the intra-abdominal pressure (measured using a rectal transducer) from the intravesical pressure (measured using a bladder transducer). If the stress incontinence is due to detrusor overactivity there are unprovoked rises in detrusor pressure at the time of stress incontinence – their absence confirms the diagnosis of GSI.

12. DISEASES OF THE LARGE INTESTINE

1. **B – Adenoma**
   Adenomas are benign neoplasms of glandular epithelium. Adenomas of the large intestine can be classified as tubular, villous or tubulovillous. Tubular adenomas are pedunculated and have a red, lobulated surface. Villous adenomas are sessile and have seaweed-like fronds. Adenomas have distinct malignant potential and are thought to be the precursor of adenocarcinomas of the colorectum. This patient's polyp is unlikely to have developed into an adenocarcinoma because it is pedunculated and small.

2. **I – Pseudomembranous colitis**
   Pseudomembranous colitis is caused by the A and B toxins produced by toxigenic strains of *Clostridium difficile*. It usually occurs several days after starting broad-spectrum antibiotic therapy and most commonly affects elderly hospitalised patients. Diarrhoea (rarely with blood) and abdominal cramps are the common symptoms. Sigmoidoscopy might reveal an erythematous, ulcerated mucosa with patchy, white membranes. In a minority of patients, however, only the proximal colon is affected and sigmoidoscopy is therefore normal.

3. **C – Amoebiasis**
   Infection with *Entamoeba histolytica* causes amoebiasis. Several of the diseases on this list can lead to colonic ulceration, but only in amoebiasis are the ulcers typically flask-shaped. The finding of periodic acid–Schiff (PAS-)positive trophozoites with ingested red cells is diagnostic of amoebiasis.

4. **F – Diverticular disease**
   A diverticulum is a blind-ending, mucosal-lined outpouching that communicates with the lumen of the organ in which it arises. The gut is the most common site of origin and, although diverticula can be found anywhere in the gut, 95% are located in the sigmoid colon. Diverticular disease is common in the elderly, the prevalence approaching 50% in the over-60s. Its pathogenesis seems to be related to the low-fibre diet eaten in Western countries, with consequent reduction in stool bulk and raised intraluminal pressure. Thickening of the bowel wall is associated with the formation of diverticula and this can lead to the development of strictures, which can simulate a carcinoma. In this patient, the diverticula have become inflamed (diverticulitis), as indicated by the pyrexia and abdominal tenderness.

5. **J – Ulcerative colitis**
   The main differential diagnosis of bloody diarrhoea in this age group lies between infective colitis and idiopathic inflammatory bowel disease. The fact that repeated stool cultures are negative makes infective colitis less likely. The colonoscopic appearances of diffuse erythema without skip lesions favour ulcerative colitis over Crohn's disease. The biopsy changes (severe chronic inflammation with crypt abscesses and crypt architectural distortion and the lack of granulomas) are typical of ulcerative colitis.

13. THE LARYNX

1. **G – Recurrent laryngeal nerve**
    This nerve provides sensory innervation to the trachea and larynx below the vocal cords and innervates all the muscles of the larynx except the cricothyroid. The superior laryngeal nerve pierces the thyrohyoid membrane and divides into an external laryngeal nerve, which supplies the cricothyroid muscle and an internal laryngeal nerve, which provides sensation to the larynx above the vocal cords.

2. **B – Cricoid cartilage**
    The conus elasticus (cricothyroid membrane) of each side meet and are strengthened in the midline anteriorly by the cricothyroid ligament. The upper free border is the vocal fold.

3. **J – Thyroid cartilage**
    The vocal fold extends from the back of the laryngeal prominence of the thyroid cartilage to the vocal process on the arytenoid cartilage. It is covered with mucous membrane and forms the vocal cord. Action of the cricothyroid muscle alters tension in the cord and the shape of the rima glottidis between the cords is altered by gliding and rotation of the arytenoid cartilages on the cricoid.

4. **A – Arytenoid cartilage**
    The aryepiglottic (quadrangular) membrane passes from the sides of the epiglottis to the anterior border of the arytenoid cartilage. The lower free border is the vestibular fold and a pouch (the laryngeal sinus) bulges laterally between the vestibular and vocal folds.

5. **C – Epiglottis**
    The epiglottis is attached to the thyroid cartilage above the vocal fold and extends upwards behind the tongue, with the piriform fossa of the pharynx recessed on each side. In swallowing, the larynx is raised, bringing the epiglottis over the superior opening.

14. NERVE SUPPLY OF THE MUSCLES OF THE LOWER LIMB

1. **H – Superior gluteal nerve**
   This nerve also supplies the gluteus minimus and tensor fascia lata. The gluteus maximus is supplied by the inferior gluteal nerve.

2. **F – Sciatic nerve**
   The semimembranosus is the most medial of the hamstring group of muscles. The sciatic nerve supplies all of them and also the ischial part of the adductor magnus muscle.

3. **B – Deep peroneal (anterior tibial) nerve**
   This nerve is a branch of the common peroneal nerve and supplies all the muscles of the anterior (dorsiflexor) group in the anterior compartment of the leg, and also the extensor digitorum brevis on the dorsum of the foot.

4. **G – Superficial peroneal (musculocutaneous) nerve**
   This nerve passes around the neck of the fibula and is vulnerable to injury at this site. It also innervates the peroneus brevis muscle.

5. **J – Tibial (posterior tibial) nerve**
   The tibial nerve innervates all the muscles of the calf.

PAPER 6

Paper 6 Questions

1. THEME: ANTIHYPERTENSIVE AGENTS

A   Amlodipine
B   Atenolol
C   Bendroflumethiazide
D   Doxazosin
E   Hydralazine
F   Indapamide
G   Losartan
H   Methyldopa
I   Moxonidine
J   Ramipril

The following patients have all presented with hypertension. Please choose the most appropriate single antihypertensive agent from the above list. Each drug may be used once, more than once or not at all.

1. A 58-year-old man is seen in his GP practice with a BP of 220/100 mmHg. He is a smoker but his total cholesterol is 4.8 mmol/l, his random blood glucose is 4.3 mmol/l, and he has no other cardiovascular risk factors. He also complains of prostatism but on per rectal examination there is a smoothly enlarged prostate and his PSA is 3.2 ng/ml.

2. An obese, 47-year-old woman is seen by her GP for hypertension (BP 170/90 mmHg). Of note, her routine investigations reveal a random blood glucose of 11.3 mmol/l and a total cholesterol of 6.9 mmol/l, and her ECG shows changes consistent with the voltage criteria of left ventricular hypertrophy.

3. A 32-year-old primigravida is seen at 24 weeks' gestation in the Antenatal Clinic complaining of increased lethargy and malaise. Her BP is 160/80 mmHg on two separate occasions. Urinary analysis shows protein +and no other abnormalities. She is started on an antihypertensive and her BP settles.

4. A 62-year-old woman who is a heavy smoker is seen in her GP surgery with episodic chest pain which is short-lived and relieved immediately by rest. A routine serum lipid profile and glucose were normal 3 months earlier. Her BP is elevated at 160/100 mmHg.

5. A 64-year-old man is seen by his GP 6 weeks after being discharged from hospital after an acute myocardial infarction. Since he was discharged he has had a persistent dry and irritating cough. He is on aspirin, metoprolol, lisinopril and GTN spray. The GP stops one of the medications and exchanges it for another agent.

2. THEME: THE MULTIDISCIPLINARY TEAM

A Chiropodist
B Community psychiatric nurse (CPN)
C Dementia support worker
D Dietician
E District nurse
F Occupational therapist
G Orthotist
H Physiotherapist
I Social worker
J Specialist nurse

For each of the following scenarios please list the members of the multidisciplinary team who should be involved in the patient's care. You may use each member once, more than once, in combination or not at all.

1. An independent 54-year-old man is seen in Out-patients with left-sided foot drop which has led to several falls. He improves with a splint and therapy.

2. A 61-year-old woman with long-standing type 2 diabetes mellitus is discharged from hospital on insulin. She has severe visual impairment secondary to her retinopathy, and peripheral sensory neuropathy. She needs assistance with most activities of daily living but is mobile with guidance about the ward.

3. A 79-year-old man with moderate cognitive impairment is seen with his wife. She feels that she can no longer cope with him at home but she is reluctant to have him 'put in a home'. He has no other medical history of note and is only on donepezil. He consistently says that he wants to stay with his wife. They have no services at present.

4. A 21-year-old man is admitted to the Emergency Department with diabetic ketoacidosis, his first presentation of diabetes mellitus. He recovers slowly over 72 hours and is seen by the various members of the multidisciplinary team before discharge home.

5. A 41-year-old schizophrenic man is admitted to the Emergency Department with a respiratory tract infection. His neighbours say that he has been acting strangely for 3 months and that he is not really looking after himself. He improves and the consultant feels that he is ready for discharge but the patient cannot get his shoes on as a result of his onychogryphosis.

3. THEME: JAUNDICE

A   Autoimmune hepatitis
B   Carcinoma of the head of the pancreas
C   Epstein–Barr virus (EBV)
D   Gallstones
E   Haemochromatosis
F   Hepatitis A virus
G   Hepatitis B virus
H   Primary biliary cirrhosis
I   Sclerosing cholangitis
J   Wilson's disease

The following patients have all presented with jaundice. Please choose the most appropriate cause from the above list. Each diagnosis may be used once, more than once or not at all.

1. A 43-year-old man presents to his GP with increasing polydypsia. On examination, he appears to be slightly 'suntanned' despite not having been in the sun for 6 months. He has spider naevi and gynaecomastia and 3-cm hepatomegaly below the right costal margin. His capillary blood glucose is 17.9 mmol/l. Routine investigations reveal: haemoglobin 8.7 g/dl, MCV 101 fl, WCC 3.9 × 10⁹/l, platelets 88 × 10⁹/l; random blood glucose 23.2 mmol/l; total bilirubin 27 μmol/l, AST 65 IU/l, ALT 51 IU/l, alkaline phosphatase 555 IU/l, albumin 31 g/l; ferritin 12770 μg/l.

2. A 38-year-old woman is seen in Medical Out-patients with a 2–month history of weight loss associated with recent onset of jaundice. On examination, she has spider naevi, Dupuytren's contracture and 4-cm hepatomegaly below the right costal margin. The diagnosis is confirmed by the presence of anti-smooth muscle and anti-LKM-1 antibodies. She improves quite rapidly with corticosteroids.

3. A 27-year-old woman with poorly controlled sickle-cell disease is admitted to hospital with severe abdominal pain, pyrexia and vomiting. On examination, she is jaundiced, has generalised abdominal pain with some localised tenderness in the right upper quadrant. Initial investigations reveal: haemoglobin 5.5 g/dl, MCV 87 fl, WCC 23.9 × 10⁹/l, platelets 411 × 10⁹/l; Na⁺ 141 mmol/l, K⁺ 4.7 mmol/l, urea 12.9 mmol/l, creatinine 112 μmol/l; total bilirubin 47 μmol/l, AST 72 IU/l, ALT 66 IU/l, alkaline phosphatase 871 IU/l, albumin 34 g/l.

4. A previously fit and well, 35-year-old man returns from India with a 1-week history of worsening abdominal pains, diarrhoea, vomiting and a fever. Over the last 72 hours he has also become jaundiced. His investigations reveal: total bilirubin 38 μmol/l, AST 332 IU/l, ALT 219 IU/l, alkaline phosphatase 238 IU/l, albumin 32 g/l, and an acute-phase IgM response confirming the presence of an RNA virus.

5. A 27-year-old man with known ulcerative colitis is seen in the
Gastroenterology Clinic for his 6-month check-up. He reports that he has been
well, with no recent acute exacerbations of his colitis. However, in the last few
months he has had occasional upper abdominal pains associated with pruritis
and, more recently, an episode of jaundice. Routine investigations reveal: total
bilirubin 18 μmol/l, AST 22 IU/l, ALT 19 IU/l, alkaline phosphatase 438 IU/l,
albumin 39 g/l. The diagnosis is confirmed on ERCP, which shows 'occasional
beading of the biliary tree'.

4. THEME: DEMENTIA

A   Alzheimer's disease
B   Creutzfeldt–Jakob disease
C   Huntington's disease
D   Hypothyroidism
E   Lewy body disease
F   Neurosyphilis
G   Normal-pressure hydrocephalus
H   Pick's disease
I   Pseudodementia
J   Vascular dementia

The following patients have all presented with dementia. Please choose the most appropriate cause from the above list. Each diagnosis may be used once, more than once or not at all.

1. A 48-year-old man presents to his GP with increasing confusion and memory problems and abnormal movements of his limbs. His wife is very concerned about him as she remembers that his father had a similar problem in his late 40s and died very soon after they were married.

2. A previously fit and well 69-year-old woman presents to her GP with a 6-month history of insidious worsening of her memory. She has until recently been very independent but can now no longer find her way to the local shops. Her mini-mental state examination (MMSE) score is 24/30 but examination and routine investigations, including FBC, U&Es, random blood glucose, LFTs, corrected Ca^{2+}, thyroid functions tests, ESR and radiographs are all within normal limits. Her CT head scan shows cerebral atrophy but nothing else of note. She makes some improvement with donepezil.

3. A 71-year-old woman presents to Medicine for the Elderly Out-patients with a 3–4-month history of confusion, falls and urinary incontinence. Her abridged mental test score (AMTS) is 6/10 and she is noted to have a dyspraxic gait. Her blood tests, including FBC, U&Es, random blood glucose, LFTs, corrected Ca^{2+}, thyroid functions tests, VDRL and ESR are all within normal limits, as is her chest radiograph and ECG. Her CT head scan shows ventricular dilatation disproportionate to her degree of cerebral atrophy.

4. An 84-year-old man is admitted to hospital with acute on chronic confusion. His wife, who has been caring for him at home with no social services, feels that she can no longer cope. He is treated for a urinary tract infection and improves but his AMTS remains at 4–5/10. His CT head scan shows mild to moderate cerebral atrophy but subsequent investigations confirm positive serum and CSF *Treponoma pallidum* haemagglutination assay (TPHA) and fluorescent *Treponema* absorption (FTA) tests.

5. A 62-year-old woman presents to Medicine for the Elderly Out-patients with a 6–8-month history of increasing speech problems. She is noted to be confusing and muddling her words and phrases. Her MMSE is 28/30. Subsequent CT head shows marked atrophy of the temporal regions.

5. THEME: ANTIBIOTICS

A   Benzylpenicillin
B   Cefotaxime
C   Cefuroxime
D   Ciprofloxacin
E   Clarithromycin
F   Doxycycline
G   Flucloxacillin
H   Metronidazole
I   Trimethoprim
J   Vancomycin

The following patients have all presented with sepsis. Please choose the most appropriate antibiotic therapy from the above list. You may use the antibiotics once, more than once, in combination or not at all. (The patients have no known drug allergies.)

1. A 29-year-old man with poorly controlled type 1 diabetes mellitus is admitted to the Emergency Department with a hot, painful, red left calf and pyrexia. On examination, he is well but has a temperature of 39.5 °C and is tachycardic at 120 bpm. He has a marked right lower limb cellulitis that is spreading over the anterolateral aspect of his shin.

2. A 59-year-old man and his wife return from a holiday in St Petersburg with diarrhoea and vomiting. The husband has noted 'sulphur' on his breath and both admit to offensive, watery stools, urgency and frequency.

3. A 19-year-old man presents to the Genitourinary Medicine Clinic with a urethral discharge and dysuria. Gonococcal cultures and microscopy are negative but the diagnosis is confirmed as *Chlamydia trachomatis* after antibody tests are reported as positive.

4. A 78-year-old woman is re-admitted to hospital 1 week after discharge with profuse, offensive, watery diarrhoea. She was previously admitted with pneumonia and had required several courses of antibiotics.

5. A 17-year-old girl is admitted to hospital with a severe headache that has been getting worse over a period of 2 days. She has marked photophobia, neck stiffness and temperature of 39.2 °C but no associated rash. Lumbar puncture confirms Gram-positive intracellular diplococci in the CSF.

6. THEME: AUTOANTIBODIES

A   Anti-ACH receptor
B   Anti-amphiphysin
C   Anti-Hu
D   Anti-Jo-1
E   Anti-MAG
F   Anti-myeloperoxidase (p-ANCA)
G   Anti-proteinase-3 (c-ANCA)
H   Anti-tissue-transglutaminase (anti-tTG)
I   Anti-Ri
J   Anti-Yo

The following patients have all presented with conditions now defined by specific autoantibodies. Please choose the most appropriate autoantibody for each of the patients from the above list. You may each autoantibody once, more than once or not at all.

1. A 59-year-old man presents to Medical Out-patients with increasing pains and weakness in his muscles (especially around his shoulders) associated more recently with a rash around his eyes and lesions over his knuckles. On direct questioning, he also admits to recent significant weight loss and haemoptysis.

2. A 39-year-old woman presents to her GP with increasing shortness of breath, haemoptysis, rhinorrhoea and ankle oedema. She is admitted to hospital, where a working diagnosis of Wegener's granulomatosis is made.

3. A 64-year-old lifelong smoker with carcinoma of the lung presents to the Emergency Department with a 2-week history of increasing falls and dizziness. On examination, as well as the signs related to his lung cancer he has marked bilateral cerebellar signs.

4. A 21-year-old woman presents to her GP with a 3-month history of increasing malaise, 'nasty smelly' motions that are difficult to flush away and weight loss. On examination she looks clinically anaemic and has lost 10 kg since her last visit 6 months ago.

5. A 31-year-old woman presents to her GP with increasing weakness. She tells the GP that she finds it difficult to finish meals and do simple tasks like washing herself as she finds it physically exhausting. Her diagnosis is confirmed by a Tensilon® test and serum autoantibodies.

7. THEME: CONSTIPATION

A   Colonic carcinoma
B   Constipation-predominant irritable bowel syndrome
C   Diabetes mellitus
D   Diverticular disease
E   Hypercalcaemia
F   Hypothyroidism
G   Iatrogenic (drug therapy)
H   Idiopathic megacolon
I   Pelvic-nerve/spinal-cord injury
J   Simple constipation

The following patients have all presented with constipation. Please select the most appropriate diagnosis from the above list. Each diagnosis may be used once, more than once or not at all.

1. A 66-year-old woman is seen in Surgical Out-patients with a long history of alternating constipation and loose stool, associated with left iliac fossa pain. She now complains of having 3 months of constipation. She tells you that she had a barium enema 1 year ago and although she cannot recall the diagnosis she was told to eat a high-fibre diet.

2. A 40-year-old woman with chronic back pain presents in the Emergency Department with a 5-day history of lower abdominal pain and urinary incontinence. She has not opened her bowels for a similar period. On examination, she has a palpable bladder and when she is catheterised 1100 ml of urine is drained. There is poor sphincter tone and absent perianal sensation.

3. A 62-year-old man is referred to a surgical clinic with a 6–week history of constipation. His bowels open once every 2 days, passing small, hard stools after a lot of straining. Previously, he opened his bowels every morning, with soft stool. He has also noticed some vague, cramping, lower abdominal pain. Examination, including proctosigmoidoscopy is normal. Investigations reveal: haemoglobin 9.8 g/dl, MCV 73.3 fl.

4. A 14-year-old boy presents in the Emergency Department with lower abdominal pain. His mother informs you that he has had severe constipation since infancy and encopresis, for which he was regularly admitted for manual evacuation at the children's hospital. On examination, there is a large indentable mass arising from the pelvis.

5. A 66-year-old woman with chronic back pain presents in the Emergency Department with colicky lower abdominal pain. She has not opened her bowels for 4 days. Her problems started after an upper gastrointestinal endoscopy for dyspepsia, when she was diagnosed with gastric erosions. She was discharged on a variety of new medications (which she has not brought with her today).

8. THEME: DISORDERS OF THE FEMALE BREAST

A   Breast abscess
B   Carcinoma of the breast
C   Cystosarcoma phylloides
D   Duct papilloma
E   Fat necrosis
F   Fibroadenoma
G   Fibroadenosis
H   Galactocoele
I   Mammary duct ectasia
J   Mammary fistula

The following women all have conditions of the breast. Please select the most appropriate diagnosis from the above list. Each diagnosis may be used once, more than once or not at all.

1. A 35-year-old woman presents having had several years of cyclical pain in both breasts and a recent finding of feeling a lump in the right breast. On examination, there is diffuse nodularity in both axillary tails, which are slightly tender on palpation. Fine-needle aspiration of a prominent nodule on the right results in aspiration of 5 ml of clear, brownish fluid, with resolution of the lump. Cytology shows cellular debris with no malignant cells.

2. A 52-year-old woman presents with a painless lump in the left breast that she noticed 5 weeks ago. On examination, a hard, irregular 3-cm lump is palpable in the upper outer quadrant. There are no obvious skin changes but the breast appears slightly asymmetric with respect to the right side when the arms are raised above the patient's head.

3. A 28-year-old woman presents 3 weeks after the birth of her first child with pain in the right breast. On examination, she has a large, 6-cm diameter, very tender swelling adjacent and medial to the nipple.

4. A 43-year-old woman presents with a 3-week history of bloodstained nipple discharge. Examination is unremarkable, with no lumps palpable in either breast.

5. An 18-year-old woman presents after noticing a painless lump in her left breast 2 weeks ago. On examination, a discrete, hard, highly mobile 1-cm lump is palpable in the medial breast. There are no skin changes or nipple discharge. Fine-needle aspiration cytology shows benign cells.

9. THEME: UROGENITAL RADIOLOGY – RENAL TRACT ABNORMALITIES

*Using the radiographic images **A–J on pages 351–353**, please match the diagnoses with the correct image. You may use each image once, more than once or not at all.*

1. Horseshoe kidney.   ☐

2. Renal transplant.   ☐

3. Staghorn calculus.   ☐

4. Vesical calculus.   ☐

5. Duplex ureters.   ☐

10. THEME: MUSCULOSKELETAL CAUSES OF BACK PAIN

A   Ankylosing spondylitis
B   Metastatic carcinoma
C   Osteoporosis
D   Prolapsed intervertebral disc
E   Pyogenic spondylitis
F   Scheuermann's disease
G   Spinal stenosis
H   Spinal tuberculosis
I   Spondylolisthesis
J   Spondylosis

The following patients have all presented with back pain of musculoskeletal origin. For each, please select the most appropriate diagnosis from the above list. Each diagnosis may be used once, more than once or not at all.

1. A 45-year-old care worker presents with acute back pain and right-sided buttock pain and sciatica after lifting a patient into bed. On examination, he has reduced right-sided straight-leg raising. Neurological examination is normal.

2. A 70-year-old man presents in the Emergency Department with severe lower thoracic back pain of 3 weeks' duration. He has attended his GP several times and is now on maximal doses of co-proxamol and Voltarol®. The pain, initially only felt on movement, is now constant day and night and he is unable to sleep. Neurological examination is normal.

3. A 13-year-old girl complains of thoracolumbar backache. Her mother has also noted that she has become increasingly round-shouldered. On examination, the patient has a fixed smooth thoracic kyphosis. Neurological examination is normal.

4. A 60-year-old man complains of a 5-year history of backache. The pain, which originally started after an acute injury, now occurs almost daily, especially after lifting or standing/sitting for prolonged periods. It is felt in the lumbar region and buttock. On examination there is mild tenderness over the lumbar spine and reduced movement. Neurological examination is normal.

5. A 60-year-old man complains of a 6-month history of back pain and an aching pain and weakness in both calves when walking. The pain starts with ambulation and resolves only after resting for some time following exercise, especially if leaning forwards. All foot pulses are present. Neurological examination is normal.

11. THEME: BLEEDING PER VAGINA IN PREGNANCY

A   Abruptio placentae
B   Atonic uterus
C   Disseminated intravascular coagulation (DIC)
D   Local cervical pathology, eg cervical ectropion
E   Marginal bleed
F   Obstetric tear
G   Placenta praevia
H   Retained products of conception (RPOC)
I   Uterine rupture
J   Vasa praevia

From the above list please choose the condition most likely to cause the clinical picture described. Each condition may be used once, more than once or not at all.

1. A 30-year-old primiparous woman has just had a spontaneous vaginal delivery. The antenatal period was complicated by idiopathic polyhydramnios. She starts bleeding heavily per vagina immediately after delivery. The third stage of labour appears to be complete.

2. A 30-year-old multiparous woman is in labour. She has had one previous child by emergency lower segment Caesarean section. Her labour is initially uneventful but becomes prolonged, and cervical dilation arrests at 8 cm. She suddenly experiences brisk vaginal bleeding, which is accompanied by a fetal bradycardia. On vaginal examination, the presenting part is no longer palpable in the pelvis.

3. A 30-year-old primiparous woman has recently had a spontaneous vaginal delivery. She had been induced for moderately severe pre-eclampsia. All stages of labour appeared to be complete. Despite all appropriate measures she has a major post-partum haemorrhage. Examination under anaesthesia reveals an empty uterus. Her bleeding per vagina continues and it is noted that she is now also bleeding from her cannulation sites.

4. A 30-year-old primiparous woman is at 32 weeks' gestation. Her antenatal period has been uneventful until she awakes one night with moderate vaginal bleeding associated with abdominal pain and uterine contractions. On arrival at hospital her pulse and blood pressure are normal, as is the fetal heart, but there is uterine tenderness with palpable contractions. Speculum examination is unremarkable except for a small amount of fresh blood in the vagina.

5. A 30-year-old primiparous woman is induced at 42 weeks for postmaturity. After prostaglandin treatment, an artificial rupture of membranes (ARM) is performed at 3-cm cervical dilatation. Her antenatal period has been uneventful up to this point. On examination, there is a longitudinal lie with a cephalic presentation with two-fifths of the head palpable per abdomen. Immediately after the ARM, there is brisk vaginal bleeding, which continues until emergency lower segment Caesarean section is required.

12. THEME: DISEASES OF THE LUNG AND PLEURA

A   Adenocarcinoma of the bronchus
B   Emphysema
C   Lobar pneumonia
D   Malignant mesothelioma
E   *Pneumocystis carinii* pneumonia
F   Pulmonary hypertension
G   Sarcoidosis
H   Small-cell carcinoma of the bronchus
I   Squamous-cell carcinoma of the bronchus
J   Tuberculosis

From the above list, please select the disease that each of the following patients is most likely to have. Each diagnosis may be used once, more than once or not at all.

1. A 70-year-old vagrant man presents with a 2-week history of productive cough, fever and worsening dyspnoea. On examination, he is extremely unwell, with cyanosis, tachycardia and hypotension. His chest radiograph shows complete consolidation of the left lower lobe.

2. A 35-year-old black woman presents with a 6-month history of shortness of breath, night sweats and weight loss. Her chest radiograph shows bilateral hilar lymphadenopathy. Transbronchial biopsy shows non-necrotising epithelioid granulomas within the interstitium. A special stain for acid-fast bacilli is negative.

3. A 62-year-old male smoker presents with haemoptysis for 2 weeks. In addition, he has severe pain in the left shoulder and left arm. His chest radiograph shows a large mass at the apex of the left lung. Sputum cytology reveals malignant keratinised cells.

4. A 35-year-old, HIV-positive man develops shortness of breath accompanied by a dry cough. His chest radiograph shows bilateral reticulonodular shadowing. Sputum culture is negative. Transbronchial biopsy shows alveoli filled with a foamy eosinophilic material and numerous boat-shaped organisms that stain positively with a silver stain.

5. A 65-year-old man, a lifelong heavy smoker, presents with recent onset of haemoptysis and dyspnoea. On examination, he has a moon face and truncal obesity. Biochemical investigations show hypokalaemia. His chest radiograph shows a large mass at the hilum of the right lung.

13. THEME: ANATOMY OF THE ALIMENTARY TRACT

A   Appendix
B   Duodenojejunal flexure
C   First part of duodenum
D   Hepatic flexure of the colon
E   Ileocaecal valve
F   Jejunum
G   Mesentery of the sigmoid colon
H   Pylorus
I   Second part of the duodenum
J   Splenic flexure of the colon

For each of the following descriptions, please choose the most appropriate structure from the above list. Each structure may be used once, more than once or not at all.

1.   Lies to the left of the second lumbar vertebra. ☐

2.   Is in contact with the fundus of the gallbladder. ☐

3.   Has mucosa characterised by prominent villi. ☐

4.   Lies on the lower pole of the right kidney. ☐

5.   Overlies the bifurcation of the left common iliac artery. ☐

14. THEME: OPENINGS IN THE BASE OF THE SKULL

A   Anterior condylar canal
B   Carotid canal
C   Foramen lacerum
D   Foramen ovale
E   Foramen spinosum
F   Inferior orbital fissure
G   Jugular foramen
H   Optic canal
I   Posterior condylar canal
J   Superior orbital fissure

For each of the following descriptions, please choose the most appropriate skull-base opening from the above list. Each opening may be used once, more than once or not at all.

1. Transmits the nerve supplying the stylopharyngeus muscle.

2. Transmits the nerve supplying the intrinsic muscles of the tongue.

3. Transmits the nerve supplying the upper incisor teeth.

4. Transmits the nerve supplying the superior oblique muscle.

5. Transmits the nerve supplying the medial pterygoid muscle.

Paper 6 Answers

1. ANTIHYPERTENSIVE AGENTS

1. **D – Doxazosin**
   This man has essential hypertension and is a smoker but has no other apparent cardiovascular risk factors. He should be encouraged to stop smoking. In view of his prostatic symptoms he required a per rectal examination and a serum PSA to exclude malignant disease. They are within normal limits and so he should be started on doxazosin.

2. **J – Ramipril**
   This obese woman has diabetes mellitus, hypercholesterolaemia and should be started on an ACE inhibitor. She will also need a statin and dietetic advice on a diabetic diet and weight loss.

3. **H – Methyldopa**
   Pregnancy-induced hypertension is an interesting therapeutic dilemma. Most antihypertensive agents are not licensed for use in pregnancy, mainly because of the theoretical risk to the fetus and ethical issues about the introduction of untested agents in this group of patients. Methyldopa, which is an extremely effective agent, has a long history of use in pregnancy, so is still used. It can cause autoimmune haemolytic anaemia and this needs to be screened for with regular monitoring of the full blood count.

4. **B – Atenolol**
   This woman has developed unstable angina associated with hypertension, a common combination. To treat both disorders, a β-blocker or a calcium-channel blocker could be used. However a β-blocker has positive prognostic effects and, if tolerated, is the treatment of choice. She should also have other risk factors addressed and, in particular, needs to be encouraged to stop smoking.

5. **G – Losartan**
   This man has been on an ACE inhibitor, which has caused his dry cough. Although at the present time there are few research data on the effects of angiotensin-II inhibitors in ischaemic heart disease they have been proposed as replacement agents when an ACE inhibitor is not tolerated.

NB: In recent years, target blood pressures have changed quite considerably, particularly in the presence of other cardiovascular risk factors such as ischaemic heart disease, stroke disease, diabetes and smoking. Blood pressure in this situation should be reduced to around 140/80 mmHg. As with the scenarios above, the agents used should be tailored to the patients' needs and co-morbidity but, most importantly, need to be effective at reducing the blood pressure to acceptable targets.

2. THE MULTIDISCIPLINARY TEAM

1. **G, H – Orthotist and physiotherapist**
   This man has a mononeuropathy (due to a common peroneal nerve palsy) causing left-sided foot drop. This might be idiopathic or due to a systemic disorder such as diabetes mellitus or to a systemic vasculitis such as Wegener's granulomatosis. It could also herald a lumbar spine problem. The treatment includes a foot splint to maintain the ankle in 'neutral' and stop the foot 'catching' on the floor and leading to falls. He should also benefit from some physiotherapy.

2. **A, D, E, F, I, J – Dietician, district nurse, chiropodist, occupational therapist, social worker and specialist nurse**
   This patient is chronologically quite young (61 years) but due to her poorly controlled type 2 diabetes mellitus has multiple disabilities and is biologically quite old. She needs a lot of help to maintain her independence at home and pre-discharge planning is vital in such a case. Almost all members of the multidisciplinary team have a role to play in her care and this case shows the importance of good multidisciplinary team work.

3. **A, D, F, H, I – Dietician, chiropodist, occupational therapist, physiotherapist and social worker**
   This situation is not uncommon in medicine for the older patient. Carers often reach a point of 'despair' where they feel isolated and undersupported as well as guilty for thinking about placing their loved one in care. With good community support and services, however, both partners can enjoy a far better quality of life.

4. **E, J – District nurse and specialist nurse**
   This patient needs empathetic education and support to help him come to terms with his new diagnosis. The diabetic specialist nurse is the patient's main contact during his hospital stay and often bears the brunt of feelings of denial or anger. With good education and a strong multidisciplinary team, however, patients can be helped through this difficult period.

5. **B, I – Community psychiatric nurse (CPN) and social worker**
   This man will also need strong multidisciplinary team support both before and after discharge if he is to continue living independently.

3. JAUNDICE

1. **E – Haemochromatosis**
    This man has developed chronic liver disease secondary to haemochromatosis. This can be a primary, idiopathic disorder that is inherited in an autosomal recessive manner. Although it more commonly occurs in association with alcohol excess, alcohol is a contributory rather than a causative agent. Secondary haemochromatosis occurs in patients who ingest excessive amounts of iron or, more commonly, receive multiple blood transfusions. Haemochromatosis leads to excess iron within the body that is deposited in various organs, most commonly the liver (leading to cirrhosis and hepatocellular carcinoma), the pituitary (hypogonadism), the myocardium (cardiomyopathy) and the pancreas (diabetes mellitus). The suntanned appearance is due to melanin (not iron) deposition in the skin.

2. **A – Autoimmune hepatitis**
    This woman has developed autoimmune hepatitis, defined by the presence of the anti-smooth muscle and anti-LKM-1 antibodies (liver/kidney-microsomal antibodies). This is an autoimmune disorder that has two peaks of incidence. There can be a childhood illness that is characterised by the presence of the anti-LKM antibodies and is closely associated with other autoimmune disorders such as vitiligo, thyroid disease and diabetes mellitus. It is characterised clinically by a rapidly progressive liver condition with cirrhosis. The second peak occurs in young adults and this form can be more insidious in its progress. It is associated with the presence of anti-smooth muscle antibodies and, to a lesser extent, antimitochondrial and anti-LKM-1 antibodies. It responds well to corticosteroids but it can relapse rapidly on their withdrawal.

3. **D – Gallstones**
    Sickle-cell disease predisposes patients to the development of gallstones because of the repeated episodes of haemolysis. The cholecystitis has precipitated a sickle crisis in this patient, and she therefore needs intravenous antibiotics (cefuroxime and metronidazole), fluids, blood transfusion and analgesia.

4. **F – Hepatitis A virus**
    This man has developed an acute hepatitis secondary to a hepatitis A virus infection. This RNA virus is endemic in areas of poverty and poor public health and is spread by the faecal–oral route. Hepatitis A virus and hepatitis E virus cause an acute viral illness associated with diarrhoea, fever and jaundice. They do not have a chronic phase and are usually self-limiting but rarely can progress to fulminant liver failure.

5. **I – Sclerosing cholangitis**
    This gentleman has developed sclerosing cholangitis, which is an idiopathic condition leading to acute and chronic inflammation within the biliary tree and subsequent fibrosis and strictures. It can be a primary idiopathic condition but is commonly associated with inflammatory bowel disease (ulcerative colitis more commonly than Crohn's disease) and HIV infection. In about 50% of affected patients, the disease runs a benign course; other patients might require a liver transplant.

4. DEMENTIA

1. **C – Huntington's disease**
    Huntington's chorea is an autosomal dominant disorder characterised by early onset of progressive cognitive impairment and chorea. The gene defect has recently been localised to chromosome 4. The disorder leads to progressive destruction within the caudate nucleus and putamen and leads to loss of GABA (γ-aminobutyric acid) and acetylcholine synthesis in these important extrapyramidal areas. The disorder is incurable and symptomatic treatment, education, genetic screening and support for both patient and family remain the mainstay of therapy.

2. **A – Alzheimer's disease**
    Alzheimer's disease is the commonest of all the dementia syndromes, although more recently, with the advent of newer imaging techniques, such as positron emission tomographic (PET) scanning, subsyndromes of the condition are now being defined. Alzheimer's dementia is characterised by insidious worsening of global cognitive impairment, with early memory impairment, problems with language skills and visuospatial problems, leading to the patient getting lost even in well-known surroundings. Depression and other psychiatric symptoms can be early features, although delusions and hallucinations occur in only 10–15% of cases. The acetylcholinesterase inhibitors are a relatively new group of medications that are now being used for these patients, particularly early on in the condition, although research has suggested that they might also have a role in the more severely cognitively impaired, as well as in Lewy-body dementia.

3. **G – Normal-pressure hydrocephalus**
    This patient has presented with the classic triad of normal-pressure hydrocephalus, namely cognitive impairment, gait dyspraxia and urinary incontinence. The label 'normal pressure' is a misnomer as the CSF pressure varies in peaks and troughs, which can be demonstrated on the insertion of an intraventricular manometer. This condition is treated by insertion of a ventriculoperitoneal shunt.

4. **F – Neurosyphilis**
    Neurosyphilis is a relatively uncommon cause of dementia in the UK but syphilis serology tests are still often included in dementia screens. The VDRL (Venereal Disease Research Laboratory) test can give a false-positive result in the elderly due to old age or coexisting chronic inflammatory conditions or in the Afro-Caribbean population due to previous yaws or pinta infection. If the VDRL is positive, the more specific *Treponema pallidum* haemagglutination assay (TPHA) and fluorescent *Treponema* absorption (FTA) tests should be done to exclude or refute the diagnosis of syphilis. If they are subsequently found to be positive, a lumbar puncture should be performed to confirm the presence of a positive CSF VDRL, which if significantly positive confirms active neurosyphilis. Patients with confirmed neurosyphilis should be treated with an appropriate course of penicillin. In late presentations of the condition (which is the most common situation in the older population) the treatment is unlikely to reverse the condition but will stop its progression.

5. **H – Pick's disease**
    This woman presents with typical features of Pick's disease, or lobar dementia. This form of dementia typically presents with relatively well-preserved cognition in the early stages of the disease but either focal frontal or temporal signs due to focal atrophy of these lobes. Patients with frontal pathology present with personality changes, disinhibition, inertia and lack of planning and self-regard. Temporal features principally focus around speech and language difficulties, including word-finding and reduced-vocabulary problems. As the disease progresses, patients develop a progressive aphasia and can develop an 'associative agnosia', an inability to recognise and name everyday objects, items and animals.

5. ANTIBIOTICS

1. **A, G – Benzylpenicillin and flucloxacillin**
    This patient has developed an acute cellulitis of the shin. The most likely causative organisms are streptococcal or staphylococcal species and the most appropriate first-line therapy includes benzylpenicillin and flucloxacillin. Patients with penicillin allergy could be given a cephalosporin or a macrolide.

2. **H – Metronidazole**
    This couple have developed giardiasis, which is treated with high-dose metronidazole (2 g/day for 3 days).

3. **E, F – Clarithromycin and doxycycline**
    This young man has developed a *Chlamydia* urethritis, which should be treated with tetracycline and then a macrolide if symptoms recur. As with all sexually transmissible disease, he should be counselled with regard to the use of condoms and recent sexual contacts need to be traced.

4. **H or J – Metronidazole or vancomycin**
    This older woman has developed *Clostridium difficile* diarrhoea, caused by the multiple courses of antibiotics she was treated with during her original admission with a chest infection. Patients require oral metronidazole or vancomycin because studies have shown that the intraluminal concentration of the drug is the important factor in the treatment and administering the drugs by intravenous or rectal routes are not as effective. Both metronidazole and vancomycin are poorly absorbed in the gastrointestinal tract and are therefore the drugs of choice.

5. **A or B – Benzylpenicillin or cefotaxime**
    This young woman has developed bacterial meningitis, which, according to the Gram stain, is due to a streptococcal infection. The most appropriate empirical antibiotic in this case would be cefotaxime as it has better CSF penetration than cefuroxime but benzylpenicillin could be used once the Gram stain result is known.

6. AUTOANTIBODIES

Like tumour markers, 'specific' antibody markers of autoimmune disease have become increasingly prevalent in clinical practice over the last decade. While their usefulness and specificity in the diagnosis and management of these complex disorders is still being explored, a close eye must be kept on this ever-expanding field. In order to illustrate the complexity and growth of this field, we have included examples of several newer antibodies which represent areas where the antibodies are being commonly employed.

1. **D – Anti-Jo-1**
   This patient has presented with features of dermatomyositis – proximal muscle weakness, a pathognomonic heliotrope rash around the eyes, and lesions over the knuckles (known as 'Gottron's papules' and named after Heinrich Adolf Gottron, 1890–1974, a German dermatologist). There are also features suggestive of a bronchogenic carcinoma (there is a well-recognised association of dermatomyositis with malignancy in middle-aged and older patients). Dermatomyositis has several associated autoantibodies, many of which appear with the closely related polymyositis. These antibodies are known as 'myositis-specific antibodies' (MSA) and include anti-Mi-2 and anti-Jo-1. In addition, these patients often have non-specifically positive antinuclear antibody titres.

2. **G – Anti-proteinase-3 (c-ANCA)**
   Wegener's granulomatosis (named after Friedrich Wegener, 1907–1990, a German pathologist and high-ranking Nazi) is a necrotising vasculitis of the small and medium-sized blood vessels, classically affecting the upper and lower respiratory tracts and the kidneys. Like many of these complex disorders, several non-specific inflammatory markers can be present, but the presence of cytoplasmic antineutrophil cytoplasmic antibody (c-ANCA), now called 'anti-proteinase-3' is specifically linked to the diagnosis and progression of this disease.

3. **C, I – Anti-Hu and anti-Ri**
   Perhaps the most common use of the autoantibodies in recent years has been in the diagnosis and characterisation of the paraneoplastic syndromes. This group of disorders is linked to many of the common malignancies, including lung, breast and ovarian tumours: the paraneoplastic cerebellar syndrome is associated with anti-Hu antibodies (small-cell carcinoma of the lung); anti-Yo antibodies are associated with breast and ovarian carcinoma; and anti-Ri antibodies are associated with all three malignancies. Other paraneoplastic syndromes and their antibodies include paraneoplastic sensory neuropathy (anti-amphiphysin – breast and small-cell carcinoma of the lung; anti-myelin-associated glycoprotein (anti-MAG) – macroglobulinaemias; and presynaptic anti-acetylcholine receptor antibodies (anti-ACHR) – Lambert–Eaton syndrome).

4. **H – Anti-tissue-transglutaminase (anti-tTG)**
   This patent has features of coeliac disease, as suggested by the history of steatorrhoea, weight loss and anaemia. Several sets of autoantibodies have been associated with this condition over the past 20 years but the most specific to date are anti-endomysial antibodies and the more recently characterised anti-tissue transglutaminase antibodies (anti-tTG). More recently still, anti-tTG antibodies have been found in patients with inflammatory bowel disease and it is recommended that anti-endomysial antibodies are requested in unison with anti-tTG titres.

5. **A – Anti-ACH receptor**
    This patient has features suggestive of myasthenia gravis. Myasthenia gravis is characterised by fatiguability, which clinically is manifest by an inability to complete everyday tasks due to increasing weakness as the task progresses. The disorder is characterised by the presence of post-synaptic antibodies directed against the alpha subunit of the acetylcholine receptor (the receptor comprises five subunits, two alpha, and single beta, gamma and delta units). The Tensilon® test is used as a diagnostic test. The patient is given an intravenous dose of edrophonium (Tensilon®), which is an acetylcholinesterase inhibitor. The patient is asked to perform a given task and this is timed pre- and post-Tensilon®, and objective measurements of muscle strength are also made. A patient with the disorder is expected to improve post-Tensilon®. The test is not specific or sensitive enough in isolation and should be used in conjunction with testing for immune markers. The edrophonium has cholinergic side-effects, including bradycardia and excess salivation, bowel movement and tear production.

7. CONSTIPATION

1. **D – Diverticular disease**
   The history could indicate either this diagnosis or one of constipation-predominant irritable bowel disease. The fact that she has had no intervention after her barium enema excludes a carcinoma and, indeed, a high-fibre diet is generally recommended for patients with diverticular disease.

2. **I – Pelvic-nerve/spinal-cord injury**
   This patient has signs of cauda equina compression. This is a neurosurgical emergency that is usually caused by a central disc protrusion compressing the lumbosacral nerve roots below the level of the cona medullaris at L1. The clinical signs are those of lower motor neurone lesions of the affected levels and can include bilateral limb signs if higher up, or only bowel and bladder dysfunction if lower segments are involved. Such debilitating disturbances can become permanent without prompt intervention.

3. **A – Colonic carcinoma**
   A change in bowel habit such as that presented should always prompt a search for a carcinoma. In this case there is a microcytic anaemia, which strongly suggests the diagnosis. In reality, a change in bowel habit to diarrhoea with rectal bleeding is more strongly suggestive than a change to constipation. The patient should undergo urgent colonoscopy (or barium enema if this is not available).

4. **H – Idiopathic megacolon**
   This is a characteristic history of this ill-understood and fairly uncommon disorder in which there is a grossly distended rectum/colon with associated severe constipation and overflow (especially evident as encopresis or incontinence at night). The diagnosis can be made on barium enema. Treatment is behavioural, psychological, medical (laxatives) and surgical (regular disimpaction, sometimes bowel resection). Megacolon can also occur in children as a result of Hirschsprung's disease and in a variety of other rare syndromes. It can arise in adulthood secondary to a variety of causes or idiopathically (ie cause unknown).

5. **G – Iatrogenic (drug therapy)**
   A variety of drugs can cause constipation and should always be considered in elderly people who are on several drugs. In this case, the likely offender is an opioid-containing analgesic which has been prescribed in place of an NSAID after her diagnosis of gastric erosions.

8. DISORDERS OF THE FEMALE BREAST

1. **G – Fibroadenosis (fibrocystic disease)**
   This is a diffuse and painful benign condition of the breast that occurs in women aged 25–45. The condition is characterised by exacerbations and remissions that are usually cyclical with the menses. The disorder probably results from abnormal expression of physiological proliferative and involutionary changes. There are four main pathological processes: adenosis, epitheliosis, fibrosis and cyst formation. The diagnosis is made on the basis of the history and examination and mammography/ultrasound, with or without cyst aspiration and cytology.

2. **B – Carcinoma of the breast**
   The age of the patient, the history and the findings on examination should point strongly to this diagnosis. Other symptoms can include nipple bleeding, deep or superficial tethering of the lump, skin changes (eg *peau d'orange* or ulceration), and a finding of enlarged axillary nodes or evidence of systemic spread to bone or liver. The diagnosis can usually be confirmed by mammography.

3. **A – Breast abscess**
   This is a disorder of the puerperium in which a cracked nipple leads to ascending infection with the pyogenic organism, *Staphylococcus aureus*. The patient should stop feeding with the affected breast and antibiotics should be prescribed (flucloxacillin). Drainage or aspiration is usually required. If the lump had no features of inflammation, a galactocoele would have been the most likely diagnosis.

4. **D – Duct papilloma**
   The most likely diagnosis here is duct papilloma. This should be suspected from the age of the patient (younger than carcinoma) and the solitary symptom of recurrent bloodstained nipple discharge without any discrete lump. A true papilloma is usually single and occurs in a major duct in the subareolar area. The tumour consists of hyperplastic columnar epithelium with a rich blood supply (hence the presentation). They are entirely benign.

5. **F – Fibroadenoma**
   This is evidenced by the very young age of the patient and the characteristic features on examination of a hard, discrete, highly mobile lump (they are sometimes referred to as a 'breast mouse' on account of the mobility). Although these tumours are completely benign, most women are anxious to have them surgically removed.

9. UROGENITAL RADIOLOGY – RENAL TRACT ABNORMALITIES

1. **(P5–P7) C – Horseshoe kidney**
   This IVU shows a horseshoe kidney. This congenital abnormality arises as a result of failure of the two embryonic kidneys to separate as they ascend from their pelvic origin to their final thoracolumbar position. Horseshoe kidneys are one of the commonest congenital defects of the renal tract, occurring in about 1 in 400 people worldwide. They often remain asymptomatic but complications include obstruction at the pelvi-ureteric junction, increased incidence of urinary tract infection and renal stones. There is also some evidence of an increased incidence of renal carcinoma.

2. **(P5–P7) B – Pelvic renal transplant**
   This IVU demonstrates contrast in the bladder but apparently no functioning kidneys. If you look carefully you can see that there is a functioning right-sided pelvic kidney – this is a transplanted kidney. Clinically, you can usually feel this kidney as a pelvic mass.

3. **(P5–P7) J – Right staghorn calculus**
   This plain radiograph shows large, right-sided renal stone, commonly known as a 'staghorn' calculus. These are often associated with recurrent infections with *Proteus* and other urease-producing organisms. Hydrolysis of urea leads to the production of ammonium, causing the production of alkaline urine and increased phosphate levels. This environment results in the formation of the stones, which in turn are thought to protect the organisms against the effects of antimicrobials.

4. **(P5–P7) D – Vesical calculus**
   This plain radiograph of the pelvis shows two large vesical (ie bladder) calculi. Adult bladder calculi are commonly associated with bladder outflow-tract obstruction and secondary urinary stasis, but can also arise as a result of chronic infection, inflammation (eg post-irradiation) or the presence of foreign bodies within the bladder. They are relatively uncommon in the Western world and are more commonly seen in the developing countries of South-East Asia, the Middle East and North Africa, where they are a disease principally of young boys.

5. **(P5–P7) G – Duplex kidneys**
   This IVU shows duplication of both kidneys and ureters, known as a 'duplex system'. This congenital duplication can lead to recurrent infections, reflux and pelvicalyceal obstruction. It can be asymptomatic but often presents in childhood with recurrent urinary tract infections. It is more common in girls than in boys and surgical correction might be required if the condition is associated with complications.

IMAGES: pages 351–353

10. MUSCULOSKELETAL CAUSES OF BACK PAIN

1. **D – Prolapsed intervertebral disc**
    This is a fairly characteristic description of an acute disc injury, although this can also occur with trivial injuries, even with coughing or sneezing. Neurological signs are present in some cases when the nerve root is compressed by the herniating disc but often there is only nerve root irritation with pain in the affected dermatome (as in this case). This is usually sciatic because L4/5 and L5/S1 are the most common levels of injury. Most herniations are posterolateral and therefore lead to unilateral symptoms. A posterior (central) disc herniation can, however, lead to the surgical emergency of cauda equina compression.

2. **B – Metastatic carcinoma**
    The history of relentlessly progressive, severe and nocturnal pain, especially in this age group, should prompt a search for cancer as a cause. Common primary sites are breast, lung, prostate, kidney, thyroid and lymphoma. Primary tumours of bone, especially myeloma, should also be considered.

3. **F – Scheuermann's disease**
    This condition, also known as adolescent kyphosis, is twice as common in girls as boys and presents as described. The condition is thought to arise from damage to the vertebral growth plates in children who outgrow their bone strength during the pubertal growth spurt. The condition can usually be confirmed radiographically and is usually treated conservatively (physiotherapy).

4. **J – Spondylosis**
    This is the most common cause of back pain and probably the most common cause of lost hours at work in the Western world. The site is usually lumbar and the condition can probably be considered to be synonymous with osteoarthritis of the spine. The accepted pathogenetic sequence is initial degenerative disc disease, leading to loss of disc height with subsequent lumbar instability and secondary osteoarthritis in the posterior facet joints. Treatment of this chronic condition is largely supportive.

5. **G – Spinal stenosis**
    The description given is characteristic of this syndrome, which is caused by narrowing of the spinal canal and subsequent compression of canal contents. Disc degeneration, spondylosis and spondylolisthesis are the main aetiological factors. The syndrome must be distinguished from other causes of limb pain on exercise, especially vascular claudication and osteoarthritis of the hip or knees.

11. BLEEDING PER VAGINA IN PREGNANCY

1. **B – Atonic uterus**
    The only common causes of primary post-partum haemorrhage (blood loss >500 ml in the first 24 hours) are atonic uterus, retained products of conception and obstetric tears. By far the most common of these is atonic uterus in the absence of any risk factors. This woman has had idiopathic polyhydramnios and so atonic uterus is even more likely, as overdistension of the uterine wall leads to ineffective myometrial contraction after delivery of the placenta.

2. **I – Uterine rupture**
    Intrapartum bleeding is only likely to be due to placental abruption, uterine rupture or undiagnosed placenta praevia. Her major risk factor is a previous lower segment Caesarean section and with a prolonged, obstructed labour she is at risk of uterine rupture. Uterine rupture only tends to occur with previous lower segment Caesarean section or uterine trauma (eg perforation) or with the use of oxytocin. Uterine rupture, abruption and placenta praevia can be associated with vaginal bleeding and fetal bradycardia if serious enough but uterine rupture is the only condition in which the presenting part can move out of the pelvis as it disappears through the scar rupture into the peritoneal cavity.

3. **C – Disseminated intravascular coagulation (DIC)**
    The common causes of primary post-partum haemorrhage are atonic uterus, retained products of conception and obstetric tears. The 'complete' third stage does not exclude retained products of conception but the empty uterus at her examination under anaesthesia does. Her major risk factor is moderately severe pre-eclampsia, which is associated with disseminated intravascular coagulation in itself. The original bleeding is most likely to be associated with atonic uterus but the prolonged, major post-partum haemorrhage leads to the consumption of clotting factors and platelets. Spontaneous bleeding from puncture sites is a classic feature of coagulopathy.

4. **A – Abruptio placentae**
    Antepartum haemorrhage can be due to placenta praevia, abruptio placentae, marginal bleed or local cervical pathology (eg cervical polyp/erosion/carcinoma). Local cervical pathology classically causes post-coital bleeding and is usually easily visible on speculum examination, which was not the case here. Abdominal pain and uterine contractions are most likely to be due to myometrial irritation from retroplacental bleeding in association with abruptio placentae, sometimes sufficient to trigger premature labour. Most abruptions are not major and do not lead to maternal or fetal compromise but they can both extend and recur. Antepartum haemorrhage with placenta praevia or marginal bleeds is usually painless.

5. **J – Vasa praevia**
    Antepartum haemorrhage immediately after artificial rupture of the membranes is highly suggestive of either placenta praevia or vasa praevia. It could be due to a coincidental abruption but this is unlikely with the timing and is more common with the sudden decompression of polyhydramnios. Given the engaged presenting part (only two-fifths palpable), a major placenta praevia is highly unlikely, as it would obstruct the pelvis. Though a minor degree of placenta praevia is possible, this is a classic story for rupture of an aberrant placental vessel that happens to traverse the cervical os (vasa praevia).

12. DISEASES OF THE LUNG AND PLEURA

1. **C – Lobar pneumonia**
    Pneumonia is defined as inflammation of the lung parenchyma and is usually caused by bacterial infection. It presents as an acute illness characterised by cough, purulent sputum, pleuritic chest pain and fever. Bacterial pneumonia can present as one of two anatomical and radiographic patterns known as 'bronchopneumonia' and 'lobar pneumonia'. In bronchopneumonia there is patchy distribution of the inflammation, typically with involvement of more than one lobe. In contrast, lobar pneumonia involves an entire lobe, and there are physical signs and radiological changes indicating consolidation of that lobe. More than 90% of lobar pneumonias are caused by *Streptococcus pneumoniae*. Patients at increased risk of developing lobar pneumonia include the elderly and those with immunosuppression, debilitation, malnutrition or chronic disease.

2. **G – Sarcoidosis**
    Sarcoidosis is a multisystem disease of unknown aetiology that is characterised by non-necrotising granulomas in many organs. It usually affects young adults and is more common in black people. The most common presentation is with respiratory symptoms such as dyspnoea or with abnormalities on chest radiography. Bilateral hilar lymphadenopathy is a characteristic feature and is found in 75–90% of patients. Other organs commonly affected include the eye and the skin. Transbronchial biopsy is the most useful investigation, showing granulomas in 90% of patients with pulmonary sarcoidosis, even if there is no radiological evidence of lung involvement. The main differential diagnosis from the other diseases listed is tuberculosis. However, the lack of caseation within the granulomas, together with the absence of stainable acid-fast bacilli, mean that sarcoidosis is much more likely.

3. **I – Squamous-cell carcinoma of the bronchus**
    A heavy smoker who presents with haemoptysis and dyspnoea is likely to have carcinoma of the bronchus unless proved otherwise. This patient also has symptoms that indicate involvement of the lower part of the brachial plexus, namely pain in the shoulder that radiates down the arm. This occurs with a tumour at the apex of the lung that erodes the ribs and the first thoracic nerve root and is known as a 'Pancoast tumour'. Highly keratinised cells in sputum are indicative of atypical squamous cells (it is squamous cells that normally produce keratin), so the most likely diagnosis in this case is squamous-cell carcinoma of the bronchus.

4. **E – *Pneumocystis carinii* pneumonia**
    Pneumocystis carinii is a ubiquitous organism that does not cause disease in normal individuals but causes a severe pneumonia in immunosuppressed patients, including those with HIV. The organism cannot be grown in culture, so diagnosis requires cytological or histological identification. Useful cytological preparations include bronchial washings or lavage. Transbronchial biopsy shows foamy eosinophilic material in the alveolar spaces. On both cytology and histology, the organism is seen as a boat-shaped or cup-shaped structure on silver staining. *P. carinii* pneumonia is one of the AIDS-defining diagnoses.

5. **H – Small-cell carcinoma of the bronchus**

    As mentioned above, haemoptysis in a smoker is a sinister symptom and should be considered as indicative of bronchial carcinoma unless proved otherwise. The fact that this patient has a moon face, truncal obesity and hypokalaemia is strongly suggestive of Cushing's syndrome. Patients with carcinoma of the bronchus quite often present with paraneoplastic endocrinopathies. Cushing's syndrome, in which there is ectopic production of ACTH by the tumour cells, is one example. The type of bronchial carcinoma most likely to cause paraneoplastic Cushing's syndrome is small-cell carcinoma because this is derived from neuroendocrine cells.

13. ANATOMY OF THE ALIMENTARY TRACT

1. **B – Duodenojejunal flexure**
    The root of the small-intestinal mesentery passes from the flexure obliquely downwards to the right sacroiliac joint, crossing the left psoas muscle, the aorta, the inferior vena cava, the right gonadal vessels, the right psoas and the right ureter, to reach the ileocaecal junction.

2. **C – First part of the duodenum**
    The pylorus lies to the right of the first lumbar vertebra. The first part of the duodenum is short and passes upwards and to the right before descending, the second part lying anterior to the hilum of the right kidney.

3. **F – Jejunum**
    The jejunum has prominent villi for absorption, in contrast to the duodenum and colon where these are absent. The duodenum is characterised by Brunner's glands, which are mucous glands with coiled pits that extend into the submucosa.

4. **D – Hepatic flexure of the colon**
    The ascending colon is largely retroperitoneal, the flexure turns medially to become the transverse colon. The colon, its mesentery and the greater omentum overlie the small gut.

5. **G – Mesentery of the sigmoid colon**
    The sigmoid colon is attached by an inverted V-shaped mesentery to the pelvic wall. The apex of the V overlies the left ureter anterior to the bifurcation of the left common iliac artery and the left sacroiliac joint.

14. OPENINGS IN THE BASE OF THE SKULL

1. **G – Jugular foramen**
    The stylopharyngeus is the only muscle supplied by the glossopharyngeal nerve. This nerve and the vagus and accessory nerves, together with the internal jugular vein and the inferior petrosal sinus, pass through the jugular foramen.

2. **A – Anterior condylar canal**
    All the intrinsic and extrinsic muscles of the tongue except the palatoglossus are supplied by the twelfth cranial nerve. This nerve also carries fibres from the ventral ramus of the first cervical nerve that supply the geniohyoid and thyrohyoid muscles. The twelfth nerve passes through the anterior condylar canal; the posterior condylar canal transmits an emissary vein.

3. **F – Inferior orbital fissure**
    The fissure transmits the infraorbital nerve, this being the continuation of the maxillary nerve out of the orbit. It supplies the lower eyelid and conjunctiva, the side of the nose and the upper lip, and through its anterior superior alveolar branch, the canine and incisor teeth, the lower lateral wall of the nose and the maxillary air sinus.

4. **J – Superior orbital fissure**
    The superior oblique muscle is supplied by the abducent nerve. The fissure is divided by the common tendinous attachment of the extraocular muscles into a narrow lateral part, transmitting the lacrimal, frontal and trochlear nerves, and a larger medial part transmitting the superior division of the oculomotor, the nasociliary, the inferior division of the oculomotor and the abducent nerves, from lateral to medial. The optic nerve and the ophthalmic artery pass into the orbit through the optic canal.

5. **D – Foramen ovale**
    The medial pterygoid muscle is supplied by the mandibular division of the trigeminal nerve; this supplies the muscles of mastication, and also the tensor tympani and tensor veli palatini. The foramen spinosum, situated just posterior and lateral to the foramen ovale, transmits the middle meningeal vessels.

PAPER 7

Paper 7 Questions

1. THEME: SECONDARY HYPERTENSION

A Acromegaly
B Chronic reflux nephropathy
C Coarctation of the aorta
D Conn's syndrome
E Cushing's syndrome
F Diabetic nephropathy
G Phaeochromocytoma
H Polycystic kidney disease
I Raised intracranial pressure
J Renal artery stenosis

The following patients have all presented with secondary hypertension. Please choose the most appropriate cause from the above list. Each cause may be used once, more than once or not at all.

1. A 29-year-old woman attends her GP with headaches and dizziness. Her BP is measured at 230/110 mmHg on three separate occasions despite treatment and she is referred to the hospital. Routine investigations reveal: Na^+ 131 mmol/l, K^+ 2.4 mmol/l, urea 3.9 mmol/l, creatinine 87 μmol/l. Further investigations reveal reduced plasma renin with a markedly raised aldosterone, despite correction of the hypokalaemia with spironolactone.

2. A 34-year-old man is seen in Medical Out-patients with visual 'blurring' and a BP of 170/100 mmHg. He is noted to have frontal bossing and bitemporal hemianopia and his capillary blood glucose is 13.7 mmol/l.

3. A 24-year-old woman is seen by her GP with vague abdominal pains and headaches. On examination, she is plethoric, her BP is 185/110 mmHg and abdominal examination reveals hepatosplenomegaly. Blood tests reveal: haemoglobin 17.9 g/dl, haematocrit 56.3, WCC 11.1 × 10^9/l, platelets 499 × 10^9/l; Na^+ 131 mmol/l, K^+ 5.8 mmol/l, urea 21.9 mmol/l, creatinine 419 μmol/l.

4. A 61-year-old man with known ischaemic heart disease and peripheral vascular disease is started on an ACE inhibitor by his GP for hypertension. Three weeks later he is admitted with increasing confusion and vomiting. Investigations reveal: haemoglobin 14.9 g/dl, MCV 88 fl, WCC 13.6 × 10^9/l, platelets 317 × 10^9/l; Na^+ 131 mmol/l, K^+ 7.3 mmol/l, urea 37.8 mmol/l, creatinine 858 μmol/l.

5. A 37-year-old woman is admitted to hospital with an episode of sweats, palpitations and headache, associated with a BP of 240/130 mmHg. Her initial blood tests, including FBC, U&Es and cardiac enzymes are all normal, but her BP is poorly controlled despite treatment with several agents. The diagnosis is later confirmed by raised urinary VMA (vanillyl mandelic acid) levels and adrenal venous sampling, which shows raised serum catecholamines from left and right adrenal veins.

2. THEME: AUTOSOMAL DOMINANT DISORDERS

A Achondroplasia
B Dystrophia myotonica
C Familial hypercholesterolaemia
D Gilbert's syndrome
E Hereditary spherocytosis
F Huntington's disease
G Marfan's syndrome
H Neurofibromatosis
I Osteogenesis imperfecta
J Romano–Ward syndrome

The following patients have all presented with autosomal dominant disorders. Please choose the most appropriate disorder from the above list. Each option may be used once, more than once or not at all.

1. A 31-year-old man is seen in the Neurology Out-patient Department with increasing weakness in all four limbs. On examination, he has bilateral ptosis with weakness and wasting of the facial muscles and a 'prolonged' handshake.

2. A 24-year-old woman is admitted to the Emergency Department with a 6-hour history of severe central chest pain. The ECG confirms an anterolateral myocardial infarct. Of note, her father and brothers have had ischaemic heart disease since their early 20s.

3. A 39-year-old woman is seen in Medical Out-patients with increasingly troublesome skin eruptions. On examination, she has several café-au-lait spots and multiple skin lesions. Of note, her grandfather had a similar condition and became wheelchair-bound due to a spinal tumour.

4. A 41-year-old man is admitted to the Emergency Department with collapse secondary to *torsade de pointes*, which spontaneously reverts. His repeat ECG shows a prolonged QTc interval. He is on no medications and subsequent serum Ca^+, Mg^+ and K^+ are all normal.

5. A 28-year-old woman is admitted to hospital with a left lower lobe pneumonia and Gram-positive diplococci are found in the sputum. Routine investigations show: haemoglobin 13.7 g/dl, MCV 87.3 fl, WCC 19.9×10^9/l with a neutrophilia, platelets 344×10^9/l; Na^+ 137 mmol/l, K^+ 4.9 mmol/l, urea 4.3 mmol/l, creatinine 97 μmol/l; total bilirubin 42 μmol/l, AST 21 IU/l, alkaline phosphatase 112 IU/l, albumin 34 g/l.

3. THEME: INFECTIVE DIARRHOEA

A Amoebiasis
B *Bacillus cereus*
C *Campylobacter jejuni*
D *Clostridium difficile*
E *Cryptosporidium*
F *Escherichia coli*
G *Gardia lamblia*
H *Salmonella enteritidis*
I *Shigella flexneri*
J *Vibrio cholerae*

The following patients have all presented with infective diarrhoea. Please choose the most appropriate cause from the above list. Each cause may be used once, more than once or not at all.

1. A 9-year-old girl is seen in the Emergency Department having recently returned home from a holiday in the Punjab. She has diarrhoea associated with blood and mucus and is opening her bowels 3–4× per hour.

2. A 17-year-old boy is seen at home by his GP with a 24-hour history of severe cramping abdominal pains associated with diarrhoea and fever after eating some poorly cooked chicken at a barbeque. He is admitted to hospital, where the diagnosis is confirmed on stool microscopy which shows motile curved Gram-negative rods.

3. A 35-year-old woman is seen by her GP with a 12-hour history of profuse diarrhoea and vomiting after eating lukewarm rice and vegetables from a Chinese takeaway. She improves after 24 hours. Subsequent stool cultures reveal a Gram-positive but aerobic bacterium in 'curled hair' colonies.

4. An 84-year-old man is re-admitted to hospital 2 weeks after a prolonged hospital stay with recurrent chest infections. He has offensive, profuse diarrhoea with abdominal pain. He is treated empirically with oral vancomycin and improves. The diagnosis is later confirmed by a positive toxin test in the stool.

5. A 78-year-old woman is admitted to hospital with severe vomiting and diarrhoea. Routine investigations confirm that she has disseminated intravascular coagulation and acute renal failure. She sadly dies 2–3 days later despite treatment with intravenous antibiotics. Several other people from her nursing home are admitted with a similar clinical picture. The outbreak is traced to some contaminated beef. The organism is seen to produce *Shiga*-like toxin 1.

4. THEME: PERIPHERAL SENSORY NEUROPATHY

A   Alcohol excess
B   Amiodarone
C   Amyloidosis
D   Demyelination
E   Diabetes mellitus
F   Hypothyroidism
G   Isoniazid
H   Paraneoplastic
I   Uraemia
J   Vitamin B$_{12}$ deficiency

The following patients have all presented with symptoms of a peripheral sensory neuropathy. Please choose the most appropriate cause from the above list. Each cause may be used once, more than once or not at all.

1. A 62-year-old man with known mitral valve disease is admitted to hospital with severe sunburn. On examination, he is noted to have 'little lesions across his cornea' but is otherwise well. He tells the ward doctor that he has been experiencing pins and needles in his hands and feet for some time and closer examination confirms a loss of joint-position sense, vibration and light touch in his hands and feet.

2. A 24-year-old man is seen in Medical Out-patients with paraesthesiae and numbness in his feet. He has been unable to drive for the last few weeks as he cannot feel the pedals in the car and he has been having episodes of blurred vision. The diagnosis is confirmed by an MRI scan of his cervical cord and brain and delayed visual-evoked responses.

3. A 79-year-old woman presents to her GP with worsening numbness in her hands and , associated with swelling of her ankles. Subsequent investigations confirm a nephrotic syndrome and the underlying diagnosis is confirmed when the renal biopsy appears apple-green under polarised light when stained with Congo red.

4. A 37-year-old woman with vitiligo presents to her GP with weight gain, increasing lethargy and malaise, associated with tingling in her hands. Routine investigations reveal: haemoglobin 11.2 g/dl, MCV 99 fl, WCC 7.8 × 10^9/l, platelets 303 × 10^9/l; Na$^+$ 127 mmol/l, K$^+$ 4.4 mmol/l, urea 4.7 mmol/l, creatinine 87 μmol/l.

5. A 35-year-old vegan woman presents to her GP with increasing lethargy, malaise and numbness in her feet. Routine investigations show: haemoglobin 4.1 g/dl, MCV 122 fl, WCC 2.1 × 10^9/l, platelets 59 × 10^9/l; Na$^+$ 135 mmol/l, K$^+$ 4.8 mmol/l, urea 3.9 mmol/l, creatinine 79 μmol/l.

5. THEME: PYREXIA OF UNKNOWN ORIGIN (PUO)

A   Brucellosis
B   Cytomegalovirus
C   Epstein–Barr virus
D   Histoplasmosis
E   Hodgkin's lymphoma
F   Infective endocarditis
G   Lyme disease
H   Renal-cell carcinoma
I   Sarcoidosis
J   Tuberculosis

The following patients have all presented with pyrexia of unknown origin. Please choose the most appropriate cause from the above list. Each cause may be used once, more than once or not at all.

1. A 64-year-old man is admitted to hospital with weight loss and abdominal pains, a swinging temperature and night sweats. Routine investigations show: haemoglobin 9.7 g/dl, MCV 72.3 fl, WCC 11.9 × 10^9/l, platelets 375 × 10^9/l; Na$^+$ 132 mmol/l, K$^+$ 3.9 mmol/l, urea 7.9 mmol/l, creatinine 127 μmol/l, random blood glucose 6.1 mmol/l; blood cultures negative. His chest radiograph shows multiple, large, round lesions in both lung fields.

2. A 14-year-old schoolgirl is seen by her GP with tender lymph nodes. She is pyrexial. She is admitted to hospital, where initial investigations are unremarkable, including blood cultures. Her blood film confirms 'atypical lymphocytes and monocytes'.

3. A 31-year-old schoolteacher returns from a holiday caving in France. He is non-specifically unwell with myalgia and a low-grade pyrexia. He also has a dry cough. Initial investigations, including FBC, U&Es, LFTs and blood film are unremarkable.

4. A 24-year-old Afro-Caribbean woman is seen in Medical Out-patients with fevers and a dry cough. Her chest radiograph reveals bilateral hilar lymphadenopathy and the diagnosis is confirmed with bronchoscopy and bronchoalveolar lavage.

5. A 51-year-old rambler presents to the Emergency Department 2–3 weeks after a walking holiday in the New Forest. He complains of arthritis, myalgia and headache. On examination, he has a low-grade fever and a spreading red rash but no other focal signs.

6. THEME: COMMON CAUSES OF RIGHT ILIAC FOSSA PAIN

A   Acute appendicitis
B   Crohn's disease
C   Irritable bowel syndrome
D   Mesenteric adenitis
E   Non-specific abdominal pain
F   Pelvic inflammatory disease
G   Perforated caecal carcinoma
H   Torsion of an ovarian cyst
I   Ureteric colic
J   Urinary tract infection

The following are descriptions of patients with common causes of right iliac fossa pain. Please select the most appropriate diagnosis from the above list. Each diagnosis may be used once, more than once or not at all.

1. A 42-year-old woman is referred to Out-patients with a 3-year history of right iliac fossa pain. The pain is often post-prandial and associated with bloating and a variable bowel habit, both in terms of consistency and frequency of stool. She has no weight loss or rectal bleeding. Barium enema examination performed 1 year ago was normal, as were all recent blood tests and an abdominal radiograph performed by her GP.

2. A 19-year-old woman is seen in the Emergency Department with a 2-day history of right iliac fossa pain. She has no gastrointestinal, urinary or gynaecological symptoms. On examination, she is afebrile and there is slight tenderness but no guarding or rebound in the right iliac fossa. Initial blood tests, an abdominal radiograph and pelvic ultrasound are all normal. She is admitted for observation but is discharged 2 days later after the pain resolves.

3. A 9-year-old girl is seen in the Emergency Department with a 24-hour history of right iliac fossa pain. She admits to general malaise and fever associated with a sore throat and a 'cold' for 2 days prior to onset of the pain. On examination, she is pyrexial (temperature 39 °C), has pharyngitis and has palpable, tender, soft jugulodigastric lymph nodes. Examination of the abdomen reveals tenderness in the right iliac fossa. Her WCC is 6.2×10^9/l.

4. A 19-year-old woman is referred to the on-call surgical team with a 3–day history of worsening right iliac fossa pain, fever and nausea. Her GP suspects appendicitis. On questioning, she has had a pale-yellow vaginal discharge for 1 week and dyspareunia. On examination, her temperature is 37.9 °C and there is tenderness and guarding in the right iliac fossa. On pelvic examination, in addition to evident vaginal discharge, she has cervical excitation and some right adnexal tenderness. Her WCC is 13.2×10^9/l.

5. A 23-year-old woman presents in the Emergency Department with a 4-hour history of sudden-onset, severe, right iliac fossa pain. She has tenderness and guarding localised to the right iliac fossa and suprapubic region.

7. THEME: ARTERIAL BLOOD GASES

A   Compensated respiratory acidosis with metabolic alkalosis; type-II respiratory failure
B   Metabolic acidosis; no respiratory problem
C   Metabolic acidosis; type-I respiratory failure
D   Metabolic alkalosis; no respiratory problem
E   Metabolic alkalosis; type-I respiratory failure
F   Mixed respiratory and metabolic acidosis; type-II respiratory failure
G   Respiratory acidosis; no metabolic problem
H   Respiratory alkalosis; no metabolic problem; no respiratory problem
I   Uncompensated metabolic acidosis; respiratory alkalosis; no respiratory failure
J   Uncompensated metabolic acidosis with respiratory alkalosis; type-I respiratory failure

The following patients have all presented with disorders leading to acid–base and/or respiratory problems. Please choose the most appropriate description of their arterial blood gas profile from the list of descriptions given above. You may use each option once, more than once or not at all.

1. A 31-year-old woman is brought into the Emergency Department by the police after being told her husband has just been killed in a car accident. She has a previous history of mild asthma, is hyperventilating and crying but is not wheezy. Her arterial blood gases on room air are: pH 7.52, $PaCO_2$ 2.4 kPa, $PaCO_2$ 15.8 kPa, HCO_3^- 24.6 mmol/l, base excess +1.6 mmol/l.

2. A 63-year-old man with long-standing COPD is being assessed for long-term oxygen treatment in the Chest Clinic. His arterial blood gases on oxygen via nasal prongs set at 2 litres/minute are: pH 7.38, $PaCO_2$ 8.9 kPa, $PaCO_2$ 9.4 kPa, HCO_3^- 34.6 mmol/l, base excess +8.1 mmol/l.

3. A 24-year-old primigravida is seen in the Emergency Department with increasing shortness of breath for the past 4–5 hours. Her arterial blood gases on room air are: pH 7.28, $PaCO_2$ 2.9 kPa, $PaCO_2$ 7.8 kPa, HCO_3^- 16.6 mmol/l, base excess –9.1 mmol/l.

4. A 27-year-old woman presents in the Emergency Department after taking a large overdose of 'painkillers'. Her arterial blood gases on room air are: pH 7.29, $PaCO_2$ 2.3 kPa, $PaCO_2$ 12.8 kPa, HCO_3^- 16.6 mmol/l, base excess –4.1 mmol/l.

5. A 77-year-old man with a 3-month history of weight loss and increasing dysphagia to solids and liquids presents in the Emergency Department with weakness and 'severe' vomiting for 10 days. His arterial blood gases on room air are: pH 7.65, $PaCO_2$ 4.9 kPa, $PaCO_2$ 11.8 kPa, HCO_3^- 55.6 mmol/l, base excess +21.8 mmol/l.

8. THEME: UROGENITAL RADIOLOGY – CLINICAL SCENARIOS

*The patients below have all presented with urogenital conditions. Using the radiographic images **A–J on pages 351–353**, please match their clinical presentations with the correct image. You may use each image once, more than once or not at all. There may be more than one image appropriate for each of the diagnoses.*

1. A 39-year-old woman with a history of recurrent urinary tract infections presents to the Emergency Department with a 12-hour history of severe, worsening, right-sided loin pain, rigors and vomiting. The FY2 doctor notes that her previous two mid-stream urine results both confirm the presence of a species of *Proteus*.

2. A 28-year-old Egyptian woman with a previous history of schistosomiasis infections, presents to her GP with increasing lower abdominal pain, dysuria and episodes of frank haematuria.

3. A 54-year-old man presents to his GP with a 3-month history of weight loss, non-specific loin pains and occasional night sweats. On examination, he looks chronically unwell, anaemic and cachectic and has a ballotable mass in one loin.

4. A 22-year-old woman is being investigated for recurrent urinary tract infections and episodic haematuria. Of note, her BP is 180/110 mmHg despite several antihypertensive medications and she has a 'ruddy' complexion. She has 'easily' ballotable kidneys bilaterally.

5. A 19-year-old man presents to his GP with a 3–4-month history of worsening, left-sided loin pain. Of note, the pain is worse when he drinks alcohol. He denies having any other urological symptoms. Examination is unremarkable, as is his dipstick urine test. The diagnosis is confirmed by IVU and he is cured with surgical correction.

9. THEME: THE PAINFUL KNEE

A   Anterior cruciate injury
B   Chondromalacia patellae
C   Infrapatellar bursitis
D   Meniscal tear
E   Osgood–Schlatter disease
F   Osteoarthrosis
G   Osteochondritis dessicans
H   Pre-patellar bursitis
I   Recurrent dislocation of the patella
J   Rheumatoid arthritis

The following are descriptions of patients with a painful knee (or knees). Please select the most appropriate diagnosis from the above list. Each diagnosis may be used once, more than once or not at all.

1. A 16-year-old girl complains of pain, principally in front of the knee, especially on ascending and descending stairs.

2. A 63-year-old patient complains of chronic pain and swelling of the knee. On examination, there is marked deformity, with valgus, especially apparent on standing.

3. A 23-year-old rugby player has a twisting injury of the knee after which the knee is 'locked' in partial flexion. On examination, there is a small effusion and extension is limited. McMurray's test is positive.

4. A 40-year-old carpet-layer presents with anterior knee pain and a painful swelling.

5. A 13-year-old adolescent presents after school athletics with anterior knee pain and a lump over the tibial tuberosity.

10. THEME: UPPER AIRWAYS OBSTRUCTION

A Acute epiglottitis
B Anaphylactic reaction
C Angioneurotic oedema
D Bilateral recurrent laryngeal nerve paralysis
E Carcinoma of the larynx
F Diphtheria
G Fracture of the larynx
H Fracture of the mandible/mid-facial fracture
I Inhaled foreign body
J Inhalation or ingestion of irritants
K Ludwig's angina
L Papilloma of the larynx
M Reduced conscious level
N Thyroid carcinoma

The following patients have all presented with stridor or with breathlessness. Please select the most appropriate diagnosis from the above list. Each diagnosis may be used once, more than once or not at all.

1. A 16-year-old girl presents with facial oedema, dyspnoea and stridor. She is apyrexial and has no past medical history.

2. A 25-year-old man presents with a history of anterior neck injury, sustained while participating in karate. He is developing increasing hoarseness. On examination, he has surgical emphysema of the neck.

3. A 75-year-old woman presents with a history of dyspnoea and stridor. She has noticed a swelling in the neck for the previous 2 months. On examination, she has a right-sided, hard, anterior neck mass that is fixed to the larynx. A lateral soft-tissue radiograph of the neck shows compression of the trachea and severe narrowing of the airway.

4. A 4-year-old boy is admitted with a 6-hour history of fever, sore throat and stridor. His temperature is 39.5 °C. The child's condition deteriorates and he has to be intubated.

5. A 45-year-old builder is rescued by the fire service after a gas explosion in a building. He is alert and orientated but has stridor, hoarseness and a cough productive of black sputum. He has burns to the face and upper torso and a fractured right femur.

11. THEME: GYNAECOLOGICAL PROCEDURES

A   Anterior vaginal repair
B   Colposcopy
C   Colposuspension
D   Endometrial ablation
E   Hysteroscopy
F   Laparoscopy
G   Large loop excision of the transformation zone (LLETZ)
H   Posterior vaginal repair
I   Total abdominal hysterectomy
J   Vaginal hysterectomy

From the above list please choose the procedure that is most appropriate for the clinical picture described. Each procedure may be used once, more than once or not at all.

1. A 28-year-old nulliparous woman has no clinical symptoms but receives an interval cervical smear result suggestive of moderate dyskaryosis.

2. A 60-year-old multiparous woman describes frequency and urinary incontinence on coughing and laughing. Examination reveals only first-degree uterovaginal prolapse. Her mid-stream urine is unremarkable and conservative measures fail to improve her symptoms. Urodynamic investigation gives a diagnosis of genuine stress incontinence (GSI).

3. A 47-year-old woman has a 6-month history of heavy, irregular periods. There has been no intermenstrual or post-coital bleeding. Her examination is completely normal and she has had a normal cervical smear in the last 2 years. A transvaginal ultrasound scan reveals a 2 cm × 3 cm serosal fibroid, endometrial thickness of 14 mm and normal ovaries. She has failed to respond to medical therapy (cyclical progestagens).

4. A 30-year-old woman has increasing dysmenorrhoea and deep dyspareunia over a period of 12 months. On examination, there is marked tenderness in the posterior fornix and the uterus feels fixed and retroverted. She has already tried 3 months of empirical treatment on high-dose progestagens for presumed endometriosis, but the symptoms have not improved. Her transvaginal ultrasound scan is unremarkable.

5. A 58-year-old multiparous woman has a feeling of 'something coming down' into the vagina that has been getting worse over the last 2 years. She describes mild frequency but no urgency or urinary incontinence. There are no bowel symptoms and she is not currently sexually active. Examination reveals a moderate cystocoele but no obvious uterovaginal prolapse, rectocoele or enterocoele.

12. THEME: DISORDERS LEADING TO ABNORMAL COAGULATION

A   Autoimmune thrombocytopenic purpura
B   Disseminated intravascular coagulation (DIC)
C   Essential thrombocythaemia
D   Haemophilia A
E   Haemophilia B
F   Sickle-cell disease
G   Systemic lupus erythematosus
H   Thrombotic thrombocytopenic purpura
I   Vitamin K deficiency
J   von Willebrand's disease

From the above list, please select the disorder that each of the following patients is most likely to have. Each diagnosis may be used once, more than once or not at all.

Patient	Bleeding time	Prothrombin (PT) ratio	Activated partial thromboplastin time (APTT)	Factor VIII:C levels	Factor IX levels	Platelet count
1	Normal	Normal	Increased	Very low	Normal	Normal
2	Normal	Increased	Increased	Normal	Normal	Normal
3	Increased	Normal	Increased	Low	Normal	Normal
4	Increased	Increased	Increased	Low	Low	Very low
5	Normal	Normal	Increased	Normal	Low	Normal

13. THEME: ANATOMY OF THE FEMORAL REGION

A   Femoral artery
B   Femoral canal
C   Femoral nerve
D   Femoral vein
E   Iliopsoas muscle
F   Inguinal ligament
G   Pectineal ligament (Cooper's ligament)
H   Pubic tubercle
I   Reflected pectineal part of the inguinal ligament
J   Saphenous opening

For each of the following descriptions, please choose the most appropriate structure from the above list. Each structure may be used once, more than once or not at all.

1. Lateral relation of the femoral artery.

2. Medial relation of the neck of the femoral canal.

3. Posterior relation of the femoral canal.

4. The site where a femoral hernia becomes subcutaneous.

5. The structure above and medial to the opening of the femoral canal.

14. THEME: MUSCLE ATTACHMENTS OF THE LOWER LIMB

A   Adductor longus
B   Adductor magnus
C   Biceps femoris (long head)
D   Gastrocnemius
E   Iliopsoas
F   Peroneus longus
G   Semitendinosus
H   Soleus
I   Tibialis posterior
J   Vastus lateralis

For each of the following attachments please choose the most appropriate muscle from the above list. the muscles may be used once, more than once, in combination or not at all.

1. Lesser trochanter of the femur.

2. Linea aspera of the femur.

3. Above and posterior to the lateral femoral condyle.

4. The upper two-thirds of the lateral surface of the fibula.

5. The tuberosity of the navicular.

Paper 7 Answers

1. SECONDARY HYPERTENSION

1. **D – Conn's syndrome**
   This young woman has hypertension associated with hypokalaemia. This might be due to Conn's syndrome (primary hyperaldosteronism) or to Cushing's syndrome. The subsequent investigations after correction of her hypokalaemia reveal hyperaldosteronism and reduced plasma renin activity, indicating Conn's syndrome. Causes include adrenal adenomas and bilateral adrenal hyperplasia, which are treated by surgical excision or with spironolactone and antihypertensive agents respectively.

2. **A – Acromegaly**
   This man has several features of acromegaly, including frontal bossing and bitemporal hemianopia. He also has hypertension and proximal myopathy. The diagnosis should be confirmed by dynamic pituitary testing which will show poorly suppressible, elevated growth hormone levels, and MRI of the pituitary fossa. The treatment is usually by neurosurgical excision of the tumour, either transnasally or transfrontally, with postoperative radiotherapy.

3. **H – Polycystic kidney disease**
   This woman has signs of polycythaemia (plethoric), hypertension and large upper abdominal masses. Blood tests confirm the polycythaemia and reveal renal impairment. This is the clinical picture of polycystic kidney disease. Adult polycystic kidney disease is an autosomal dominant disorder which can present in early adulthood with local symptoms such as urinary infections (recurrent), haematuria, abdominal pain, renal failure or renal stones and systemic symptoms, including polycythaemia, anaemia, hypertension and subarachnoid haemorrhage (due to the association with berry aneurysms).

4. **J – Renal artery stenosis**
   This patient has known ischaemic heart disease and pulmonary vascular disease which imply that he has generalised atherosclerosis. Significant pulmonary vascular disease is associated with a 25–30% risk of significant renal artery stenosis and is a contraindication to starting an ACE inhibitor unless the kidneys and renal arteries are imaged. Renal artery stenosis and aortic stenosis are both contraindications to starting on ACE inhibitors as this causes a rapid deterioration in both of these conditions.

5. **G – Phaeochromocytoma**

This patient has poorly controlled blood pressure despite the addition of several antihypertensive agents. Subsequent investigations show a raised 24-hour urinary VMA (vanillyl mandelic acid) and raised serum catecholamines on adrenal venous sampling. VMA is a metabolite of adrenaline and noradrenaline (epinephrine and norepinephrine) excreted in the urine. Other investigations include a radio-labelled ^{131}I-MIBG (metaiodobenzylguanidine) scan, which is preferentially taken up at sites of sympathetic overactivity, and a CT scan of the abdomen to visualise the tumour. The treatment includes an α- and a β-blocker, always starting with α-blockade and then β-blockade (if required). If started in the other way round, unopposed α activity is potentially life-threatening. Definitive surgical excision of the tumour is usually curative, although expert endocrine opinion, surgery and anaesthesia are required.

2. AUTOSOMAL DOMINANT DISORDERS

1. **B – Dystrophia myotonica**
   This man has bilateral ptosis and facial weakness associated with a 'prolonged handshake', all features of dystrophia myotonica. Myotonica means 'continued muscle contraction after cessation of voluntary effort' and is characteristically seen when asking the patient to perform a given task and then asking them to stop (eg 'squeeze my fingers ... and now stop'. – the patient is not able to let go). The syndrome is characterised by mild intellectual impairment, frontal balding, cataracts, cardiomyopathy and conduction system defects. The disorder becomes apparent between the ages of 20 and 40 and is insidiously progressive.

2. **C – Familial hypercholesterolaemia**
   This patient has the commonest autosomal dominant disorder in the Western world, familial hypercholesterolaemia. This condition causes premature macrovascular atherosclerosis and subsequent ischaemic heart disease, stroke and peripheral vascular disease. Management is with high-dose statins and family screening. All secondary risk factors (eg hypertension, diabetes mellitus and smoking) should also be addressed.

3. **H – Neurofibromatosis**
   This patient has developed several stigmata of neurofibromatosis, including the skin tumours and café-au-lait spots (more than five is considered pathological). The disorder has been divided into a peripheral syndrome, type-I neurofibromatosis (chromosome 17) and a central syndrome, type-II neurofibromatosis (chromosome 22).

4. **J – Romano–Ward syndrome**
   This patient has developed *torsades de pointes* secondary to a prolonged QTc interval caused by his Romano–Ward syndrome. Other causes include Jevell–Lange–Nielson (autosomal recessive), hypocalcaemia, hypomagnesaemia and hypokalaemia, severe bradycardia (tachy-brady syndrome), ischaemic heart disease and drugs, including antipsychotics, antihistamines and anti-arrhythmics (eg amiodarone).

5. **D – Gilbert's syndrome**
   This patient has a severe streptococcal pneumonia and an associated hyperbilirubinaemia with otherwise normal liver function tests. This is caused by Gilbert's syndrome, which is a benign condition leading to hyperbilirubinaemia in times of stress. The underlying cause needs to be treated and the patient should be told about the condition in order to stop 'overzealous' doctors subjecting them to further liver function tests and imaging! Their family should also be screened.

3. INFECTIVE DIARRHOEA

1. **I – *Shigella flexneri***
   This girl has developed shigellosis or bacillary dysentery, which is one of the commonest causes of infant and childhood mortality worldwide. The four species of *Shigella* cause a spectrum of disease from a mild, even asymptomatic infection, up to a life-threatening dysentery with bloody diarrhoea associated with mucus and pus. They are spread by the faecal–oral route. *Shigella dysenteriae* is found in tropical areas and causes severe enteritis with systemic complications due to the production of an enterotoxin, cytotoxin and neurotoxin. It requires antibiotic treatment. In the UK, *S. sonnei* and *S. flexneri* are more common and cause a more benign, self-limiting condition.

2. **C – *Campylobacter jejuni***
   This young man has developed *Campylobacter* food poisoning, one of the commonest causes of food poisoning in the UK. It is associated with meat, chicken and dairy products. It is usually a self-limiting condition but can occasionally cause severe systemic upset and require antibiotic treatment with ciprofloxacin or clarithromycin.

3. **B – *Bacillus cereus***
   This woman has developed an acute gastroenteritis due to a *Bacillus cereus* infection. This Gram-positive bacillus causes a rapid onset of vomiting and diarrhoea within 2–6 hours of ingestion of affected foods. It is characteristically associated with poorly heated/reheated rice, which leads to germination and multiplication of the bacilli and toxin production. The disorder is self-limiting and the symptoms last only 24–48 hours.

4. **D – *Clostridium difficile***
   This man has developed *Clostridium difficile* diarrhoea as a result of his prolonged admission and antibiotic treatment for his recurrent infections. Several studies have shown experienced nurses to be 90% sensitive in their diagnosis of *C. difficile* so if the charge nurse says '*C. Diff* diarrhoea' … it invariably is! Treatment includes oral (ie not parenteral) metronidazole or vancomycin because it is the intraluminal concentration of the antibiotic that is important. Other management includes supportive treatment with intravenous or oral fluids.

5. **F – *Escherichia coli***
   This group of patients have developed an *Escherichia coli* infection. The various strains of this organism produce several different toxins, including an enterotoxin that is secreted by the non-invasive ETEC (enterotoxigenic *E. coli*) group. This usually causes a self-limiting condition lasting for a few days but can cause a more severe illness with cholera-like symptoms and signs. The more severe cytototoxin-producing group of organisms includes the strain *E. coli* O157, which produces the *Shiga*-like toxin that can lead to a severe diarrhoeal illness associated with acute renal failure and disseminated intravascular coagulation – the haemolytic–uraemic syndrome. This is particularly common in children and the elderly and is often fatal without early treatment.

4. PERIPHERAL SENSORY NEUROPATHY

1. **B – Amiodarone**
    This man has been placed on amiodarone, which has led to several side-effects, including a peripheral sensory neuropathy. Amiodarone is principally used in older patients with poorly controlled paroxysmal atrial fibrillation, sustained atrial fibrillation or paroxysmal ventricular tachyarrhythmia, although, more recently, implantable defibrillator devices have superseded this role. It has numerous side-effects, including:
    - Skin effects – photosensitivity (patients can claim free suntan lotion!), a slate-grey pigmentation and erythema multiforme.
    - Pulmonary fibrosis (very uncommon at doses below 400 mg per day).
    - Dysthyroid disease – amiodarone affects the thyroid's physiology at several levels and can cause hypo- or hyperthyroid disease, which might or might not be clinically manifest.
    - Hepatitis – again, this might or might not be clinically manifest.
    - Microcorneal deposits.

    Most of the side-effects are totally reversible on withdrawal of the drug but, as with all drug therapies, patients must be warned of the important side-effects on starting the drug.

2. **D – Demyelination**
    This young man has developed episodic visual blurring and symptoms of a peripheral sensory neuropathy. His investigations will show plaques of demyelination within the cervical cord, brainstem, periventricular white matter and cerebellum. The delayed visual-evoked responses also help to confirm the diagnosis of multiple sclerosis. The treatment of this condition will depend on the patient's wishes and on the pattern of subsequent disease.

3. **C – Amyloidosis**
    This patient has developed amyloidosis, leading to a nephrotic syndrome and a peripheral sensory neuropathy (although it is a relatively uncommon cause of neuropathy). The diagnosis is confirmed by the appearance of amyloid proteins in biopsy tissue, usually taken from the gums or rectum. The classic appearance is of an apple-green coloration under polarised light after staining with Congo red.

4. **F – Hypothyroidism**
    This woman with vitiligo has clinical and investigative evidence of hypothyroidism. She has weight gain, lethargy and symptoms of a sensory neuropathy, a macrocytosis and hyponatraemia. The diagnosis should be confirmed with thyroid function tests and the patient should be started on thyroxine-replacement therapy, titrated slowly against the clinical and biochemical response.

5. **J – Vitamin B$_{12}$ deficiency**
    This woman has developed vitamin B$_{12}$ deficiency, as evidenced by the symptoms of anaemia, the peripheral sensory neuropathy and the confirmatory investigations, including a gross macrocytosis in association with a pancytopenia. Although her vegan diet is the most likely cause, she needs an autoantibody screen to exclude pernicious anaemia and related autoimmune diseases such as thyroid disease. She will also require vitamin B$_{12}$ and folate levels, as well as glucose, thyroid function tests and liver function tests; a history should also be taken to exclude alcohol excess and drug side-effects. Treatment consists of a loading course of hydroxycobalamin (three 1-mg doses over 1 week) and then single repeat doses every 3 months.

5. PYREXIA OF UNKNOWN ORIGIN (PUO)

1. **H – Renal-cell carcinoma**
   This man has a microcytic anaemia and mild renal impairment and his chest radiograph shows multiple, large lesions or cannonball metastases. This presentation is consistent with renal-cell carcinoma. The diagnosis can be confirmed on renal ultrasound scan, urine cytology and CT scan of the abdomen.

2. **C – Epstein–Barr virus**
   This schoolgirl has developed a severe EBV infection. Sepsis and viral infections cause tender lymphadenopathy, in contrast to the non-tender lymphadenopathy that characteristically occurs in haematological malignancy. EBV infection is confirmed by the 'monospot' test and the Paul–Bunnell test. The monospot confirms the presence of the associated atypical mononuclear cells on the blood film. The Paul–Bunnell test confirms the presence of heterophile IgM antibodies. These lead to agglutination of sheep red blood cells in vitro. Rising EBV IgM titres are also commonly used for diagnosis in hospitalised patients.

3. **D – Histoplasmosis**
   This man has developed a primary histoplasmosis infection. The infection is caused by a fungus with spores that can survive in moist soil or in bat and/or bird droppings for several years. It is a 'classic' infection of cavers who explore caves in endemic areas. The primary infection is often asymptomatic but can present with a PUO, a flu-like illness and a dry cough. Secondary complications in the lung include secondary bacterial infection, pleural effusions and pleurisy. A chronic pulmonary infection can develop which is almost identical to pulmonary TB.

4. **I – Sarcoidosis**
   This Afro-Caribbean woman has developed pulmonary sarcoidosis, as evidenced by the bilateral hilar lymphadenopathy seen on chest radiography and the clinical presentation. The diagnosis is confirmed on bronchoscopy and biopsy and bronchoalveolar lavage, which will show non-caseating granulomatous infiltration with inflammatory cells and T-helper cells.

5. **G – Lyme disease**
   This patient has developed Lyme disease, a spirochaete infection spread by ticks (which live on the deer of the New Forest). There are three distinct phases of the disease.
   1. A non-specific, flu-like illness associated with myalgia, arthralgia, fever and lymphadenopathy, and characterised by a spreading red rash (erythema chronicum migrans).
   2. The second stage develops weeks to months later, with meningo-encephalitis, cranial nerve and peripheral neuropathies and cardiac problems.
   3. A chronic progressive episodic arthritis (this phase does not seem to occur in the UK).

   The treatment is with penicillin or tetracycline.

6. COMMON CAUSES OF RIGHT ILIAC FOSSA PAIN

It is possible to name at least 20 causes of right iliac fossa pain. The list given in this question includes some of the more common ones. In general, like so much in medicine, it is more common to see a common condition presenting atypically than a rare condition presenting typically. For example, a urinary tract infection, while usually associated with suprapubic pain, can also present with right iliac fossa pain. For a complete list, consider the contents of the abdomen anatomically from front to back in the region of the right iliac fossa:

- Anterior abdominal wall, eg rectus sheath haematoma
- Peritoneal viscera – caecum, small intestine, appendix, right fallopian tube and ovary, bladder
- Retroperitoneal structures – kidney, ureter, iliac artery (leaking aneurysm), iliac vein thrombosis, undescended testis (torsion), psoas muscle (abscess).

1. C – Irritable bowel syndrome

The long history and typical symptoms fulfilling the Rome criteria suggest this 'non-diagnosis' which should only be made when an organic cause for the patient's symptoms has been excluded (as in this case). As in this case, patients are typically middle-aged women.

2. E – Non-specific abdominal pain

This is the commonest eventual diagnosis in patients presenting with right iliac fossa pain. The description should only be employed for patients in which ALL other relevant causes of pain have been excluded by investigation.

3. D – Mesenteric adenitis

The patient described is typical of this condition, in which mesenteric lymph node enlargement causes abdominal pain in response to a systemic illness, usually viral. In this case the patient has a viral upper respiratory tract infection. Evidence of such infections should always be sought, especially in children, to avoid unnecessary appendicectomy.

4. F – Pelvic inflammatory disease

The patient might be assumed to have appendicitis were it not for the symptoms and signs, which are typical of pelvic inflammatory disease. The cause is bacterial infection of the tubes/ovaries (salpingo-oophoritis) and this is usually contracted primarily via sexual transmission. Organisms include *Neisseria gonorrhoeae* and *Chlamydia trachomatis*.

5. H – Torsion of an ovarian cyst

The history, in particular the sudden onset of pain without gastrointestinal disturbance, suggests this diagnosis, which is a common differential diagnosis in a young woman. The diagnosis can usually be confirmed by pelvic ultrasound examination, and the patient often requires surgery. A similar presentation is seen with haemorrhage into and rupture of an ovarian cyst.

7. ARTERIAL BLOOD GASES

Arterial blood gases seem to cause medical undergraduates no end of pain and misery. This is because the data are often decontextualised, ie viewed in isolation, and they have no real schema on which to attack the data. On a practical point, if you are interested in the acid–base balance you can obtain the necessary information from a venous blood sample. It is only when respiratory function is compromised that a set of arterial gases are required.

1. **H – Respiratory alkalosis; no metabolic problem; no respiratory problem**
   This patient's gases suggest that she is hyperventilating in response to the devastating news about her husband. There are no metabolic or respiratory problems. She might require sedatives to help her sleep and help with the anxiety and she should be discharged to a place with support and comfort (ie to family or friends).

2. **A – Compensated respiratory acidosis with metabolic alkalosis; type-II respiratory failure**
   This man's gases are typical of a relatively well patient with COPD. He has long-standing type-II respiratory failure (causing the hypoxaemia and hypercapnia) with metabolic compensation by the kidneys (leading to retention of bicarbonate). He is well controlled on his oxygen therapy and should be given the long-term oxygen treatment at home.

3. **J – Uncompensated metabolic acidosis with respiratory alkalosis; type-I respiratory failure**
   The history and gases suggest that this pregnant woman has had a significant pulmonary embolism. There is evidence of a metabolic acidosis (most likely due to lactic acidosis) and a respiratory alkalosis (as she hyperventilates secondary to the hypoxaemia). There is also evidence of type-I respiratory failure.

4. **I – Uncompensated metabolic acidosis; respiratory alkalosis; no respiratory failure**
   Patients who overdose on aspirin demonstrate both metabolic and respiratory derangement. The salicylate is an acid, which leads to a metabolic acidosis. However, in the early phase of the overdose the salicylate will cross the blood–brain barrier and stimulate the respiratory centres in the brainstem, so the initial derangement is a respiratory alkalosis. The gases will therefore show a respiratory alkalosis, closely followed by a metabolic acidosis, the latter becoming the increasingly dominant derangement with time (as in this case).

5. **D – Metabolic alkalosis; no respiratory problem**
   The history and gases are highly suggestive of an obstructing lesion, either in the lower oesophagus or the stomach. In a man of this age, gastric outlet obstruction due to a gastric malignancy is the probable cause. The gases show a severe metabolic alkalosis with no respiratory compromise. Other causes include chronic vomiting and/or diarrhoea and the milk-alkali syndrome, in which patients ingest large amounts of alkalotic antacid preparations (eg calcium carbonate) and milk due to dyspepsia. Hypokalaemic metabolic alkalosis is a side-effect of loop and thiazide diuretics.

8. UROGENITAL RADIOLOGY – CLINICAL SCENARIOS

1. **(P5–P7) J, G – Right staghorn calculus and duplex kidneys**
   This patient has symptoms suggestive of a urinary tract infection and renal colic. This is due to presence of a large, right-sided staghorn calculus, which in turn has been caused by her recurrent *Proteus* urinary tract infections. A duplex system will also predispose the patient to recurrent infections.

2. **(P5–P7) D – Vesical calculus**
   This patient has developed bladder or vesical calculi secondary to her previous schistosomiasis infection. Schistosomiasis (also known as 'bilharzia' after the German parasitologist, Theodor Maximilian Bilharz, who first described the disease in Egypt in 1851) is a parasitic flatworm infection caused by several different species. The life cycle of the worm involves eggs being shed by infected humans in faeces and urine into fresh water. Here they hatch into 'miracidia', which then infect freshwater snails. Within the snails they develop and are released as free-swimming 'cercariae' back into the fresh water. The cercariae are attracted and are able to penetrate human skin. Here they lose their swimming tails, becoming 'schistosomulum', which are subsequently are carried via the venous and portal systems to the liver where they mature into adult worms. It is the worms of the *Schistosoma haematobium* species, which then migrate to the venus plexuses around the lower urinary tract. Mature adult worms then produce eggs, which pass through the ureteric and bladder wall into the urine. Other species, including *S. mansoni* and *S. japonicum* remain in the mesenteric and rectal veins and their eggs pass through the intestinal wall into the faeces.

3. **(P5–P7) F – Displaced left-sided kidney**
   This patient has signs and symptoms suggestive of a renal carcinoma. Renal carcinoma is a relatively common malignancy, being the sixth most common cause of cancer death in the Western world. It is more common in whites and in men (male to female ratio 2 : 1) and is commonest in the fourth to sixth decades. There is a genetic link, with many patients having an identifiable defect within the short arm of chromosome 3. Risk factors include a strong family history (because of the chromosome abnormalities), von Hippel–Lindau syndrome (40% of patients with this condition develop renal-cell carcinoma), cigarette smoking, obesity (particularly in women), some causes of chronic renal failure (chronic analgesic abuse, polycystic kidney disease) and dialysis, renal transplantation, unopposed oestrogens and environmental exposure to asbestos and petrol-related products.

4. **(P5–P7) A – Polycystic kidneys**
   This patient has bilaterally enlarged kidneys, a ruddy complexion (inferring that she has polycythaemia), recurrent urinary tract infections, haematuria and poorly controlled hypertension. These signs and symptoms are suggestive of adult polycystic kidney disease. The haematuria might be due to the urinary tract infection, bleeding into the cysts, calculi or renal-cell carcinoma. Patients often describe loin pain, which has similar causes. There can be a dull ache due to the enlargement of the kidneys but more severe, acute pain might be due to uro-sepsis, stones or bleeding into the cysts. The diagnosis is confirmed by ultrasound or CT scan of the renal tract.

5.   **(P5–P7) H – Obstructed left kidney**
      This young man has developed symptoms of an obstructed pelvi-ureteric junction.
      Classically, this causes loin pain that can be worse after drinking alcohol. Other
      associated features include signs and symptoms of urinary tract infection, but
      haematuria is not usually associated with this condition. In young men it is commonly
      an idiopathic condition but other causes (that need to be excluded) include
      congenital defects of the ureteric insertion, chronic reflux and recurrent infection,
      calculi, transitional-cell carcinoma and extrinsic compression by an abdominal aortic
      aneurysm or retroperitoneal fibrosis. Surgical correction (pyeloplasty) is usually
      curative but in severe cases nephrectomy can be required. (His left-sided symptoms
      exclude the similar right-sided lesion shown in radiograph **E**).

IMAGES: pages 351–353

9. THE PAINFUL KNEE

1. B – Chondromalacia patellae
Softening of the articular cartilage of the patella is often associated with anterior knee pain in teenage girls. It is thought to result from mal-tracking of the patella during flexion and extension. On clinical examination, pain can be elicited by the patella femoral crepitation test. Treatment is rest, analgesia and physiotherapy.

2. J – Rheumatoid arthritis
This can occasionally start in the knee as a monoarticular synovitis. With the passage of time, the joint can become increasingly deformed. Although deformity can also occur (with chronic pain and swelling) in osteoarthritis, a valgus deformity is characteristic of rheumatoid, in contrast to the varus deformity that is frequently seen with severe osteoarthritis.

3. D – Meniscal tear
The description given is characteristic of this very common injury. McMurray's test (rotating the knee during various degrees of flexion and extension) aims to catch the torn meniscal fragment between the articular surfaces of the knee and then induce it to snap free with a palpable and audible click. (**NB:** While you should know the principle of this test, it can be very difficult to convincingly demonstrate in less than very experienced hands. It is also very painful for the patient if positive!)

4. H – Pre-patellar bursitis
The occupation gives this away. Commonly called 'housemaid's knee', this is now more common in people with occupations that require them to kneel to work. Treatment is avoidance and bandaging (and, occasionally, aspiration).

5. E – Osgood–Schlatter disease
This is a traction injury of the tibial apophysis for the patellar ligament. The presentation and findings are characteristic and the radiological findings diagnostic. Treatment is restriction of activity to permit eventual spontaneous recovery.

10. UPPER AIRWAYS OBSTRUCTION

1. **C – Angioneurotic oedema**
    This is a condition of unknown aetiology that most commonly affects young females. Management is by close observation, antihistamines and intravenous steroids/adrenaline (epinephrine) nebulisers. Should the condition deteriorate, the patient might require orotracheal intubation. It is distinguished from anaphylactic shock by the absence of a precipitating allergen (eg antibiotics, bee stings).

2. **G – Fracture of the larynx**
    This man has fractured his thyroid cartilage. He is in danger of developing a haematoma of the larynx that could obstruct the airway and so he should be admitted to hospital for observation. If the situation deteriorates, tracheostomy might be required as an emergency procedure. A lateral, soft-tissue view of the neck or tomography of the larynx should be performed and if the cartilages are displaced the larynx should be repaired surgically; otherwise, scarring can leave lasting damage necessitating a permanent tracheostomy.

3. **N – Thyroid carcinoma**
    This patient has findings consistent with anaplastic carcinoma of the thyroid. This is one of the less common thyroid malignancies and it has a uniformly terrible prognosis because of direct invasion of vital neck structures such as the airway, as in this case. A palliative tracheostomy can relieve symptoms and temporarily prolong life.

4. **A – Acute epiglottitis**
    The rapid onset of the stridor and the high temperature give the clue to the diagnosis. The infecting organism is *Haemophilus influenzae* type B, which responds to broad-spectrum antibiotics. If there is any but the mildest degree of stridor, the child must be taken to the operating theatre and anaesthetised on the operating table with a surgeon scrubbed up and the instruments opened so that tracheostomy or cricothyroidotomy can be performed in the event of the anaesthetist being unable to intubate. In this condition the epiglottis is red and swollen and protrudes above the tongue (the 'rising sun' sign), but patients must NEVER be examined to visualise this as to do so can precipitate complete respiratory obstruction. With immunisation, such infections are becoming rarer. The differential diagnosis is acute laryngotracheobronchitis, and in the third world in an unimmunised population, diphtheria.

5. **J – Inhalation or ingestion of irritants**
    In this case the patient has smoke inhalation, with burns to the upper airway. The supraglottic airway is extremely susceptible to obstruction as a result of exposure to heat. When a patient is admitted to hospital after a burn injury, the doctor should be alert to the possibility of airway involvement. Clinical indications of inhalation injury include facial burns, singeing of the nasal hairs, carbon deposits in the oropharynx, carbonaceous sputum, hoarseness and a carboxyhaemoglobin level greater than 10%. The symptom of stridor is an indication for immediate orotracheal intubation. A similar pattern of airway obstruction can be caused by ingestion of corrosives, such as strong acids or alkalis.

11. GYNAECOLOGICAL PROCEDURES

1. B – Colposcopy

A cervical smear result with either moderate or severe dyskaryosis (ie a high-grade smear) is an initial indication for colposcopy. This allows colposcopic assessment of the cervix to see if this agrees with the cytological diagnosis. It is common for punch biopsy to be performed to gain a histological diagnosis (eg CIN 1, 2 or 3). It is usually on the basis of histological proof of high-grade CIN or persistent low-grade CIN that a large loop excision of the transformation zone (LLETZ) is performed (though, more rarely, a 'see and treat' LLETZ might be performed).

2. C – Colposuspension

The two commonest causes of stress incontinence are genuine stress incontinence (GSI) and detrusor overactivity. GSI is diagnosed on urodynamic studies, when there is demonstrable stress incontinence without aberrant detrusor activity. It must always be performed before any bladder-neck surgery. The only procedures that might be helpful from the list are an anterior vaginal repair and colposuspension. Anterior vaginal repair only has a small effect on stress incontinence and is mainly used when the symptoms are predominantly of prolapse (a cystocoele). Therefore, when the main complaint is incontinence, colposuspension is still a widely used and highly effective treatment for GSI.

3. E – Hysteroscopy

Abnormal vaginal bleeding in women over 40 needs to be investigated as the risks of endometrial pathology (polyp, hyperplasia and carcinoma) increase with age. Intermenstrual bleeding and post-coital bleeding can be suggestive of cervical pathology. Their absence and a recent, normal cervical smear and a normal cervix on examination usually rule out the need for colposcopy. Endometrial ablation and hysterectomy might be required eventually if conservative medical therapy fails but the next logical procedure is a diagnostic hysteroscopy (with curettage) to assess the endometrial cavity. Serosal fibroids are not implicated in menorrhagia because they do not affect the size of the cavity, in contrast to submucosal fibroids, and are therefore best left alone.

4. F – Laparoscopy

The symptoms and signs are highly suggestive of endometriosis and it is good practice to try empirical treatment in these cases – up to 80% improve with medical treatment. When there has been no improvement after treatment, either the endometriosis is resistant to medical suppression or the diagnosis is wrong (ie it could instead be pelvic inflammatory disease, adhesions or ovarian pathology). Diagnostic laparoscopy is therefore indicated to assess for pelvic pathology and obtain a diagnosis – it might also be therapeutic (eg adhesiolysis). A form of hysterectomy might ultimately be a treatment for endometriosis but this is not indicated at this stage (this is usually a last resort).

5. A – Anterior vaginal repair

Prolapse of the pelvis can be divided into anterior-compartment prolapse (bladder into vagina – cystocoele), middle-compartment prolapse (uterus into vagina) and posterior compartment prolapse (bowel or rectum into vagina – entero- or rectocoele). The appropriate surgery is usually an anterior vaginal repair, vaginal hysterectomy or posterior vaginal repair, respectively. Mild urinary symptoms are extremely common after the menopause and are often exacerbated by an anterior prolapse. The appropriate operation here is an anterior vaginal repair to restore the bladder to its anatomical position. This is often performed with a vaginal hysterectomy as multiple compartment defects are common, but in this case there is no clinical evidence of other defects.

12. DISORDERS LEADING TO ABNORMAL COAGULATION

1. **D – Haemophilia A**
   Haemophilia A is an X-linked inherited coagulation disorder with a prevalence of about 1 in 5000 of the male population. Patients with haemophilia A have reduced levels of factor VIII:C in the blood, resulting in abnormal coagulation and excessive bleeding. The extent of the bleeding depends on how severe the reduction in factor VIII:C is, the most severe disease occurring with levels of less than 1% of normal. Factor VIII is involved in the intrinsic coagulation pathway, the integrity of which is tested by measurement of the APTT time. In haemophiliacs, the reduction in factor VIII results in disruption of the intrinsic coagulation pathway and the APTT time is therefore prolonged. The PT ratio, which measures the integrity of the extrinsic pathway, and the bleeding time, which tests the ability of platelets to aggregate and form a platelet plug, are unaffected in haemophilia.

2. **I – Vitamin K deficiency**
   Vitamin K is a fat-soluble vitamin that is essential for the production of clotting factors II, VII, IX and X. Factor VII is involved in the extrinsic pathway, factor IX in the intrinsic pathway and factors II and VII in the final common pathway. Consequently, both the intrinsic and extrinsic pathways are defective in patients with vitamin K deficiency and the PT ratio and APTT time are both prolonged. The bleeding time is not affected as platelet numbers and function are normal. Vitamin K deficiency occurs as a result of inadequate stores, such as in haemorrhagic disease of the newborn, and secondary to fat malabsorption, such as in bile duct obstruction. Oral anticoagulant drugs are vitamin K antagonists.

3. **J – von Willebrand's disease**
   von Willebrand's disease is due to a deficiency or abnormality of von Willebrand factor. This factor plays a role in adhesion of platelets to damaged subendothelium as well as stabilising factor VIII:C in plasma. Consequently, in von Willebrand's disease there is defective platelet function (even though platelet numbers are normal) coupled with rapid destruction of factor VIII:C, leading to factor VIII:C deficiency. The laboratory test profile is therefore similar to that of haemophilia A (namely prolonged APTT time and normal PT ratio), together with evidence of abnormal platelet aggregation, namely prolonged bleeding time. Von Willebrand's disease has been classified into three types with different clinical features and inheritance pattern.

4. **B – Disseminated intravascular coagulation (DIC)**
   In disseminated intravascular coagulation (DIC) there is widespread activation of coagulation by release of procoagulant material and by generalised platelet aggregation or diffuse endothelial damage. This leads to consumption of platelets and coagulation factors and secondary activation of fibrinolysis with production of fibrin degradation products. The clinical consequence of this sequence of events is initial thrombosis followed by widespread bleeding. The bleeding time, PT ratio and APTT time are all prolonged while the levels of clotting factors and the platelet count are reduced. Causes of DIC include septicaemia, haemolytic transfusion reactions, severe trauma, burns, liver disease and obstetric conditions such as placental abruption.

5. **E – Haemophilia B**

Haemophilia B, also known as Christmas disease, is caused by deficiency in factor IX. The inheritance and clinical features are similar to those of haemophilia A but the incidence is much lower. Not surprisingly, patients with haemophilia B have low levels of factor IX and normal levels of factor VIII:C. In all other aspects, the laboratory test profile of the two diseases is identical.

13. ANATOMY OF THE FEMORAL REGION

1. **C – Femoral nerve**
   The femoral vein lies medial to the artery and these vessels lie within the femoral sheath, formed by the pelvic fascia posteriorly and the transversalis fascia anteriorly, and passing into the thigh deep to the inguinal ligament. The femoral nerve is outside of the sheath.

2. **I – Reflected pectineal part of the inguinal ligament**
   The reflected part of the inguinal ligament passing onto the superior pubic ramus is a medial relation of the canal, the femoral vein being the lateral relation. The femoral canal lies within the femoral sheath together with the femoral vessels.

3. **G – Pectineal ligament (Cooper's ligament)**
   The ligament passes along the superior pubic ramus. Although of no anatomical note, the pectineal ligament is useful surgically to stitch into femoral hernia repairs. The anterior relation of the neck of the hernia is the inguinal ligament.

4. **J – Saphenous opening**
   The femoral canal passes from its neck over the pectineal ligament and pectineus muscle, to the saphenous opening. Femoral hernias emerging at this site are directed proximally over the inguinal ligament, because the superficial fascia is attached to the lower margin of the saphenous opening.

5. **H – Pubic tubercle**
   The pubic tubercle is an important surface marking because it gives attachment to the medial end of the inguinal ligament. The saphenous opening is 1 cm lateral to and 3 cm below this point and is overlain by the groin crease (the exposure of the saphenous opening for venous surgery is in the crease). The superficial inguinal ring is above and medial to the pubic tubercle. This anatomy, although clearly demonstrable in thin people, can be more difficult to identify in the obese, and consequently the differentiation between femoral and inguinal hernias can be tricky in these patients.

14. MUSCLE ATTACHMENTS OF THE LOWER LIMB

1. **E – Iliopsoas**
    The psoas major arises from the intervertebral discs of the lumbar vertebrae, the adjacent vertebrae and their transverse processes, and fibrous arches crossing over the lumbar vertebral bodies. The iliacus is attached to the upper two-thirds of the iliac fossa and these two muscles converge to pass underneath the inguinal ligament and are attached to the lesser trochanter and the adjacent femoral shaft below it.

2. **A, B, J – Adductor longus, adductor magnus and vastus lateralis**
    The adductor muscles are attached proximally to the inferior pubic ramus, the adductor magnus gaining an additional attachment with the hamstring muscles to the ischial tuberosity. The vastus lateralis arises by an aponeurosis from the lateral side of the greater trochanter and the gluteal tuberosity, as well as the lateral lip of the linea aspera. It joins the rectus femoris, vastus medialis and vastus intermedius to form the quadriceps muscle. These four portions are attached to the upper border and sides of the patella, forming a single musculotendinous expansion. From the apex of the patella, a strong tendon descends to attach to the tibial tubercle.

3. **D – Gastrocnemius**
    This is the attachment of the lateral head; the medial head has an equivalent attachment on the corresponding femoral condyle. The muscle is the most superficial in the calf. It descends to join the tendon of the soleus in the mid-calf, forming the tendo calcaneus – this is attached to the middle of the posterior surface of the calcaneus.

4. **F – Peroneus longus**
    The tendon descends behind the lateral malleolus, separated from it by the tendon of peroneus brevis. They cross the lateral surface of the calcaneus, separated by the peroneal tubercle. The peroneus longus gains attachment to the sides of the base of the first metatarsal and adjacent area on the medial cuneiform bone. The peroneus brevis is attached to the tuberosity on the base of the fifth metatarsal.

5. **I – Tibialis posterior**
    The upper attachment is to the posterior surface of the interosseous membrane and adjoining surfaces of the tibia and fibula. The tendon passes deep to that of flexor digitorum longus, grooving the back of the medial malleolus before passing under the flexor retinaculum. In the sole it is attached to the tuberosity of the navicular, and also to all other tarsal bones except the talus.

PAPER 8

Paper 8 Questions

1. THEME: HYPONATRAEMIA

A Addison's disease
B Bendroflumethiazide
C Bronchogenic carcinoma
D Herpes encephalitis
E Hypothyroidism
F *Legionella* pneumonia
G Meningococcal meningitis
H Paroxetine
I Pseudohyponatraemia
J Subarachnoid haemorrhage

The following patients have all presented with hyponatraemia. Please choose the most appropriate cause from the above list. Each cause may be used once, more than once or not at all.

1. A 31-year-old woman is seen in Medical Out-patients after an admission with severe acute pancreatitis. She is a teetotaller. Examination during her hospital stay revealed multiple eruptive xanthomata and despite her being well on discharge, her Na$^+$ is 127 mmol/l.

2. A 26-year-old man is admitted to hospital with a severe headache and photophobia. On examination, he is looking unwell and is pyrexial (37.4 °C) but he has no rash. A CT head scan is unremarkable, other than showing raised intracranial pressure. The diagnosis is confirmed on electroencephalography (EEG) and a polymerase chain reaction test of his CSF.

3. A 32-year-old woman is admitted to hospital with confusion and a headache. On examination, she is very agitated and has a GCS of 13/15, but there is no obvious meningism or photophobia. Respiratory examination reveals a mild expiratory wheeze and she has an oxygen saturation of 87% on air. Routine blood tests show haemoglobin 12.9 g/dl, MCV 87 fl, WCC 7.9 × 10^9/l (with a relative lymphopenia), platelets 322 × 10^9/l; Na$^+$ 117 mmol/l, K$^+$ 3.9 mmol/l, urea 3.9 mmol/l, creatinine 88 μmol/l.

4. A 71-year-old woman who has previously been treated for polymyalgia rheumatica presents in the Emergency Department with low blood pressure, a decreased random blood glucose and marked hyponatraemia. Her mid-stream urine is positive for nitrites and leucocytes. She improves with intravenous dextrose, cefuroxime, gentamicin and hydrocortisone.

5. An 82-year-old woman with vitiligo presents to the Emergency Department with confusion, having been found on the floor by neighbours. On examination, she is described as 'pudgy and overweight', her temperature is 34.3 °C and she is bradycardic. Her ECG shows sinus bradycardia with prominent J-waves. Routine blood tests reveal: haemoglobin 11.7 g/dl, MCV 103 fl, WCC 13.9 × 10⁹/l, platelets 199 × 10⁹/l; Na⁺ 125 mmol/l, K⁺ 3.7 mmol/l, urea 12.9 mmol/l, creatinine 133 μmol/l.

2. THEME: SHORTNESS OF BREATH

A   Asbestosis
B   Asthma
C   Atypical pneumonia
D   Chronic obstructive pulmonary disease
E   Fibrosing alveolitis
F   Histiocytosis
G   Pulmonary embolism
H   Sarcoidosis
I   Streptococcal pneumonia
J   Wegener's granulomatosis

The following patients have all presented with shortness of breath. Please choose the most appropriate cause from the above list. Each diagnosis may be used once, more than once or not at all.

1. A 49-year-old woman with known rheumatoid arthritis presents to her GP with a 3-month history of increasing exertional dyspnoea. On examination, she has several signs of chronic rheumatoid arthritis and on respiratory examination she is found to have fine bibasal inspiratory crepitations.

2. A 61-year-old man who has previously been fit and well is admitted to hospital with a 36–hour history of worsening shortness of breath. On examination he is confused and unwell. Examination of his chest reveals a mild expiratory wheeze but he is unable to co-operate with a peak flow rate. His chest radiograph is relatively unremarkable but his arterial blood gases show signs of marked type-I respiratory failure.

3. A 68-year-old man who is still very active and running marathons has noticed increased wheeze and shortness of breath on training runs. On examination he is relatively well but his peak flow rate is only 300 litres/minute (predicted rate is 480 litres/minute). He is given some inhalers and steroids and returns 10 days later. He feels a lot better and the peak flow rate is now 500 litres/minute.

4. A 71-year-old woman who was recently diagnosed with carcinoma of the breast is admitted to hospital with acute onset of shortness of breath. On examination she is tachypnoeic, tachycardic and has an oxygen saturation of 86% on air. Her chest radiograph is unremarkable.

5. A 29-year-old Afro-Caribbean woman is seen by her GP with increasing shortness of breath on exercise. The GP notes a painful lesion over her shin. A chest radiograph reveals bilateral hilar lymphadenopathy and pulmonary infiltrates.

3. THEME: HEPATOMEGALY

A Alcoholic hepatitis
B Amyloidosis
C Autoimmune hepatitis
D Haemochromatosis
E Hepatitis A virus infection
F Hepatitis B virus infection
G Multiple metastases
H Polycystic kidney disease
I Primary biliary cirrhosis
J Sarcoidosis

The following patients have all presented with hepatomegaly. Please choose the most appropriate cause from the above list. The options may be used once, more than once or not at all.

1. A 29-year-old woman whose grandmother died suddenly of 'stroke' presents in the Emergency Department with confusion. On examination, she is unwell and hypertensive, with a blood pressure of 210/120 mmHg but cardiovascular and respiratory examinations are otherwise unremarkable. Abdominal examination reveals 5-cm hepatomegaly and bilateral ballotable kidneys. Investigations show: Na^+ 129 mmol/l, K^+ 6.9 mmol/l, urea 31.2 mmol/l, creatinine 729 μmol/l.

2. A 24-year-old man has returned from Cambodia with acute jaundice. In the last 2 weeks he has become feverish, with diarrhoea and vomiting. On examination, he is clinically icteric, and has tender, 4-cm hepatomegaly below the costal margin. Investigations show: haemoglobin 13.2 g/dl, MCV 86 fl, WCC 4.1×10^9/l (lymphocytes 2.3×10^9/l), platelets 349×10^9/l; total bilirubin 52 μmol/l, AST 1397 IU/l, ALT 1298 IU/l, alkaline phosphatase 296 IU/l, albumin 31 g/l; INR 1.3. Serological tests confirm an RNA virus.

3. A 58-year-old man known to have alcohol problems presents to his GP with lethargy and malaise. On examination, he looks 'suntanned' and he has spider naevi, Dupuytren's contracture and gynaecomastia. He has 5 cm of hepatomegaly below the right costal margin and possible ascites. He has a capillary blood glucose reading of 16.4 mmol/l.

4. A 67-year-old man presents to his GP with weight loss and constipation. On examination he is cachectic and abdominal examination reveals 6–cm hepatomegaly and a left upper quadrant mass. An ultrasound scan of the abdomen reveals several hyperechogenic areas in the right lobe of the liver.

5. A 48-year-old woman presents to her GP with a 1-year history of pruritis, which is now associated with increasing jaundice. On examination, she is icteric and has 3-cm hepatomegaly. Blood tests reveal anti-smooth muscle antibodies.

4. THEME: PUPILLARY DEFECTS

A   Afferent pupillary defect
B   Argyll Robertson pupil
C   Cataract
D   Fixed, dilated pupil
E   Fixed, dilated pupils
F   Holmes–Adie pupil
G   Horner's syndrome
H   Iridectomy
I   Opiate narcosis
J   Pinpoint pupils

The following patients have all presented with pupillary defects. Please choose the most appropriate cause from the above list. Each cause may be used once, more than once or not at all.

1. A 79-year-old woman with metastatic carcinoma is brought in by ambulance to the Emergency Department with a decreased level of consciousness. She was recently converted to MST from regular oramorph but her husband has continued to give her the oramorph. She recovers a little with an intravenous dose of naloxone.

2. A 19-year-old student is seen for a routine medical on attending his new medical school. The doctor notices that his left pupil is larger than the right and is very slow to react to light. She also finds it difficult to elicit tendon reflexes on the left.

3. A 69-year-old man is admitted to hospital with acute on chronic confusion due to a chest infection. Neurological examination shows an irregular, small pupil on the right. A CT head scan shows atrophy but no focal abnormality. A CSF screen for treponemal disease is positive.

4. A 49-year-old man with hypertension and diabetes mellitus presents in the Emergency Department with a sudden severe headache associated with 'closure' of his right eye. Subsequent MRI and angiography show a ruptured posterior communicating artery aneurysm, which is repaired neurosurgically.

5. A 61-year-old, 'heavy smoker' presents to his GP with a 3-month history of weight loss, haemoptysis and a hoarse voice. More recently he has noticed that his left eye looks 'closed'.

5. THEME: AUTOANTIBODIES

A   Acetylcholine-receptor antibody
B   c-ANCA
C   Anti-endomysial antibody
D   Anti-GBM antibody
E   IF antibody
F   Jo-1 antibody
G   LKM antibody
H   Antimitochondrial antibody
I   p-ANCA
J   Scl-70 antibody

The following patients have all presented with disorders associated with characteristic autoantibodies. Please choose the most appropriate autoantibody from the above list. Each antibody may be used once, more than once or not at all.

1. A 64-year-old woman with well-controlled Graves' disease presents to her GP with a 3-month history of increasing lethargy. On examination, she is clinically euthyroid but looks pale. Routine blood tests confirm that she is euthyroid and gave the following results for other tests: haemoglobin 6.1 g/dl, MCV 114 fl, WCC 3.3 × 10⁹/l, platelets 104 × 10⁹/l. The blood film shows hypersegmented neutrophils.

2. A 17-year-old girl presents to her GP with a 3-month history of steatorrhoea, weight loss and lethargy. On examination she is thin, with a BMI of 17 kg/m²; examination is otherwise unremarkable. Investigations show: haemoglobin 8.7 g/dl, MCV 104 fl, WCC 4.9 × 10⁹/l, platelets 293 × 10⁹/l; U&Es, thyroid function tests and LFTs all normal.

3. A 42-year-old woman presents to her GP with worsening pruritis, malaise and recent onset of jaundice. On examination, she is noted to have early Dupuytren's contracture, spider naevi and 2–3-cm hepatomegaly. Later investigations confirm a diagnosis of primary biliary cirrhosis.

4. A 73-year-old man presents to his GP with increasing weakness around the upper and lower limbs. Examination reveals proximal muscle weakness associated with a heliotrope rash. Routine investigations reveal: ESR 92 mm/hour and creatine kinase 21 000 IU/l and the diagnosis is confirmed on EMG. A chest radiograph reveals a large left apical mass.

5. A 64-year-old man with known carcinoma of the lung presents to his GP with a 3-week history of increasing weakness of his upper and lower limbs and intermittent dysphagia to solids and liquids. On examination there is demonstrated 'fatiguability' but this slowly improves. Diagnosis is confirmed on EMG.

6. THEME: THE ACUTE ABDOMEN

A Acute (severe) pancreatitis
B Biliary peritonitis
C Perforated appendix
D Perforated caecum
E Perforated duodenal ulcer
F Perforated sigmoid disease
G Perforated small intestine
H Primary bacterial peritonitis
I Ruptured abdominal aortic aneurysm
J Superior mesenteric artery occlusion
K Urinary peritonitis

The following are descriptions of patients with an acute abdomen. Please select the most appropriate diagnosis from the above list. Each diagnosis may be used once, more than once or not at all.

1. A 62-year-old man presents with an 8-hour history of increasing upper abdominal pain that is radiating to the back and is associated with nausea and vomiting. On examination, he is dehydrated and clinically jaundiced and has widespread tenderness and guarding.

2. A 72-year-old woman with rheumatoid arthritis presents with a rapid onset of severe abdominal pain that was initially localised to the epigastrium but which is now present all over the abdomen, together with nausea and vomiting. She had been complaining of dyspepsia in the 4 weeks leading up to this presentation. On examination she has a rigid abdomen.

3. A 66-year-old woman with a long history of constipation and left iliac fossa pain presents with a 2-day history of increasingly severe left iliac fossa pain associated with nausea and vomiting. On examination there is widespread peritonism, maximal in the left iliac fossa.

4. An 83-year-old woman presents with a 48-hour history of colicky abdominal pain, abdominal distension and absolute constipation. She is admitted and undergoes further investigation with a gastrograffin enema. During the night you are called to the ward to find the patient moribund, with a rigid abdomen.

5. An 81-year-old man is brought to the Emergency Department by ambulance, having woken with severe abdominal and back pain associated with collapse. On examination, he has a reduced level of consciousness and a distended abdomen. His pulse is 130 bpm and BP 82/52 mmHg.

7. THEME: HEMISCROTAL PAIN

A   Acute epididymo-orchitis
B   Haematocoele
C   Strangulated inguinoscrotal hernia
D   TB orchitis
E   Testicular seminoma
F   Testicular teratoma
G   Testicular torsion
H   Torsion of an epididymal cyst
I   Torsion of hydatid of Morgagni
J   Varicocoele

The following are descriptions of patients with hemiscrotal pain. Please select the most appropriate diagnosis from the above list. Each diagnosis may be used once, more than once or not at all.

1. A 9-year-old boy presents with sudden onset of severe right scrotal pain and nausea. On examination, the right testis is swollen and lying higher than the testis. Examination reveals the right scrotum to be hot, erythematous and very tender, preventing detailed palpation of the scrotal contents.

2. A 25-year-old man is seen in the Emergency Department with a 24-hour history of severe right scrotal pain and swelling. Direct questioning reveals some frequency of micturition and dysuria for several days. On examination, he is febrile (38.6 °C) and the right hemiscrotum is swollen and tender, the overlying skin being red and hot. The WCC is 14.8×10^9/l; and urine dipstick testing shows leucocytes +++ and nitrites +.

3. A 30-year-old man presents with a history of dull, left-sided scrotal ache that has been present for several months. On examination, both testes are normal but the left hemiscrotum appears larger than the right, with a soft, compressible swelling that feels like a bag of worms and is only evident when the patient stands up.

4. A 42-year-old man undergoes a routine vasectomy after having completed his family. The operation is performed as an in-patient because he has a prosthetic heart valve. The following day you are called to the ward because the patient has woken with left-sided scrotal pain and swelling. On examination, the testis is impalpable in an enlarged, tender left hemiscrotum which does not transilluminate.

5. A 33-year-old man presents to his GP with swelling of his left hemiscrotum. He had experienced some dull aching in the scrotum and had been feeling generally unwell for several weeks. The left testis is slightly enlarged and feels hard and irregular in shape. Blood tests show a raised β-hCG but a normal α-FP.

8. THEME: MISCELLANEOUS RADIOGRAPHIC IMAGES – RADIOLOGICAL DIAGNOSIS

*Using the radiographic images **A–J on pages 354–356**, please match the radiological diagnoses with the correct image. You may use each image once, more than once or not at all. There may be more than one image appropriate for each of the diagnoses.*

1. Ectopic calcification.

2. Bone fracture.

3. Loss of the joint space.

4. Cortical thickening.

5. Cortical erosion.

6. Gas in the soft tissue.

9. THEME: ARTERIAL BLOOD GASES

	pH	PaO$_2$ (kPa)	O$_2$ Saturation (%)	PaCO$_2$ (kPa)	HCO$_3^-$ (mmol/l)	Base excess (mmol/l)
A	7.05	13.5	100	2.7	7.1	−19.9
B	7.21	5.9	76	7.3	14.6	−10.5
C	7.38	7.9	87	6.9	35.9	+12.8
D	7.42	13.1	98	4.9	25	+0.7
E	7.48	14.9	100	2.3	24.6	+0.8
F	7.49	8.4	88	2.6	19	−4.9
G	7.66	13.2	98	5.5	67	+21.8

The following patients have all presented with conditions causing derangement of their arterial blood gases. Please choose the most appropriate set of arterial blood gases for each of the patients from the above list. You may use each profile once, more than once or not at all.

1. A 31-year-old man with known severe peptic ulcer disease presents to his local Emergency Department with profuse vomiting. The medical SpR makes a diagnosis of gastric outflow tract obstruction, which is confirmed at upper gastrointestinal endoscopy.

2. A previously fit and well 17-year-old boy presents in his local Emergency Department in a stuporose state. His mother tells the doctors that he has been losing weight recently and 'drinking and weeing for England'. His initial observations and investigations show: pulse 120 bpm, regular, BP 90/60 mmHg, temperature 39.8 °C, capillary blood glucose >48 mmol/l.

3. A 67-year-old woman presents to the Emergency Department with a 12-hour history of increasing shortness of breath and sharp, left-sided chest pain. Of note, she recently underwent an emergency laparotomy for a perforated diverticular abscess. On examination, she is obviously distressed, is hyperventilating and has a loud left-sided pleural rub in the mid-zone.

4. A 64-year-old man with known COPD is seen in the Chest Clinic for assessment for long term oxygen therapy. On questioning, he remains severely limited by his airways disease but is managing well on his nebulisers and inhalers and is relatively well, with no new symptoms.

5. A 23-year-old 'brittle' asthmatic is 'blue-lighted' into the Emergency Department with a severe asthma attack. On arrival he is deeply cyanosed, unable to speak or perform a peak flow and has a near-silent chest. Within 5 minutes of arrival he has a near respiratory arrest and is electively paralysed and ventilated by the attending anaesthetist.

10. THEME: SKIN ULCERATION

A   Anthrax
B   Basal-cell carcinoma
C   Chancrous ulcer
D   Gummatous ulcer
E   Ischaemic ulcer
F   Marjolin's ulcer
G   Neuropathic ulcer
H   Pyoderma gangrenosum
I   Squamous-cell carcinoma
J   Tuberculous ulcer
K   Venous ulcer

The following are descriptions of patients with ulcers. Please select the most appropriate diagnosis from the above list. Each diagnosis may be used once, more than once or not at all.

1. A 42-year-old man presents 3 weeks after unprotected intercourse with a shallow, indurated, painless round ulcer on his penis. The ulcer has a raised, hyperaemic edge and there is associated shotty inguinal lymphadenopathy.

2. An 80-year-old man presents with a 0.5-cm, ovoid ulcer with a central scab and a rolled edge on the inner canthus of the right eye. He thinks that it has been present for some years, causing only itching and occasional very slight bleeding.

3. A 66-year-old retired Royal Marine with a large scar from a burn sustained in the war in Oman presents with a painless, 3-cm area of irregular ulceration within the region of scarring. It is surrounded by a raised edge and has a bloodstained discharge from the base. There is no regional lymphadenopathy.

4. A 58-year-old woman is referred by her GP with an 'extensive' enlarging ulcer above the medial malleolus of the left leg which has now become infected. On examination, there is a 12-cm, irregular, shallow ulcer with a sloping edge and granulation tissue at the base with a seropurulent exudate. There is surrounding erythema, induration and pigmentation.

5. A 42-year-old farmer presents with toxaemia in the Emergency Department. A small ulcer with a black base and indurated edge is noticed on his forearm and there is axillary lymphadenopathy. He describes the ulcer as starting as a small papule, which then broke down to form the ulcer.

11. THEME: EARLY PREGNANCY

A   Anembryonic pregnancy (blighted ovum)
B   Complete miscarriage
C   Ectopic pregnancy
D   Hydatidiform mole (complete)
E   Hydatidiform mole (incomplete)
F   Incomplete miscarriage
G   Inevitable miscarriage
H   Missed (delayed) miscarriage
I   Septic miscarriage
J   Threatened miscarriage

From the above list please choose the diagnosis most likely to describe the clinical picture. Each diagnosis may be used once, more than once or not at all.

1. A 28-year-old woman, gravida 1, para 0 (G1P0), has had 6 weeks of amenorrhoea, moderate vaginal bleeding and lower abdominal cramps. A pregnancy test is positive. Examination reveals no abdominal or vaginal tenderness and the cervical os is closed. A transvaginal ultrasound scan (TVS) reveals a 20 mm × 20 mm area in the endometrial cavity suggestive of retained products of conception (RPOC).

2. A 28-year-old woman, gravida 1, para 0 (G1P0), has had 6 weeks of amenorrhoea, mild vaginal bleeding and lower abdominal cramps. A pregnancy test is positive. Examination reveals mild lower abdominal tenderness and also mild tenderness on vaginal examination, but the cervical os is closed with no excitation. TVS reveals an empty uterus and free fluid in the rectovaginal pouch. Over the next 48 hours her β-hCG levels go from 1200 IU/l to 1370 IU/l.

3. A 28-year-old woman, gravida 1, para 0 (G1P0), has had 6 weeks of amenorrhoea, moderate vaginal bleeding and lower abdominal cramps. A pregnancy test is positive. Examination reveals no abdominal or vaginal tenderness and the cervical os is closed. TVS reveals an empty uterus and no free fluid in the rectovaginal pouch. Over the next 10 days her pregnancy test becomes negative.

4. A 28-year-old woman, gravida 1, para 0 (G1P0), has had 7 weeks of amenorrhoea, mild vaginal bleeding and mild lower abdominal cramps. A pregnancy test is positive. Examination reveals no abdominal or vaginal tenderness and the cervical os is closed. TVS reveals an intrauterine pregnancy with a measurement (crown–rump length) equivalent to 6 weeks. There is no fetal heart activity. There is no free fluid in the rectovaginal pouch.

5. A 28-year-old woman, gravida 1, para 0 (G1P0), has had 7 weeks of amenorrhoea, mild vaginal bleeding and mild lower abdominal cramps. The pregnancy test is positive. Examination reveals no abdominal or vaginal tenderness but the uterus feels about 12 weeks' gestation and the cervical os is closed. TVS reveals a large volume of cystic spaces in the endometrial cavity and no fetal pole.

12. THEME: DISEASES OF THE HEART

A Atrial myxoma
B Congestive cardiomyopathy
C Constrictive pericarditis
D Cor pulmonale
E Fibrinous pericarditis
F Hypertrophic cardiomyopathy
G Infective endocarditis
H Mitral valve stenosis
I Myocarditis
J Ventricular aneurysm

From the above list, please select the disease that each of the following patients is most likely to have. Each diagnosis may be used once, more than once or not at all.

1. Three days after an anterior myocardial infarct, a 63-year-old man develops a sharp chest pain which is worse on movement and on lying down. Auscultation reveals a pericardial rub and his ECG shows 'saddle-shaped' ST-segment elevation in several leads.

2. A 75-year-old woman with a long history of COPD develops pitting oedema of both ankles. On examination, she has a palpable liver and moderate ascites. An echocardiogram shows right ventricular hypertrophy.

3. A 19-year-old man collapses while playing football and cannot be resuscitated. He had no previous history of ischaemic heart disease, hypertension or valve abnormalities. At post-mortem examination the heart weighs 800 g and shows marked left ventricular hypertrophy. The ventricular septum is particularly thick.

4. A 59-year-old man presents with a 1-week history of pyrexia, fatigue, night sweats and muscle pains. Four days before the onset of these symptoms he had had a dental extraction and had forgotten to tell the dentist about his past history of rheumatic fever. On examination, his temperature is 38.5 °C and he has a diastolic murmur. Blood cultures grow *Streptococcus viridans*.

5. A 65-year-old woman suffers a large anteroseptal myocardial infarct. Six months later she presents in acute left ventricular failure, her chest radiograph showing a left ventricular 'bulge'. Echocardiography shows that the bulge expands during systole.

13. THEME: ANATOMY OF THE INGUINAL REGION

A Conjoint tendon
B Deep inguinal ring
C External oblique muscle
D Inferior epigastric vessels
E Inguinal ligament
F Internal oblique muscle
G Reflected pectineal part of the inguinal ligament
H Superficial inguinal ring
I Transversalis fascia
J Transversus abdominis muscle

For each of the following descriptions, please choose the most appropriate structure from the above list. Each structure may be used once, more than once or not at all.

1. Inferior relation of the medial end of the inguinal canal.

2. The structure through which a direct inguinal hernia enters the inguinal canal.

3. The structure through which an indirect inguinal hernia enters the inguinal canal.

4. Superior relation of the inguinal canal.

5. Medial relation of the neck of an indirect inguinal hernia.

14. THEME: VESSELS OF THE NECK

A Common carotid artery
B External jugular vein
C Facial artery
D Internal carotid artery
E Internal jugular vein
F Maxillary artery
G Subclavian artery
H Superficial temporal artery
I Thoracic duct
J Vertebral artery

For each of the following descriptions, please choose the most appropriate vessel from the above list. Each vessel may be used once, more than once or not at all.

1. Lies adjacent to the transverse process of the seventh cervical vertebra. ☐

2. A posterior relation of the opening between the sternal and clavicular heads of sternocleidomastoid muscle. ☐

3. Grooves the upper surface of the first rib. ☐

4. Crossed from lateral to medial by the hypoglossal nerve. ☐

5. Palpable just above the zygomatic arch. ☐

Paper 8 Answers

1. HYPONATRAEMIA

1. **I – Pseudohyponatraemia**
   This patient has signs and symptoms consistent with hypertriglyceridaemia, as evidenced by the recent pancreatitis and the eruptive xanthomata. Her hyponatraemia is in fact 'pseudohyponatraemia' due to the excess triglycerides.

2. **D – Herpes encephalitis**
   This young man has developed hyponatraemia secondary to raised intracranial pressure and secondary SIADH. All causes of raised intracranial pressure, atypical pneumonias, bronchogenic carcinoma, diffuse pulmonary fibrosis and TB can cause SIADH. The diagnosis is confirmed by paired serum and urinary osmolalities, which will show a relatively concentrated urine in the presence of dilute serum. SIADH can only be diagnosed in the presence of a normal blood pressure, euvolaemia and euthyroidism.

3. **F – *Legionella* pneumonia**
   This patient has signs and symptoms of an atypical pneumonia, most likely to be due to *Legionella pneumophila*. This infection commonly causes a SIADH with marked hyponatraemia, exacerbating the associated confusion.

4. **A – Addison's disease**
   This patient has been on long-term steroids for polymyalgia rheumatica and this has led to secondary Addison's with hypotension, hypoglycaemia and hyponatraemia. Patients require hydrocortisone replacement, which initially should be given intravenously or intramuscularly.

5. **E – Hypothyroidism**
   This elderly woman has presented with hypothermia, bradycardia, a macrocytic anaemia and hyponatraemia. Her clinical appearance and these results suggest hypothyroidism. The hyponatraemia is thought to be due to a similar mechanism to SIADH although this is still unclear.

2. SHORTNESS OF BREATH

1. E – Fibrosing alveolitis
This woman has developed fibrosing alveolitis secondary to her rheumatoid arthritis. This is a similar picture to idiopathic pulmonary fibrosis and can also be associated with finger clubbing. Other respiratory or pulmonary manifestations of rheumatoid disease in the chest include pleuritic chest pain, exudative pleural effusions and intrapulmonary nodules.

2. C – Atypical pneumonia
This man has signs, symptoms and investigation results compatible with an atypical pneumonia. This group of pneumonias are atypical for four reasons; They have an ATYPICAL:

- Presentation and symptoms – multisystem involvement and atypical respiratory findings, including shortness of breath, dry cough and wheeze.
- Signs – often the respiratory findings are 'unimpressive' and the chest is often clear, but the patient looks unwell and is very dyspnoeic. The patient can also have multisystem signs, including confusion, drowsiness, jaundice and rashes.
- Investigations – the white cell count can be normal but have an abnormal differential. Atypical infections can also cause SIADH and hyponatraemia, autoimmune haemolytic anaemia (AIHA), thrombocytopenia and hepatic jaundice. The chest radiograph is often unremarkable but might show diffuse alveolar shadowing resembling pulmonary oedema. The arterial blood gases typically show type-I respiratory failure. The atypical organisms are difficult to culture in the laboratory and antibody titres are often necessary. A new urinary *Legionella* antigen test is also being used.
- Antibiotics – patients with atypical pneumonia should be treated with high-dose erythromycin or clarithromycin, rifampicin or a tetracycline.

3. B – Asthma
This man probably has exercise-induced asthma. He is unlikely to be a smoker (as he is a marathon runner) but others in his household might be smokers. He should be advised to use a prophylactic β_2-agonist before exercising but might require regular inhaled steroids if symptoms worsen or persist.

4. G – Pulmonary embolism
This patient has developed a pulmonary embolism on a background of carcinoma of the breast. Malignancy increases the risk of thromboembolic events and any middle-aged to older patient presenting with an unexplained deep vein thrombosis or pulmonary embolism needs investigation, including the PSA (in men), LFTs and a corrected Ca^{2+}, a chest radiograph, a mammogram (in women) and ultrasound of the pelvis and hepatobiliary tree. This patient requires confirmation of the diagnosis by V/Q scan or spiral CT and angiography, and long-term treatment with warfarin.

5. **H – Sarcoidosis**

This patient has developed pulmonary sarcoidosis and associated erythema nodosum. The chest radiographic findings are divided into:

Stage 0 – no changes

Stage 1 – bilateral hilar lymphadenopathy (BHL)

Stage 2 – BHL plus mid-zone changes/infiltrates

Stage 3 – diffuse pulmonary infiltrates.

All patients require specialist review and some patients with progressive disease will need steroids (with bone-sparing agents) and occasionally immunosuppression.

3. HEPATOMEGALY

1. **H – Polycystic kidney disease**
    This woman has signs of adult polycystic kidney disease (APKD), leading to renal failure and secondary polycystic enlargement of the liver. APKD can cause cystic changes and enlargement within all of the major intra-abdominal organs, including the liver, spleen, pancreas and ovaries. Her grandmother probably died of a ruptured berry aneurysm (causing a fatal subarachnoid haemorrhage).

2. **E – Hepatitis A virus infection**
    This young man has developed an acute hepatitic jaundice secondary to an acute hepatitis A virus infection. Hepatitis A virus is an RNA virus and causes an acute jaundice following a flu-like illness. This is usually a self-limiting condition. In rarer cases it can cause fulminant liver failure requiring liver transplantation. It is spread by the faecal–oral route and is endemic in areas of poverty and poor water hygiene.

3. **D – Haemochromatosis**
    This man has signs consistent with haemochromatosis, as evidenced by his 'suntan', which is due to melanin deposition within the skin, his hyperglycaemia (secondary to pancreatic infiltration) and chronic liver disease (causing the spider naevi, Dupuytren's contracture and gynaecomastia). Haemochromatosis is associated with chronic alcohol excess in 15–20% of cases but alcohol is not suggested as the primary cause. The diagnosis can be confirmed by a markedly elevated serum ferritin and by liver biopsy (if required).

4. **G – Multiple metastases**
    This man has a probable carcinoma of the colon with secondary deposits in the liver. Depending on his general health and wishes, he might be offered surgical, oncological and/or palliative-care treatment.

5. **J – Primary biliary cirrhosis**
    This middle-aged woman has developed primary biliary cirrhosis, which is classically defined by the presence of antimitochondrial antibodies but which can also be associated with an anti-smooth muscle antibody (which is more characteristic of autoimmune hepatitis).

4. PUPILLARY DEFECTS

1. **J – Pinpoint pupils**
   This patient is receiving oramorph (morphine elixir) and MST (morphine sulphate tablets) which has led to opiate narcosis. Patients can present with drowsiness, unconsciousness, pinpoint pupils, shallow breathing or even respiratory arrest. With large accidental overdoses, patients can require an intravenous infusion of naloxone or even ventilation until the effects have worn off. Pinpoint pupils and unconsciousness can also be seen in brainstem strokes.

2. **F – Holmes–Adie pupil**
   This patient has a Holmes–Adie pupil. This is a benign, idiopathic disorder in which the pupillary reflexes and ipsilateral tendon reflexes are slow and sluggish. The pupil is mid-dilated and reacts slowly to direct light.

3. **B – Argyll Robertson pupil**
   This man has an Argyll Robertson pupil due to neurosyphilis. His CSF studies confirm treponemal disease and he should receive a course of penicillin. The small, irregular Argyll Robertson pupil can be unilateral or bilateral and is now relatively rare. It can also rarely occur in diabetes mellitus.

4. **D – Fixed dilated pupil**
   This patient has developed an acute painful third nerve palsy associated with the rupture of a posterior communicating artery aneurysm. The patient has a ptosis associated with a fixed, dilated pupil which looks 'down and out' due to the unopposed actions of the superior oblique and abductor muscles (supplied by the fourth and sixth cranial nerves, respectively).

5. **G – Horner's syndrome**
   This patient has developed a left-sided Horner's syndrome in association with a left-sided apical lung cancer. Horner's syndrome is due to an interruption of the sympathetic nerve supply to the pupil, anywhere from the hypothalamus, down through the brainstem and cervical cord as it emerges at T1, and up through the neck, synapsing within the superior cervical ganglion and on to the eye. Horner's syndrome is the association of pupillary constriction (miosis) and partial ptosis, plus or minus enophthalmos. There can also be unilateral loss of sweating (anhidrosis), which is complete with central nervous causes, partial with pre-cervical ganglionic causes and absent with post-cervical ganglionic causes.

5. AUTOANTIBODIES

1. D – IF antibody

This patient has developed a macrocytic anaemia with associated pancytopenia and hypersegmented neutrophils. They all point to a diagnosis of pernicious anaemia, where autoantibodies form against intrinsic factor production and release from the gastric parietal cells, there is complex formation between the vitamin B_{12} molecule and intrinsic factor, and the complexes subsequently bind to receptors within the ileum. Pernicious anaemia is commonly associated with other autoimmune diseases, including hypothyroidism.

2. C – Anti-endomysial antibody

This young woman has developed coeliac disease, an autoimmune disorder of the upper gastrointestinal tract. Autoantibodies in this condition include antigliadin and antireticulin antibodies and the anti-endomysial antibody, which is specific for the condition. A newer specific antibody, anti-tissue transglutaminase (anti-tTG) has also been identified recently.

3. H – Antimitochondrial antibody

This patient has developed primary biliary cirrhosis, an autoimmune condition of the liver that is primarily seen in middle-aged women. There are several autoantibodies associated with the condition but the commonest, antimitochondrial antibodies (AMA), are found in over 90% of patients. Seven agenic components within the mitochondria have now been identified as precipitants of the autoimmune reaction. Anti-smooth muscle antibodies are also found in this condition, although these are more commonly seen in autoimmune hepatitis.

4. F – Anti-Jo-1 antibody

This man has developed a myositis, as evidenced by the limb weakness and associated dramatic elevation of his creatine kinase. He has a characteristic heliotrope rash around the eyes, suggesting a diagnosis of dermatomyositis, which in turn is characterised by the presence of anti-Jo-1 antibody. In later life dermatomyositis has a significant association with bronchogenic and other cancers.

5. A – Acetylcholine-receptor antibody

This man has developed Lambert–Eaton syndrome, a myasthenic syndrome classically associated with small-cell carcinoma of the lung. The autoantibodies in this condition act pre-synaptically to block the release of acetylcholine. In myasthenia gravis the antibodies act post-synaptically to block acetylcholine binding, as well as causing down-regulation of the receptors and complement-mediated lysis.

6. THE ACUTE ABDOMEN

The term 'acute abdomen' describes a non-traumatic catastrophic event that affects any of the abdominal organs. The characteristic presenting feature is acute, severe abdominal pain.

1.   A – Acute (severe) pancreatitis
This presentation is consistent with several of the diagnoses in the options list. However, the presence of jaundice pushes us towards a diagnosis of gallstone pancreatitis, when, in addition to the features of pancreatitis, there can also be features of biliary obstruction caused by a stone impacted at the ampulla of Vater. Treatment in such a case is intensive resuscitation and monitoring, as for all patients with pancreatitis, and also consideration should be given to performing an urgent ERCP to remove the stone and thus prevent further disease exacerbation.

2.   E – Perforated duodenal ulcer
This is still one of the most common causes of peritonitis despite a huge drop in incidence as a result of the widespread use of H_2-blockers and proton-pump inhibitors. The diagnosis should be suggested in this case by the history of rheumatoid arthritis with the likely use of NSAIDs. Treatment is aggressive resuscitation and then surgery (oversew).

3.   F – Perforated sigmoid disease
This is a characteristic presentation of this complication of diverticular disease. The sigmoid colon is by far the most common site, hence left iliac fossa pain. The perforation can be small and localised as a paracolic abscess or can lead to purulent or faecal peritonitis. The former can be drained radiologically, but a patient with peritonitis requires an emergency laparotomy and sigmoid colectomy (after appropriate resuscitation).

4.   D – Perforated caecum
This patient has presented with a large-bowel obstruction. The obstructing lesion is most commonly in the sigmoid colon or rectum (causes including carcinoma, diverticular disease and volvulus) but the site of maximal dilatation is the caecum. When tension in the caecal wall occludes the blood supply, the wall can become gangrenous and will eventually perforate, leading to faecal peritonitis (and often death). Tenderness in the right iliac fossa in a patient with large-bowel obstruction should therefore prompt urgent surgery.

5.   I – Ruptured abdominal aortic aneurysm
This diagnosis should be strongly suspected in a patient presenting with an acute abdomen and evidence of hypovolaemic shock. An expansile mass might not be palpable after a leak or rupture because of haematoma formation.

7. HEMISCROTAL PAIN

1. **G – Testicular torsion**
   This is evidenced by the patient's age and the classic history and examination findings. The commonest age for torsion is 10–15 years (it very rarely occurs over the age of 21). It is, however, sometimes difficult to distinguish a torsion from acute epididymo-orchitis in sexually active young males. Whilst the two can usually be clinically separated, surgical exploration is mandatory if there is any doubt over the diagnosis in order to prevent loss of the testis. (**NB:** Missed torsion is a recognised source of litigation.)

2. **A – Acute epididymo-orchitis**
   Epididymo-orchitis is an inflammation that is usually primarily of the epididymis and is most commonly of bacterial aetiology. In younger men, it is usually secondary to sexually transmitted diseases such as *Chlamydia* or gonorrhoea (torsion must be excluded – see above); it also commonly occurs in an older age group, when it is secondary to urinary tract infection with coliforms.

3. **J – Varicocoele**
   This is a bunch of dilated and tortuous veins in the pampiniform plexus (ie varicose veins in the spermatic cord). It occurs more commonly on the left and when it is large is causes an aching/dragging sensation in the scrotum.

4. **B – Haematocoele**
   This is evidenced by the history of surgery (and especially with the use of warfarin therapy, as would be the case for this patient with a prosthetic valve) and examination findings. A haematocoele is a collection of blood within the tunica vaginalis. Acute haematocoele is a common accompaniment of scrotal trauma (eg surgical, football, fighting), but a secondary haematocele can also occur with infection and tumours of the testis. In either case, it can be distinguished from a hydrocoele because it does not transilluminate. If left untreated, the resultant haematoma can form a hard, non-tender mass, which is clinically indistinguishable from a testicular tumour.

5. **E – Testicular seminoma**
   This is evidenced by the age of the patient, the history and examination findings and by the tumour markers. There are two common primary testicular tumours, teratoma and seminoma. Seminomas most commonly occur in 30–40-year-olds. In contrast, teratoma occurs in a younger age group (20–30-year-olds). Both present as a painless swelling or lump in the testis, which is palpable as a hard irregular mass in cases where a secondary hydrocoele is absent (see above). Alpha-fetoprotein is produced by yolk-sac cellular elements and is raised in teratoma but not in seminoma; β-hCG is secreted by trophoblastic cells and can be present in either tumour type.

8. MISCELLANEOUS RADIOGRAPHIC IMAGES – RADIOLOGICAL DIAGNOSIS

1. **(P8–10) A, D – Osteomyelitis and calcified thyroid nodule**
   Radiograph **A** is an AP film of the right foot and shows evidence of calcification of the dorsalis pedis artery. This is almost pathognomonic of diabetes mellitus. Radiograph **D** is a plain film of the upper thorax and cervical spine and shows the trachea grossly displaced to the left. This is associated with evidence of ectopic calcification within the soft tissues on the right side of the neck, due to a large, calcified, probably multinodular goitre.

2. **(P8–10) J – Skull fracture**
   This lateral skull radiograph shows a large frontoparietal fracture, consistent with blunt trauma.

3. **(P8–10) C, E – Cervical spondylosis and osteoarthritis of the left knee**
   Radiograph **C** shows cervical spondylosis and radiograph **E** shows the classic deformity and features of an osteoarthritic right knee joint. Loss of joint space is a radiographic characteristic of osteoarthritis. Other features to look for include periarticular sclerosis and osteophyte formation, particularly prominent in radiograph **E**.

4. **(P8–10) B – Paget's disease of bone**
   This plain radiograph of the right hip joint shows characteristic features of Paget's disease of bone. Due to the abnormal bone turnover, there is cortical thickening, which is particularly marked around the pelvic bones, with an associated abnormal traebecular pattern.

5. and 6. (P8–10) A – Osteomyelitis
   This plain radiograph of the right foot shows gross abnormalities that are consistent with osteomyelitis with soft-tissue involvement. There is marked soft-tissue swelling with a gas shadow visible within the soft tissue of the second toe. There is marked destruction of the second metacarpophalangeal joint with evidence of erosion of the head of the second metacarpal bone and proximal phalanx. The calcification within the dorsalis pedis artery is highly suggestive of diabetes mellitus.

IMAGES: pages 354–356

9. ARTERIAL BLOOD GASES

1. **G – pH 7.66, PaO$_2$ 13.2 kPa, O$_2$ saturation 98%, PaCO$_2$ 5.5 kPa, HCO$_3^-$ 67 mmol/l, base excess +21.8 mmol/l**
    This patient has developed gastric outflow tract obstruction. In the neonate this can be caused by congenital pyloric stenosis and is marked by projectile vomiting of feeds. In the young adult it is usually due to severe peptic ulcer disease. In the older adult malignancy should be excluded by oesophagogastroduodenoscopy or imaging. The vomiting causes loss of hydogen ions and this is in turn leads to a relative excess of bicarbonate ions. Other causes of metabolic alkalosis include chronic diarrhoea, ingestion of alkali (eg milk-alkali syndrome), drugs (eg diuretics) and Bartter's syndrome (a defect within the renal tubules leading to hypokalaemic hypochloraemic metabolic alkalosis).

2. **A – pH 7.05, PaO$_2$ 13.5 kPa, O$_2$ saturation 100%, PaCO$_2$ 2.7 kPa, HCO$_3^-$ 7.1 mmol/l, base excess –19.9 mmol/l**
    This young man presents with a history of polydypsia and polyuria and has now become acutely unwell with hyperglycaemia. The most likely abnormality is a severe metabolic acidosis secondary to diabetic ketoacidosis (DKA). Patients presenting with this clinical picture are often very unwell, with hypotension and shock. This leads to renal impairment and lactic acidosis which both contribute to the worsening acid-base problem. The management is based around intravenous insulin, fluid resuscitation, potassium supplementation and anticoagulation, as well as identifying and treating any underlying precipitating cause.

3. **F – pH 7.49, PaO$_2$ 8.4 kPa, O$_2$ saturation 88%, PaCO$_2$ 2.6 kPa, HCO$_3^-$ 19 mmol/l, base excess –4.9 mmol/l**
    This woman has presented with features suggestive of an acute pulmonary embolism. This will lead to type-I respiratory failure with a corresponding respiratory alkalosis (due to hyperventilation) and a metabolic acidosis (in this case this is in the early stages). Note the very similar gases in profile E. This patient is also hyperventilating but they are not hypoxic and there is no suggestion of any acidosis. The other group of patients who present with hyperventilation are those with severe metabolic acidosis, where they attempt to compensate for their acidosis by producing a respiratory alkalosis ('Kussmaul's breathing' in DKA).

4. **C – pH 7.38, PaO$_2$ 7.9 kPa, O$_2$ saturation 87%, PaCO$_2$ 6.9 kPa, HCO$_3^-$ 35.9 mmol/l, base excess +12.8 mmol/l**
    This gentleman is attending Out-patients for assessment of long-term oxygen therapy. He is relatively well and clinically stable. The arterial blood gases show that he has type-II respiratory failure with a compensated respiratory acidosis (ie a metabolic alkalosis). Patients who chronically retain carbon dioxide (producing a respiratory acidosis) compensate by retaining bicarbonate renally. The pH is normal, which means that the system is compensated.

5. **B – pH 7.21, PaO$_2$ 5.9 kPa, O$_2$ saturation 76%, PaCO$_2$ 7.3 kPa, HCO$_3^-$ 14.6 mmol/l, base excess –10.5 mmol/l**
    Asthma usually produces type-1 respiratory failure and if severe causes a lactic acidosis. However, as the patient becomes increasingly fatigued, their respiratory rate falls and they may suffer type-2 respiratory failure. This is accompanied by lactic acidosis, which in turn makes the drop in pH greater.

10. SKIN ULCERATION

Ulcers are correctly described (as in this question) in terms of their location, size, shape, edge, base and discharge and this should be remembered by the candidate faced with an ulcer as a short case. The other most favoured examiner's question is probably the definition: 'a discontinuation of an epithelial surface'.

1. **C – Chancrous ulcer (syphilitic chancre)**
    The classic description, site and short time interval after unprotected sex makes this a strong possibility. Classically called a 'Hunterian chancre' (presumably because his was the first description rather than on the basis of first-hand experience), this is the pathognomonic lesion of primary syphilis. The other ulcer in syphilis, a gummatous ulcer, occurs as a late manifestation of the infection at a site distant from that of sexual contact and as a result of a granulomatous hypersensitivity reaction.

2. **B – Basal-cell carcinoma**
    The characteristic history and ulcer description and classic site (95% are on the face) suggest this diagnosis. While the lesion grows very slowly and does not metastasise, if it is left deep erosion can occur – the so-called 'rodent ulcer'. This is a favourite of pictorial textbooks for its macabre appearance, but is now fortunately quite rare.

3. **F – Marjolin's ulcer**
    This is an eponym reserved for a squamous-cell carcinoma which arises in a long-standing area of inflammation or scarring, most commonly in practice a chronic venous ulcer or a third-degree burn. Most of the features of a squamous-cell carcinoma are present, although there will be no lymphadenopathy because deep scars have no lymphatic drainage.

4. **K – Venous ulcer**
    This is the commonest site (the gaiter area) and typical description of this ulcer, which is caused by deep venous insufficiency in the lower limb, usually as a result of previous deep vein thrombosis. In addition to lipodermatosclerosis (described) there can be other features of venous disease (eg varicose veins, other healed ulcers, limb swelling). Treatment is with graduated compression bandages/stockings (interestingly, a concept first described by Hippocrates).

5. **A – Anthrax**
    Caused by the large, Gram-positive, aerobic, spore-forming organism, *Bacillus anthracis*, this is a description of cutaneous anthrax (the most common type). The organism is found in cattle and those affected are usually dairy or beef farmers, zoo-keepers, cowboys and buffalo hunters (although these last two are rare in the UK!). Currently uncommon, it is hoped that in the light of terrorist threats this will not become a more topical subject!

11. EARLY PREGNANCY

1. **F – Incomplete miscarriage**
    Moderate to heavy vaginal bleeding is suggestive of a form of definite miscarriage compared with mild vaginal bleeding, which is more common with threatened miscarriage (per vaginal bleeding before 24 weeks with a viable intrauterine pregnancy) and ectopic pregnancy. Patient-reporting of bleeding can, however, be misleading and is only a guide. If there is no abdominal or vaginal tenderness this makes sepsis or ectopic pregnancy less likely. Retained products of conception (RPOC) on a transvaginal ultrasound scan (TVS) tells us this was an intrauterine pregnancy and that, because products were left behind, it is an incomplete miscarriage. This gives no indication of the underlying problem with the pregnancy and is purely a description of the stage of the miscarriage at presentation.

2. **C – Ectopic pregnancy**
    Any of the options on the list are possible, given the clinical history, but unless it is a very early pregnancy, both complete and incomplete miscarriages tend to have more than mild bleeding. The presence of both abdominal and vaginal tenderness makes sepsis or ectopic pregnancy more likely. An empty uterus on TVS with free fluid in the rectovaginal pouch means that there might have been haemorrhage due to ectopic pregnancy. A slow-rising β-hCG is typical with ectopic pregnancy and if an intrauterine pregnancy is present it is likely to be visible on TVS with a β-hCG of >1000 IU/l.

3. **B – Complete miscarriage**
    Again, moderate to heavy vaginal bleeding is more suggestive of a form of definite miscarriage (as in question 1) and the fact that there is no abdominal or vaginal tenderness makes sepsis or ectopic pregnancy less likely. The closed cervical os tells us only that any form of miscarriage is not actively occuring at the time of examination. An empty uterus on TVS can occur with a very early intrauterine pregnancy (too small), with ectopic pregnancy and with a complete miscarriage. The absence of free fluid in the rectovaginal pouch means there has at least been no haemorrhage due to ectopic pregnancy (less likely). The history and the rapid disappearance of β-hCG mean that a complete miscarriage is the diagnosis as there tends to be either a slow fall, stasis or a slow rise of β-hCG with ectopic pregnancy.

4. **H – Missed (delayed) miscarriage**
    This is by definition not an ectopic pregnancy. This is a non-viable embryo as fetal heart activity should be visible at 6 weeks. This is known as a 'delayed' or 'missed' miscarriage where there has been early embryonic demise. This describes the type of miscarriage rather than its stage of completion. This cannot be a threatened miscarriage (vaginal bleeding before 24 weeks with a viable intrauterine pregnancy).

5. **D – Hydatidiform mole (complete)**
    'Large for dates' in early pregnancy is usually due to wrong dates, multiple pregnancy, or pelvic masses such as fibroids or molar pregnancies. TVS descriptions of complete hydatidiform moles usually feature large amounts of cystic spaces (hydropic chorionic villi), a 'snow storm' appearance and no evidence of a fetus. This is therefore most likely to be a complete mole as the TVS images are usually less striking with partial moles and can even show some normal features.

12. DISEASES OF THE HEART

1.   E – Fibrinous pericarditis

Fibrinous pericarditis occurs at about the second or third day after a transmural myocardial infarct as an inflammatory response to the necrotic heart muscle. It is usually localised to the area of infarction. Fibrin on the pericardial surfaces manifests clinically as acute onset of pain and fever. The 'rubbing together' of the inflamed visceral and parietal pericardia leads to a pericardial friction rub on auscultation, though this tends to disappear if a pericardial effusion develops. This type of pericarditis usually resolves spontaneously.

2.   D – Cor pulmonale

This patient has symptoms and signs of right-sided cardiac failure. Given her history, this is most likely to be due to pulmonary hypertension resulting from long-standing COPD. The resultant right ventricular hypertrophy and/or right ventricular failure are known as 'cor pulmonale'. Acute cor pulmonale is most often caused by pulmonary embolism while chronic cor pulmonale is due to any lung disease that results in pulmonary hypertension. In chronic cor pulmonale the right ventricle develops compensatory hypertrophy and progressively dilates. Ultimately, it is unable to maintain cardiac output at normal levels and when this occurs, symptoms and signs of right-sided congestive cardiac failure develop (eg dependent oedema, effusions and hepatomegaly).

3.   F – Hypertrophic cardiomyopathy

'Cardiomyopathy' is a general term used to describe heart muscle disease of unknown origin. Hypertrophic cardiomyopathy (HCM), also known as 'asymmetric septal hypertrophy', is characterised by myocardial hypertrophy and disorganisation of myocytes on histology. The hypertrophy is most pronounced in the left ventricle and interventricular septum, particularly in the area immediately beneath the aortic valve. The normal weight of a heart in an adult man is 300–400 g, so in this patient the weight of the heart is at least twice normal. Because the thick-walled ventricle is abnormally stiff, left ventricular filling (and therefore emptying) is impaired, compounded in about 30% of cases by outflow obstruction, Typical presenting features include chest pain, dyspnoea, syncope, arrhythmias and sudden death.

4.   G – Infective endocarditis

Infective endocarditis is an infection of either the cardiac valves or the mural surface of the endocardium. It is usually the consequence of two factors, an abnormal endocardium (which facilitates bacterial adherence and growth) and the presence of organisms in the bloodstream (bacteraemia). This patient has an abnormal endocardium because of chronic rheumatic valvular disease and bacteraemia as a result of a dental extraction. Most cases of infective endocarditis are caused by streptococci or staphylococci, though numerous other organisms have been implicated. *Streptococcus viridans* is an α-haemolytic streptococcus that colonises the mouth and is often associated with dental disease or procedures. The hallmark of infective endocarditis is the presence of large friable vegetations containing bacteria, fibrin and platelets on the affected cardiac valve. These not only cause destruction of the valve leaflets but can also fragment, resulting in embolic phenomena. Infective endocarditis typically presents, therefore, with features of chronic infection (such as fever and night sweats), valvular damage (such as 'crashing' acute regurgitation or cardiac failure) and emboli (such as stroke and splinter haemorrhages).

5. **J – Ventricular aneurysm**

Ventricular aneurysm is a late complication of a transmural myocardial infarction. It results from replacement of the infarcted muscle by a thin layer of collagenous scar tissue that progressively stretches and bulges as the intraventricular pressure rises during systole. Complications of ventricular aneurysms include arrhythmias, left ventricular failure and mural thrombosis with systemic embolisation; rupture of the aneurysm itself is rare.

13. ANATOMY OF THE INGUINAL REGION

1. **G – Reflected pectineal part of the inguinal ligament**
   The inguinal ligament is the lower upturned edge of the external oblique muscle. It is an inferior relation of the inguinal canal, and in the medial part of the canal the inguinal ligament is reflected backwards onto the superior pubic ramus. This part is also known as the 'lacunar ligament'.

2. **I – Transversalis fascia**
   A direct inguinal hernia protrudes through a weakness in the posterior wall of the canal, beneath the conjoint tendon, and protrudes through the superficial inguinal ring alongside the spermatic cord.

3. **B – Deep inguinal ring**
   Indirect inguinal hernias pass within the spermatic cord through the deep ring, the canal and the superficial inguinal ring, and can follow the cord into the scrotum, whereas direct inguinal hernias passing through the superficial inguinal ring do not have a natural pathway to descend into the scrotum.

4. **F – Internal oblique muscle**
   The internal oblique muscle arises from the lateral two-thirds of the inguinal ligament, initially lying anterior to the deep inguinal ring. It then arches over the inguinal canal and is joined by the aponeurotic fibres of the transversus abdominis muscle to form the conjoint tendon. This passes behind the medial end of the inguinal canal to the superior pubic ramus.

5. **D – Inferior epigastric vessels**
   A direct inguinal hernia emerges medial to the vessels through Hesselbach's triangle, the other two sides being the lateral border of the rectus abdominis muscle and, below, the inguinal ligament. Pressure over the deep inguinal ring (just above the mid-point of the inguinal ligament) will control a reduced indirect inguinal hernia but, on coughing, a direct inguinal hernia will still bulge into the canal and out through the superficial inguinal ring.

14. VESSELS OF THE NECK

1. **J – Vertebral artery**
    The artery arises from the first part of the subclavian artery and passes adjacent to the seventh vertebra on its way to the vertebral arterial canal of the sixth and upper cervical transverse processes.

2. **F – Internal jugular vein**
    This is a valuable landmark for closed or open insertion of a central venous line.

3. **G – Subclavian artery**
    At this point the attachment of the scalenus anterior muscle separates it from the subclavian vein. The latter lies behind the clavicle and can be approached from above or below the bone for the insertion of venous access lines. The T1 nerve root lies posterior to the artery.

4. **D – Internal carotid artery**
    The hypoglossal nerve descends between the internal jugular vein and the internal carotid artery, before passing forwards over the internal and external carotid arteries and hyoglossus to innervate the tongue.

5. **H – Superficial temporal artery**
    The artery is palpable over the squamous temporal bone and is a useful and accessible monitor of the pulse in anaesthetised patients. It is also subject to temporal arteritis, an important diagnosis to make as soon as possible, so that treatment can be initiated before the onset of visual complications.

PAPER 9

Paper 9 Questions

1. THEME: LESIONS SEEN ON OPHTHALMOSCOPY

A   AV nipping
B   Blot haemorrhage
C   Dot haemorrhage
D   Hard exudates
E   Maculopathy
F   Optic atrophy
G   Papilloedema
H   Retinitis
I   Silver wiring
J   Soft exudates

The following patients have all presented with lesions seen on ophthalmoscopy. Please match with the most appropriate findings from the above list. The findings may be used once, more than once, in combination or not at all.

1. A 29-year-old man with poorly controlled type 1 diabetes mellitus is seen in the Diabetes Out-patient Clinic for his 6-monthly review. His latest Hb A$_{1c}$ is 9.7%. His visual acuity has dropped by two lines since his last visit and ophthalmoscopy shows severe pre-proliferative retinopathy with lesions particularly prominent around the centre of the retina, temporal to the disc. He is referred urgently to the ophthalmologist.

2. A 64-year-old, type 2 diabetic man is seen in the Diabetes Out-patient Clinic for his annual review. His visual acuity is 6/12, which is the same as it has been for the last 2 years, but ophthalmoscopy has revealed signs of background retinopathy.

3. A 49-year-old woman is seen in Medical Out-patients with resistant high blood pressure. She is on lisinopril, nifedipine and atenolol but despite these medications her BP is 200/90 mmHg, lying and standing. Ophthalmoscopy shows grade-II hypertensive retinopathy.

4. A 47-year-old woman presents at the Emergency Department with a tonic–clonic seizure. On examination, she has left-sided weakness, grade 4/5, and equivocal plantar responses. A contrast-enhanced CT head scan shows a large, right-sided space-occupying lesion with a mass effect to the left and associated oedema.

5. A 24-year-old homosexual man presents with severe diarrhoea which is later confirmed as cryptosporidiosis. He is also noted to have several violaceous lesions on his palate and chest. Three weeks later he is admitted with severe visual blurring and is seen to have a 'cottage cheese and tomato ketchup' lesion on the left retina.

2. THEME: CHEST RADIOGRAPH FINDINGS

A   Bilateral hilar lymphadenopathy
B   Cardiomegaly
C   'Double' left heart border
D   Depression of the horizontal fissure
E   Elevation of the horizontal fissure
F   Loss of the hemidiaphragm
G   Obscuration of the right heart border
H   Pleural effusion
I   Tracheal deviation to the left
J   Tracheal deviation to the right

For each of the disorders below please list the possible radiological abnormalities from the above list. You may use the options once, more than once, in combination or not at all.

1. Chronic heart failure. ☐

2. Left lower lobe collapse. ☐

3. Right apical mass. ☐

4. Right middle lobe pneumonia. ☐

5. Right lower lobe collapse. ☐

6. Sarcoidosis – stage 1. ☐

7. Right-sided tension pneumothorax. ☐

3. THEME: SPLENOMEGALY

A   Acute myeloid leukaemia
B   Chronic granulocytic leukaemia
C   Cytomegalovirus
D   Gaucher's disease
E   Hodgkin's lymphoma
F   Infective endocarditis
G   Malaria
H   Myelofibrosis
I   Thalassaemia
J   Visceral leishmaniasis

The following patients have all presented with splenomegaly. Please choose the most appropriate cause from the above list. Each diagnosis may be used once, more than once or not at all.

1. A 33-year-old woman is admitted to hospital with lethargy and a low-grade pyrexia 6 weeks after having her wisdom teeth removed. On examination, she is anaemic and has a temperature of 37.4 °C. Cardiovascular examination reveals a pansystolic murmur heard primarily at the apex. She is also noted to have a 'tippable' spleen. Urine analysis is positive for blood.

2. A 29-year-old diabetic woman who has recently had a renal transplant is admitted to hospital with a pyrexial illness, lethargy and respiratory distress. On examination she is unwell, with a temperature of 38 °C. Ophthalmoscopy reveals microvascular retinopathy with a 'cottage cheese and tomato ketchup' appearance in the left retina. She is also noted to have 3-cm hepatomegaly and 2-cm splenomegaly below the costal margins.

3. A 51-year-old man is admitted to hospital with increasing lethargy and shortness of breath. On examination, he is clinically anaemic, has a purpuric rash over his lower limbs and has 6–8-cm splenomegaly below the left costal margin. Blood tests reveal: haemoglobin 6.1 g/dl, MCV 82 fl, WCC 20.2 × 10^9/l (70% blasts), platelets 17 × 10^9/l.

4. A 23-year-old student presents to her GP with night sweats and non-tender lymphadenopathy. Of note she had a severe Epstein–Barr virus infection at the age of 14 years. On examination, she has generalised lymphadenopathy with 6-cm splenomegaly. Routine investigations reveal: haemoglobin 8.7 g/dl, MCV 87 fl, WCC 22.9 × 10^9/l (marked eosinophilia), platelets 299 × 10^9/l; ESR 89 mm/h. A lymph node biopsy confirms the presence of Reed–Sternberg cells.

5. A 49-year-old woman is admitted from Medical Out-patients with weight loss, increasing shortness of breath on exercise and spontaneous epistaxis. On examination, she is clinically anaemic and is heavily bruised with 10-cm splenomegaly. Her FBC reveals: haemoglobin 5.2 g/dl, MCV 81 fl, WCC 250 × 10^9/l, platelets 79 × 10^9/l.

4. THEME: SEIZURES

A   Astrocytoma
B   Cerebral abscess
C   Cerebral infarct
D   Cerebral metastases
E   Herpes encephalitis
F   Hypocalcaemia
G   Hyponatraemia
H   Subarachnoid haemorrhage
I   Sturge–Weber syndrome
J   Tuberose sclerosis

The following patients have all presented with seizures. Please choose the most appropriate cause from the above list. Each cause may be used once, more than once or not at all.

1. A 19-year-old woman with a deeply pigmented 'birth mark' on the left side of her face presents in the Emergency Department after having several tonic–clonic seizures during the previous 4–5 hours.

2. A 31-year-old, HIV-positive man presents in the Emergency Department with a 2-day history of worsening headaches, fever, vomiting and weakness of the left upper limb. While being examined by the doctor he has a tonic–clonic seizure. A contrast-enhanced CT scan of the head confirms a large 'ring-enhancing' lesion in the right frontoparietal region with associated mass effect and oedema.

3. A 71-year-old woman is placed on paroxetine for depression. Of note she is already on bendroflumethiazide for hypertension. Six weeks later she is brought to the Emergency Department by ambulance, having had several seizures. Her husband says that she has been increasingly confused for several days but that otherwise she has been well.

4. A 52-year-old smoker with long-standing hypertension presents in the Emergency Department with acute onset of a severe, generalised headache and a reduced level of consciousness. While in the department he has a 'violent' and prolonged tonic-clonic seizure. He is paralysed and ventilated, and a CT head scan shows hyperdense areas within the ventricles and around the brainstem.

5. A 42-year-old devout Moslem woman is brought to the Emergency Department with a collapse. On examination, she is very pale and noted to have a positive Chvostek's and Trousseau's sign. Examination is otherwise unremarkable. Her son tells the doctor that she has had three or four 'funny turns' during the last 24 hours.

5. THEME: ACUTE RENAL FAILURE

A   Anti-GBM disease
B   Benzylpenicillin
C   *Escherichia coli* O157
D   Gentamicin
E   IgA nephropathy
F   *Legionella* pneumonia
G   Multiple myeloma
H   Ramipril
I   Streptococcal pneumonia
J   Wegener's granulomatosis

The following patients have all presented with acute renal failure. Please choose the most appropriate cause from the above list. Each diagnosis may be used once, more than once or not at all.

1. A 29-year-old man presents acutely unwell in the Emergency Department. He has a decreased level of consciousness, confusion and diarrhoea. Investigations reveal: haemoglobin 11.9 g/dl, MCV 91 fl, WCC 13.6 × 10^9/l, platelets 249 × 10^9/l; Na$^+$ 124 mmol/l, K$^+$ 3.9 mmol/l, urea 11.1 mmol/l, creatinine 207 μmol/l. The diagnosis is confirmed by urinary antigen titres.

2. A 78-year-old woman is admitted with a severe cellulitis of her left shin. She is started on appropriate intravenous treatment but 5 days later investigations show: Na$^+$ 131 mmol/l, K$^+$ 6.4 mmol/l, urea 19.3 mmol/l, creatinine 516 μmol/l. She also has marked proteinuria and peripheral oedema.

3. Ten days after developing a sore throat, a 19-year-old man presents to his GP with increasing ankle oedema and lethargy. He has marked proteinuria on his dipstick urine testing and the U&Es show: Na$^+$ 130 mmol/l, K$^+$ 6.6 mmol/l, urea 14.9 mmol/l, creatinine 488 μmol/l.

4. A 38-year-old woman is admitted to hospital with a 10-day history of a flu-like illness, shortness of breath with marked haemoptysis, and ankle oedema. Her chest radiograph reveals 'patchy shadowing in both lung fields, consistent with pulmonary haemorrhage'. Urinalysis shows protein +++; U&Es show Na$^+$ 128 mmol/l, K$^+$ 6.9 mmol/l, urea 22.3 mmol/l, creatinine 516 μmol/l.

5. A 31-year-old man presents to his GP with 'nasal congestion', episodes of frank haemoptysis and a 1-week history of increasing shortness of breath and peripheral oedema. Investigations show: Na$^+$ 128 mmol/l, K$^+$ 7.2 mmol/l, urea 21 mmol/l, creatinine 736 μmol/l; ESR 129 mm/h; corrected Ca^{2+} 2.34 mmol/l. Plasma electrophoresis reveals increased β$_2$-globulin.

6. THEME: MISCELLANEOUS RADIOGRAPHIC IMAGES – CLINICAL DIAGNOSIS

*Using the radiographic images **A–J on pages 354–356**, please match the clinical diagnosis with the correct image. You may use each image once, more than once or not at all. There may be more than one image appropriate for each of the diagnoses.*

1. Osteomyelitis. ☐

2. Osteoarthritis. ☐

3. Secondary metastatic deposit. ☐

4. Paget's disease of bone. ☐

5. Acromegaly. ☐

7. THEME: DYSPHAGIA

A   Achalasia
B   Bulbar palsy
C   Chagas' disease
D   CREST syndrome
E   Gastro-oesophageal reflux disease
F   Myasthenia gravis
G   Oesophageal candidiasis
H   Oesophageal carcinoma
I   Paraoesophageal hernia
J   Pharyngeal pouch (Zenker's diverticulum)
K   Pharyngeal web
L   Pseudobulbar palsy

The following patients have all presented with difficulty swallowing (dysphagia). Please select the most appropriate diagnosis from the above list. Each diagnosis may be used once, more than once or not at all.

1. A 42-year-old man presents with a long history of epigastric burning pain which is worse at night. He also suffers from severe burning pain in the chest when drinking hot liquids. Recently he has noted some difficulty swallowing solids. Endoscopy reveals confluent circumferential erosions and stricturing in the lower oesophagus. A 24-hour ambulatory oesophageal pH measurement profile demonstrates a pH of less than 4 for 10% of the recording.

2. A 69-year-old man presents with a 3-month history of difficulty swallowing. He initially felt solids sticking at chest level but now has difficulty drinking. He has lost 8 kg in weight. Examination is unremarkable apart from his gaunt appearance.

3. A 50-year-old man from Brazil is an in-patient on the cardiology ward with heart failure. You are asked to give an opinion regarding his additional symptoms of dysphagia. He has regurgitation of solids and liquids equally, both occurring shortly after swallowing, and has hypoalbuminaemia which is leading to a worsening of his peripheral oedema.

4. An 80-year-old woman presents to the Ear, Nose and Throat Clinic with a history of progressive dysphagia. She says that, initially, food stuck at the back of her throat, causing her discomfort which was relieved on regurgitation (which was assisted by pressing on her neck).

5. A 59-year-old patient is admitted to hospital from the Emergency Department with severe upper abdominal and chest pain associated with vomiting. On questioning he admits to having had several less severe episodes previously and some dysphagia. With a working diagnosis of perforated duodenal ulcer, an erect chest radiograph is performed to look for free gas under the diaphragm. However, the radiograph shows a large bubble of gas lying in the chest behind the heart.

8. THEME: GENETIC RISK FACTORS FOR COLORECTAL CANCER

A Acromegaly
B *APC* gene
C Familial adenomatous polyposis (FAP)
D Hereditary non-polyposis colorectal cancer (HNPCC)
E K-*ras* gene
F Microsatellite instability
G Mismatch repair genes
H Peutz–Jeghers syndrome
I *TP53* gene
J Ulcerative/Crohn's colitis

The following are descriptions of patients with an increased risk of colorectal cancer. Please select the most appropriate diagnosis from the above list. Each diagnosis may be used once, more than once or not at all.

1. A hereditary autosomal dominant condition caused by germline mutations in the *APC* gene.

2. A condition in which the 40–80% of cases are caused by germline mutations in mismatch repair genes leading to DNA microsatellite instability.

3. An autosomal dominant condition characterised by perioral pigmentations, upper and lower gastrointestinal hamartomatous lesions, and small-bowel, pancreatic and colorectal cancers.

4. When it affects the colon throughout its length, this condition is associated with a 1% risk of colorectal cancer after 10 years of active disease and approximately a further 1% per year increase in risk thereafter.

5. A condition defined by clinical and pedigree criteria known as the 'Amsterdam criteria'.

9. THEME: ECG RHYTHM STRIPS

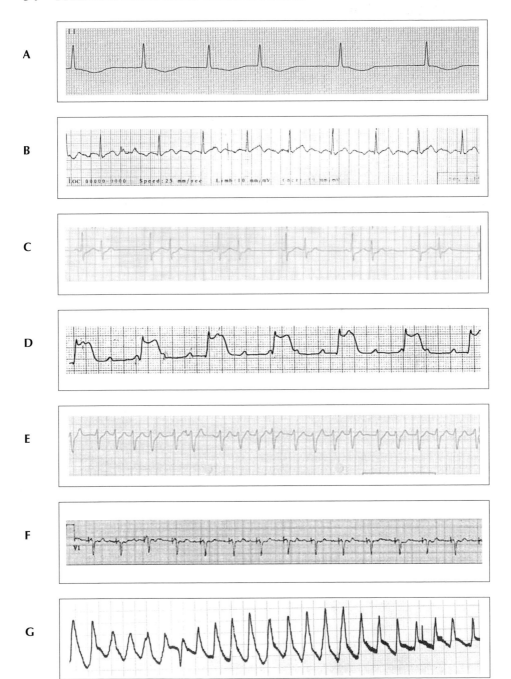

A

B

C

D

E

F

G

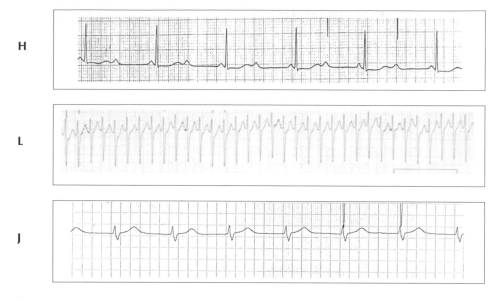

H

L

J

The following patients have all presented with abnormal cardiac rhythms. Please choose the most appropriate rhythm strip from the ECG strips above. You may use each strip once, more than once or not at all.

1. A 63-year-old man who is known to be on several 'heart tablets', including one for an irregular heart beat, presents to the Emergency Department with nausea and vomiting. On examination, he is unwell-looking and is vomiting and his intial observations show him to be hypotensive with bradycardia. The near-patient testing in the Department shows him to have a normal FBC but his U&Es show hypokalaemia and raised urea and creatinine levels.

2. A 57-year-old man presents to the Emergency Department with severe central chest pain radiating down his left arm. He is haemodynamically stable but is notably bradycardic. The ST2 doctor, who is taking her MRCP clinical examinations in a few weeks time, thinks that, clinically, he has cannon waves of his JVP.

3. A previously fit and well, 24-year-old woman presents to the Emergency Department with dizziness and a feeling of light-headedness. On examination, she is noted to have a very fast but low-volume pulse, with a blood pressure of 100/65 mmHg. Her condition improves with intravenous adenosine.

4. A 71-year-old man is seen in the Emergency Department after being mugged in the street. He has sustained several lacerations of the scalp. His rhythm strip confirms the reason for the hard 'mass' found in the upper part of the left side of his anterior chest wall.

5. A 63-year-old woman with long-standing hypertension presents to the Emergency Department with severe, generalised abdominal pain. On examination, she is acutely unwell, is distressed despite intravenous analgesia, and is 'bent double'. Clinically, she has peritonitis. The surgical ST4 doctor makes a diagnosis of an acutely ischaemic bowel secondary to an embolic event.

10. THEME: NECK LUMPS

A   Branchial cyst
B   Carotid body tumour
C   Cervical lymphadenopathy
D   Cervical rib
E   Cystic hygroma
F   Pharyngeal pouch
G   Sternomastoid tumour
H   Supraclavicular lymphadenopathy
I   Thyroglossal cyst
J   Thyroid disease

The following patients have all presented with a palpable lump in the neck. Please select the most appropriate diagnosis from the above list. Each diagnosis may be used once, more than once or not at all.

1. A 22-year-old man presents with an asymptomatic, slow-growing, painless lump in the posterior triangle of the neck above the clavicle. Direct questioning reveals a 3-month history of malaise, weight loss, pruritis and episodic night sweats. The lump is 3 cm in diameter, firm and non-tender.

2. A 68-year-old man presents with an asymptomatic, slow-growing, painless lump in the neck. On examination, he has a hard, 2-cm mass lying laterally in the anterior triangle of the neck, deep to the middle third of the right sternomastoid muscle. You notice that the patient has dysphonia.

3. An infant attends with his mother, who is concerned because he has a right torticollis. On examination, there is a swelling in the middle third of the sternomastoid muscle.

4. A 12-year-old girl presents with a history of recurrent sore throats. On examination, she has a firm, 2-cm mass lying laterally in the anterior triangle of the neck, deep to the upper third of the left sternomastoid muscle, just below the angle of the mandible. Oropharyngeal examination reveals enlarged tonsils.

5. A 26-year-old woman presents with a slow-growing, smooth, painless lump in the anterior triangle of the neck. The mass is just to the left of the midline and overlying the laryngeal cartilage and moves on swallowing.

11. THEME: INFECTIONS IN PREGNANCY

A   Cytomegalovirus
B   Group B β-haemolytic *Streptococcus (GBS)*
C   Hepatitis B
D   HIV
E   Parvovirus B19
F   Rubella
G   Syphilis
H   *Toxoplasma gondii*
I   Urinary tract infection
J   Varicella zoster virus

From the above list please choose the infection or infectious agent most likely to cause the clinical pictures described below. Each option may be used once, more than once or not at all.

1. Often asymptomatic, easy to treat but if left untreated is associated with maternal sepsis, hyperemesis gravidarum and premature labour.

2. This infection is an indication for antenatal therapy, delivery by caesarean section, neonatal therapy and refraining from breastfeeding.

3. This rare infection can cause teratogenesis in the fetus and long-term neurological sequelae for the mother. It is very easy to treat once identified.

4. If acquired in the first 20 weeks of pregnancy it can lead to mental retardation, congenital deafness and heart defects in the fetus.

5. Present in 15–20% of the pregnant population and asymptomatic.1 per 1000 neonates will suffer life-threatening sepsis as a result of this.

12. THEME: AUTOIMMUNE DISEASES

A   Addison's disease
B   Graves' disease
C   Hashimoto's thyroiditis
D   Pernicious anaemia
E   Polymyositis
F   Primary hypoparathyroidism
G   Scleroderma
H   Sjögren's syndrome
I   Systemic lupus erythematosus
J   Type-1 diabetes mellitus

From the above list, please select the disease that each of the following patients is most likely to have. Each disease may be used once, more than once or not at all.

1. A 66-year-old woman presents with increasing tiredness, dyspnoea on exercise and swollen ankles. On examination, she has pallor of the mucous membranes and pitting oedema of both ankles. Investigations show: haemoglobin 4.0 g/dl, MCV 121 fl, normal serum folate levels and grossly reduced vitamin B_{12} level.

2. A 38-year-old woman presents with a 2-month history of symmetrical joint pains in the hands and feet. More recently, she developed a rash over both cheeks and the bridge of her nose. On examination she is hypertensive. Investigations show a high ESR, reduced levels of complement and a high titre of antinuclear antibodies in the serum. Dipstick urinalysis shows the presence of protein.

3. A 45-year-old woman presents with a 3-month history of tiredness, weight gain, constipation and amenorrhoea. On examination, she has dry skin, bradycardia and a mild proximal myopathy. Investigations show: haemoglobin 8.6 g/dl with a normal MCV, a low serum T_4, a high serum thyroid-stimulating hormone (TSH) and raised serum creatine kinase.

4. A 38-year-old woman presents with a 4-month history of recurrent conjunctivitis, dry mouth, mouth ulcers and swelling in the neck. On examination she has bilateral parotid enlargement. A Schirmer's tear test shows reduced tear production. Laboratory investigations show moderately raised antinuclear antibodies, positive rheumatoid factor and anti-Ro antibodies.

5. A 52-year-old woman presents with a 3-month history of progressive difficulty in getting up from a chair, walking up stairs and combing her hair. On examination, she has severe proximal weakness of the arms and legs. Investigations show a raised serum creatine kinase, positive rheumatoid factor and antibodies to tRNA synthetase (Jo-1). Muscle biopsy shows a lymphocytic infiltrate between the muscle fibres associated with fibre necrosis and regeneration.

13. THEME: UROGENITAL ANATOMY

A   Left kidney
B   Left adrenal gland
C   Left ureter
D   Membranous urethra
E   Ovary
F   Pelvis of the right kidney
G   Prostate
H   Right adrenal gland
I   Right ureter
J   Trigone of the bladder

For each of the following descriptions, please choose the most appropriate structure from the above list. Each structure may be used once, more than once or not at all.

1. A posterior relation of the left colic artery.

2. A posterior relation of the second part of the duodenum.

3. An anterior relation of the right common iliac artery.

4. A superior relation of the deep perineal pouch.

5. A posterior relation of the obliterated umbilical ligament.

14. THEME: SURFACE MARKINGS OF THE HEART

A Left costoxiphoid angle
B Left fifth intercostal space in the anterior axillary line
C Left fifth intercostal space in the mid-clavicular line
D Left third costosternal junction
E Medial end of the second right intercostal space
F Medial end of the sixth left intercostal space
G Medial to the fourth costosternal junction
H Medial to the third left intercostal space
I Mid-sternal at the level of the fourth intercostal space
J Right sternal border

For each of the following descriptions, please choose the most appropriate markings from the above list. Each marking may be used once, more than once or not at all.

1. Surface marking of the tricuspid valve.

2. Optimal site for auscultation of the mitral valve.

3. Surface marking of the right border of the heart.

4. Optimal site for auscultation of the aortic valve.

5. Access site for intracardiac injection.

Paper 9 Answers

1. LESIONS SEEN ON OPHTHALMOSCOPY

1. **B, C, D, E, J – Blot haemorrhage, dot haemorrhage, hard exudates, maculopathy and soft exudates**
   This patient has pre-proliferative diabetic retinopathy, which is characterised by background changes (dot and blot haemorrhages and hard exudates) and cotton-wool spots (areas of retinal oedema). This patient has also developed maculopathy, which is characterised by hard exudates at its periphery, known as a 'macular star'. Maculopathy is a reason for urgent ophthalmology referral as it should be treated promptly. Failure to identify this problem can lead to rapid deterioration of the patient's acuity and blindness.

2. **B, C, D – Blot haemorrhage, dot haemorrhage and hard exudates**
   This patient has developed background diabetic retinopathy, characterised by dot haemorrhages (capillary microaneurysms), blot haemorrhages (leakage of blood into the retina) and hard exudates (lipid and protein deposits which have a yellowish or white colour and a well-defined edge). Background retinopathy heralds the onset of microvascular disease and is associated with early nephropathy. Patients should be placed on an ACE inhibitor and their glycaemic and BP control optimised.

3. **A, I – AV nipping and silver wiring**
   Hypertensive retinopathy is divided into four grades:
   Grade I – the vessels show increased tortuosity and there is 'silver wiring', which is a result of increased reflectivity of the vessels.
   Grade II – grade I changes plus arteriovenous (AV) nipping at points of crossing of the vessels.
   Grade III – this heralds the onset of retinal ischaemia and is characterised by cotton-wool spots and flame-shaped haemorrhages.
   Grade IV – grades I–III changes plus papilloedema.
   Grades III and IV are associated with 'malignant' or accelerated hypertension and require urgent medical treatment. The BP needs to be titrated down SLOWLY. Rapid reduction with antihypertensives can lead to acute cerebral infarction.

4. **G – Papilloedema**
   This patient has a large space-occupying lesion with associated oedema and mass effect, leading to raised intracranial pressure. This has caused papilloedema, which is seen as loss of the borders of the optic disc, which in turn becomes engorged, with dilatation of the surrounding vessels and small haemorrhages.

5. **H – Retinitis**
    This HIV-positive man has features of AIDS, as defined by the cryptosporidiosis,
    Kaposi's sarcoma and CMV retinitis. The retinitis has a characteristic appearance
    which has been variously described as 'cottage cheese and raspberry jam', 'scrambled
    eggs and tomato ketchup' or even 'cottage cheese and ketchup'.

2.   CHEST RADIOGRAPH FINDINGS

1.   **(P8–10) B, H – Cardiomegaly and pleural effusion**
The signs of chronic heart failure are associated with the enlarged heart (cardiomegaly) and with fluid within the spaces of the pleural cavity, ie pleural effusions, interlobar (fluid in the fissure), interlobular (fluid between the lobules, producing Kerley B lines), alveolar (causing the 'hazy' alveolar shadowing, classically in a bat-wing pattern) – and, as a result, upper-lobe diversion of the blood vessels.

2.   **(P8–10) C, F – 'Double' left heart border and loss of the hemidiaphragm**
Left lower lobe collapse classically produces a 'double left heart border' as the collapsed lobe 'falls' behind the heart. It can also cause obscuration of the left hemidiaphragm. Causes of lobar collapse include proximal obstruction due to infection, plugging of major bronchi, aspiration of foreign bodies and, most commonly, proximal obstructing tumours.

3.   **(P8–10) E, H, I – Elevation of the horizontal fissure, pleural effusion and tracheal deviation to the left**
A right apical mass can cause tracheal deviation to the left due to the trachea being 'pushed away'. However, if it causes right upper lobe collapse this will lead to tracheal deviation towards the lesion as it 'pulls' the trachea across. Lobar collapse will also lead to elevation of the horizontal fissure, and might be associated with hilar lymphadenopathy and possibly a pleural effusion.

4.   **(P8–10) G, H – Loss of the right heart border and pleural effusion**
A right middle lobe pneumonia causes loss of the right heart border and can be associated with a pleural effusion.

5.   **(P8–10) D, F – Depression of the horizontal fissure and loss of the hemidiaphragm**
Right lower lobe collapse will cause obscuration of the right hemidiaphragm and 'depression' of the horizontal fissure. Causes of lobar collapse are similar to those listed in the answer to question 2.

6.   **(P8–10) A – Bilateral hilar lymphadenopathy**
Sarcoidosis classically causes bilateral hilar lymphadenopathy, which in turn can be associated with mid-zone or more diffuse interstitial shadowing and eventually 'honeycombing'.

7.   **(P8–10) I – Tracheal deviation to the left**
Tension pneumothoraces cause mediastinal shift and tracheal deviation away from the side of the pneumothorax.

IMAGES: pages 354–356

3. SPLENOMEGALY

1. **F – Infective endocarditis**
   This patient has developed several stigmata of infective endocarditis – a mitral regurgitant murmur, low-grade fever, anaemia, dipstick-positive haematuria and a 'tippable' spleen. For the spleen to be palpable it must be at least two to three times its normal size.

2. **C – Cytomegalovirus**
   This patient with a recent renal transplant has developed a systemic CMV infection. She has the typical features of CMV retinitis and has palpable hepatosplenomegaly and evidence of pneumonitis. This diagnosis is confirmed by antibody titres, with an acute IgM response, or by tissue biopsies, which show the pathognomonic intranuclear 'owl's eye' inclusions. In the immunocompromised patient an antiviral agent such as ganciclovir should be used.

3. **A – Acute myeloid leukaemia**
   This man has a normocytic anaemia and thrombocytopenia, but a leucocytosis with predominantly blast cells. The diagnosis can be confirmed on bone marrow examination, which characteristically shows hypercellularity and blast cells. Depending on the patient's general health and wishes he should be offered chemotherapy with expert haematological and oncological follow-up.

4. **E – Hodgkin's lymphoma**
   This young woman has developed Hodgkin's lymphoma which is strongly associated with previous EBV infection. She has the characteristic 'Reed–Sternberg' cells in her lymph node biopsy, which represent abnormal lymphocytes. The disorder is classified by the affected lymphoid tissue involved above and below the diaphragm and the presence or absence of systemic symptoms such as night sweats, weight loss, malaise and lethargy, the so called 'B-symptoms'. Diagnosis is usually confirmed on the peripheral blood film and lymph node biopsy.

5. **B – Chronic granulocytic leukaemia**
   This woman has a diffusely enlarged spleen associated with a normocytic anaemia, thrombocytopenia and a 'massive' leucocytosis. This picture is in keeping with chronic granulocytic leukaemia, which is one of the five worldwide causes of a 'giant spleen'. The other four are chronic malaria, visceral leishmaniasis (kala-azar), myelofibrosis and Gaucher's disease.

4. SEIZURES

1. I – Sturge–Weber syndrome

This young woman has Sturge–Weber syndrome, the association of a diffuse facial port-wine stain or naevus in a division of the trigeminal nerve and intracranial angiomata. Patients can present at any age with seizures.

2. B – Cerebral abscess

This HIV-positive patient has developed an intracerebral abscess which could be caused by tuberculosis, toxoplasmosis, streptococcal or staphylococcal infection. Ring-enhancing lesions can also represent a primary or secondary malignant tumour or lymphomatous deposits.

3. G – Hyponatraemia

This woman has developed severe hyponatraemia due to the combination of paroxetine and bendroflumethiazide. Both of these tablets are relatively common causes of hyponatraemia.

4. H – Subarachnoid haemorrhage

This man has had a large subarachnoid haemorrhage, leading to fresh blood (which appears white in an unenhanced scan) within the ventricles. He requires nimodipine to stop secondary bleeds through vasospasm, correction of any clotting abnormalities, and an urgent neurosurgical opinion. If the GCS is 7/15 or below he should also be electively paralysed and ventilated.

5. F – Hypocalcaemia

Devout Moslem women who cover up with traditional robes have little or no exposure to sun. If they do not have adequate calcium and vitamin D intake through other sources they run the risk of osteomalacia and hypocalcaemia which rarely can be severe enough to cause seizures.

5. ACUTE RENAL FAILURE

1. **F – *Legionella* pneumonia**
   This patient has developed an atypical pneumonia secondary to *Legionella pneumophila* infection. As with many atypical pneumonias, there might be few respiratory signs or symptoms, and the patient can principally present with signs and symptoms of multisystem involvement. The renal impairment is caused by the effects of overwhelming sepsis and resulting multiorgan failure.

2. **B – Benzylpenicillin**
   This patient has developed acute renal impairment and a possible nephrotic syndrome due to the intravenous penicillin she has been placed on for her cellulitis. Drugs such as penicillin can cause acute tubulointerstitial nephritis or an immune-mediated glomerulonephritis.

3. **E – IgA nephropathy**
   This young man has developed acute renal failure 10 days after a sore throat. IgA nephropathy classically occurs 7–10 days after an acute infection, whereas post-streptococcal glomerulonephritis occurs a little later, at 14 days.

4. **A – Anti-GBM disease**
   This woman has developed anti-glomerular basement membrane disease, previously called 'Goodpasture's syndrome'. The common basement membrane antigen is found in the kidney and lung and this condition leads to an acute glomerulonephritis and pulmonary haemorrhage with subsequent nephrotic syndrome and respiratory failure.

5. **J – Wegener's granulomatosis**
   This man has both upper and lower respiratory tract symptoms associated with acute renal failure. This combination is classical of Wegener's granulomatosis, which causes a glomerulonephritis and acute renal failure. The diagnosis may be confirmed by the presence of c-ANCA and typical biopsy findings.

6. MISCELLANEOUS RADIOGRAPHIC IMAGES – CLINICAL DIAGNOSIS

1. **(P8–10) A – Osteomyelitis**
   This plain radiograph is highly suggestive of osteomyelitis, with a gas shadow in the soft tissue of the second toe. Osteomyelitis is usually caused by *Enterobacter*, *Staphylococcus* and *Pseudomonas* species in adults and arises as a result of direct spread from an overlying infection or ulcerating lesion or from a puncture wound. People with sickle-cell disease are prone to *Salmonella* infection. In children osteomyelitis is more likely to be caused by blood-borne organisms, including *Streptococcus, Staphylococcus, Enterobacter* and *Haemophilus* species.

2. **(P8–10) C, E – Cervical spondylosis and osteoarthritis**
   These plain radiographs show osteoarthritis of the cervical spine and of the right knee. Cervical spondylosis can lead to cervical myelopathy and cord compression, which in turn can require neurosurgical intervention. Osteoarthritis commonly affects the large joints of the lower limb and patients can require joint replacement.

3. **(P8–10) H, I – Left-hemisphere ring-enhancing lesion and cannonball metastases**
   Radiograph **H** shows a ring-enhancing lesion in the left temporoparietal region consistent with a metastatic deposit. Radiograph **I** shows multiple lesions in both lung fields consistent with cannonball metastases. Intracerebral metastases are common and can occur with any of the common malignancies, including breast, lung, colon and renal carcinoma, as well as malignant melanoma. Cannonball metastases usually come from gonadal, renal, breast or colonic primaries.

4. **(P8–10) B – Paget's disease of bone**
   This plain radiograph of the right hip shows the characteristic features of Paget's bone disease. Clinically, Paget's bone disease presents with arthritic and bony pain, immobility, bone deformity, fractures and, rarely, osteosarcoma. Other complications include cranial nerve compression leading to optic atrophy, blindness and deafness, cervical cord compression and high-output cardiac failure.

5. **(P8–10) F – Acromegaly**
   This lateral skull radiograph shows features suggestive of acromegaly. This patient has an enlarged, protruding mandible (prognathism) with enlargement of the pituitary fossa. The diagnosis should be confirmed using gadolinium-enhanced magnetic resonance imaging of the pituitary fossa and surrounding structures and dynamic testing of pituitary function using an oral glucose tolerance test (a large glucose load should suppress growth hormone levels in normal individuals).

IMAGES: pages 354–356

7. DYSPHAGIA

1. **E – Gastro-oesophageal reflux disease**
   This patient has gastro-oesophageal reflux disease (GORD), as evidenced by the long history of classic symptoms. The diagnosis is confirmed by endoscopy, when he has been found to have grade-III disease, ie circumferential disease leading to a stricture. The pH study confirms an increased lower oesophageal acid exposure (pH<4 for >4% of the time).

2. **H – Oesophageal carcinoma**
   The history of rapidly progressive dysphagia in a man of this age should prompt this diagnosis. The weight loss is also strongly suggestive. A histological diagnosis would be confirmed at endoscopy, and the size of the lesion by barium swallow, which usually shows the typical irregular, shouldered 'apple core' appearance.

3. **C – Chagas' disease**
   This disorder is caused by the parasite *Trypanosoma cruzi* and is endemic in large parts of rural South America, making it one of the commonest diseases in the world. Infection follows the bite of a rather unpleasant nocturnal insect (the reduviid bug) that lives preferentially in the roofs of adobe dwellings. There is a long incubation period followed by manifestations of the disorder, which are largely immune-mediated, and include cardiomyopathy and mega-oesophagus/megacolon. The oesophageal manifestations are similar to achalasia both clinically and pathologically (destruction of the myenteric plexus) and occur in 25% of cases.

4. **J – Pharyngeal pouch (Zenker's diverticulum)**
   This disorder first, described by Ludlow in 1767, is a pulsion diverticulum of the lateral pharynx at a point of congenital weakness between the crico- and thyro-pharyngeal portions of the inferior constrictors called 'Killian's dehiscence'. Food sticks in the diverticulum and causes dysphagia by compressing the upper oesophagus. Treatment is largely surgical. The condition is important to remember for the unwary endoscopist who can easily perforate the diverticulum on intubation of the patient.

5. **I – Paraoesophageal hernia**
   Unlike the very common sliding hernia (hiatus hernia) which can cause reflux disease/dyspepsia, the rolling type (although much less common) is a serious condition that requires surgical intervention. A variable portion of the stomach 'rolls' through a defect in the diaphragm to one side of the oesophagus where it can become strangulated, leading to the acute presentation described here. A barium swallow aids diagnosis. Treatment is by gastropexy, with or without an anti-reflux procedure.

8. GENETIC RISK FACTORS FOR COLORECTAL CANCER

A variety of hereditary conditions are linked with the development of colorectal cancer, and the genes responsible for tumour development continue to be elucidated. While such conditions are rare compared with sporadic tumours, representing only 5–10% of all such cancers, they are important, not just for the families that have them (screening and surveillance), but also as an example of the increasing role of genomics and genetics in medicine and surgery.

1. **C – Familial adenomatous polyposis (FAP)**
   This condition is present in <1% of all patients with colorectal cancer. The patient develops hundreds of adenomas, principally in the distal colon and rectum, from the age of approximately 10 years. Untreated, 100% of those affected will progress over time to develop colorectal cancer. Treatment is by proctocolectomy. Relatives should undergo genetic testing and close endoscopic surveillance. Depending on the exact allelic site of sequence alteration in the *APC* gene, the patient might have other abnormalities such as desmoid tumours, carcinoma of the ampulla of Vater or osteomata of the mandible.

2. **D – Hereditary non-polyposis colorectal cancer (HNPCC)**
   These are the genetic defects classically associated with this condition, in which affected individuals have a much greater than average chance of developing colorectal cancer. It represents approximately 3% of all cases of colorectal cancer. Compared with sporadic carcinomas, carcinomas develop at a younger age (typically in the 30–50-year age group), are often multiple ('synchronous lesions'), and are more commonly right-sided. The two commonest mutations are of the mismatch repair genes, *MLH1* and *MSH2*. Mutations lead to conformation abnormalities and disordered function of the mismatch repair enzymes that the genes encode, with subsequent acquisition of other DNA sequence aberrations of colorectal cancer oncogenes such as *APC*, K-*ras* and *TP53*.

3. **H – Peutz–Jeghers syndrome**
   The classic findings of this rare hereditary disorder are described here. It is one of three clinically similar hamartomatous polyposis syndromes associated with colorectal cancer, the others being even rarer (Cowden's disease and familial juvenile polyposis). The mutant genes responsible have been elucidated for most cases.

4. **J – Ulcerative/Crohn's colitis**
   These are the classically cited risks for patients with ongoing active pancolitis (the risks are similar for both disorders). The lifetime risk of developing colorectal cancer is 17 times the risk of an average-risk population (which is 1/18). Patients require regular colonoscopic surveillance after 8 years of disease, and subsequent proctocolectomy if areas of dysplasia are found on biopsies. Patients with left-sided colitis have a lower risk and should be screened after 15 years of disease.

5. **D – Hereditary non-polyposis colorectal cancer (HNPCC)**
   The condition described in answer 2 is currently defined within families affected by colorectal cancer on the basis of the Amsterdam criteria (I and II). The former, more stringent, Amsterdam I criteria require at least three relatives with histologically verified colorectal cancer; one must be a first-degree relative and of the other two, at least two successive generations must be affected and at least one relative must have received the diagnosis before the age of 50 years. Amsterdam II criteria are similar but allow for relatives with other cancers associated with HNPCC (endometrial, stomach, ovary, upper urinary tract and small bowel).

9. ECG RHYTHM STRIPS

The rhythm strips show:

A – Slow atrial fibrillation with digoxin effect
B – Atrial flutter
C – Atrial bigemini
D – Complete heart block with ST elevation
E – Fast atrial fibrillation
F – Paced rhythm
G – Torsades de Pointes
H – Second-degree heart block (2:1 block)
I – Supraventricular tachycardia (SVT)
J – Nodal rhythm

1. **A – Slow atrial fibrillation with digoxin effect**
   This patient is being treated for atrial fibrillation (the irregular heart beat) with digoxin. Hypokalaemia and renal impairment both potentiate the effects of digoxin and increase the chances of toxicity. Digoxin toxicity allegedly predisposes patients to any form of arrhythmia, both bradycardias and tachycardias. Classically, it causes bradycardia and heart block. Patients taking digoxin might show a 'digoxin effect' (the 'dig effect') on their ECG, which is independent of the serum levels. This is marked by upsloping ST segments (more commonly called the 'reverse tick sign'). This is seen in the complexes of this rhythm strip.

2. **D – Complete heart block with ST elevation**
   This rhythm strip demonstrates dissociation of the atria and ventricles, ie a regular P-wave pattern that shows no relation to the regular QRS complex pattern. This patient has presented with an acute myocardial infarction, reflected in the ST elevation in the rhythm strip. Because the rhythm strip is usually taken from lead II, the ST elevation is in keeping with an acute inferior myocardial infarction. This represents the right coronary artery territory which in the majority of people supplies the sinoatrial node (SAN) and the atrioventricular node (AVN). This patient has suffered ischaemia to the AVN, causing complete heart block. Clinically, complete heart block is associated with the right atrium contracting against a closed tricuspid valve, causing cannon waves in the JVP.

3. **I – Supraventricular tachycardia (SVT)**
   This rhythm strip shows a narrow-complex tachycardia/SVT that has been terminated using the AVN blocker, adenosine. Any patient presenting with an arrhythmia that is successfully terminated should go on to have a 12-lead ECG to look for possible underlying conduction abnormalities or signs of ischaemia.

4. **F – Paced rhythm**
   This rhythm strip demonstrates a pacing spike preceding each QRS complex. This is a 'paced rhythm' and should not cause any concern.

5. **B, E – Atrial flutter or fast atrial fibrillation**
   This patient's hypertension has predisposed her to atrial fibrillation or flutter. This in turn has caused a systemic embolism, commonly associated with stroke but which can cause ischaemia of the bowel or a limb. In this case it has led to an acutely ischaemic bowel. The treatment includes surgical resection of the affected bowel, rate control of the fast atrial fibrillation and anticoagulation with heparin and then warfarin.

10. NECK LUMPS

1. **H – Supraclavicular lymphadenopathy**
   This patient has supraclavicular lymphadenopathy. The diagnosis in a man of this age with the constitutional symptoms described is most likely to be lymphoma. The student should remember that this is also a site for metastatic carcinoma from bronchogenic, breast and some gastrointestinal malignancies (eg colorectal or stomach malignancies, leading to Virchow's node or Troisier's sign).

2. **C – Cervical lymphadenopathy**
   This is evidenced by the anatomical position given. In this case the cause of the lymphadenopathy is metastatic carcinoma from a laryngeal primary. This is one of the commonest causes of swelling of the deep cervical nodes, which lie behind the sternomastoid muscles. Primary lesions can occur in the skin of the head and neck, the lips, tongue and buccal cavity, and the larynx.

3. **G – Sternomastoid tumour**
   This condition of infancy can represent an organising haematoma or an area of fibrosis secondary to ischaemia. It is caused either by birth trauma or by some other late intrauterine event. The condition can present with a lump or torticollis.

4. **C – Cervical lymphadenopathy**
   This is evidenced by the anatomical position given. In this case the cause of the lymphadenopathy is acute inflammation, probably tonsillitis. Other acute inflammatory causes of cervical lymphadenopathy are pharyngitis/laryngitis and EBV infection. Chronic inflammatory causes include TB and sarcoid. (**NB:** You have now had all four main causes of cervical lymphadenopathy – acute inflammation, chronic inflammation, lymphoma and metastatic carcinoma.)

5. **J – Thyroid disease**
   This patient has a solitary thyroid nodule and requires investigation to exclude a papillary carcinoma (the differential diagnosis includes a dominant nodule within a multinodular goitre, simple cyst and thyroid adenoma).

11. INFECTIONS IN PREGNANCY

1. **I – Urinary tract infection**
   Many of the listed infections are asymptomatic and can cause maternal sepsis. Urinary tract infection in pregnancy is commonly asymptomatic and picked up on routine antenatal urine testing rather than as a result of symptoms. Due to the relative immunosuppression of pregnancy, once it becomes systemic it can quickly lead to sepsis if not treated. The high pyrexia and systemic prostaglandin release can cause premature labour and it is the only infection in the list that is actively associated with hyperemesis gravidarum.

2. **D – HIV**
   HIV infection has a perinatal transmission rate of about 15%, which can be reduced to approximately 1% after antenatal maternal antiretroviral treatment (azidothymidine or AZT), elective Caesarean section, neonatal antiretroviral treatment (AZT) and by not breastfeeding. Hepatitis B needs none of these as it is easily prevented by neonatal vaccination and hepatitis immunoglobulin. None of the other infections require the mother to refrain from breastfeeding.

3. **G – Syphilis**
   Syphilis, rubella, CMV, *Toxoplasma* and varicella zoster virus (very rarely) can all cause teratogenesis. Parvovirus B19 causes hydrops fetalis due to fetal anaemia. Syphilis (tertiary) is the only infection here that is likely to lead to long-term maternal neurological sequelae in an immunocompetent host and it is the only one easily treated (with high-dose penicillin). The treatment of toxoplasmosis is more complex and as all the others are viral they are also difficult to treat.

4. **F – Rubella**
   Mental retardation, congenital deafness and heart defects are the classic triad of congenital rubella if contracted during the first 20 weeks of pregnancy. CMV and toxoplasmosis can cause microcephaly, hydrocephalus and mental retardation but do not usually cause heart defects or specific deafness.

5. **B – Group B β-haemolytic *Streptococcus* (GBS)**
   Group B *Streptococcus* is a commensal organism in the vagina in up to 15–20% of woman and by definition is therefore asymptomatic. Seropositivity to parvovirus B19, CMV, rubella and varicella zoster virus is much more common (60%, 70%, 97% and 97%, respectively). *Toxoplasma* seropositivity is only found in around 10% in the UK and HIV and hepatitis B are much rarer than this. One in 1000 neonates become infected with Group B streptococci during labour and delivery and can suffer life-threatening sepsis. If a woman is found to be positive for Group B *Streptococcus* she is therefore treated with penicillin during labour to prevent transmission to the fetus.

12. AUTOIMMUNE DISEASES

1. **D – Pernicious anaemia**
   This patient has symptoms and signs suggestive of cardiac failure due to anaemia. Investigations confirm a severe macrocytic anaemia due to vitamin B_{12} deficiency. Pernicious anaemia is an autoimmune disease of the stomach in which there is chronic inflammation and atrophy of the gastric mucosa, leading to destruction of parietal cells, failure of intrinsic factor production and consequent malabsorption of vitamin B_{12}. The disease is most prevalent in elderly women and is associated with other organ-specific autoimmune diseases such as thyroid disease, Addison's disease and vitiligo. Anti-parietal cell antibodies are found in 90% of patients with pernicious anaemia, but can also be found in other conditions. Anti-intrinsic factor antibodies are more specific but are found in only 50% of cases.

2. **I – Systemic lupus erythematosus**
   SLE is a multisystem disease that has a variable clinical presentation and behaviour. Arthralgia and skin rashes are the most common features, but involvement of the kidneys, lungs, heart, CNS and eyes are also common. This patient exhibits the classic 'butterfly' rash on the cheeks, but other cutaneous manifestations can include vasculitic lesions and purpura. Renal involvement is indicated by the hypertension and proteinuria. The fundamental defect in SLE is thought to be a failure to maintain self-tolerance. Consequently, a large number of autoantibodies are produced that can damage tissues, either directly or in the form of immune-complex deposits. Antinuclear antibodies are present in 90% of patients with SLE, but other antibodies such as rheumatoid factor and antiphospholipid antibodies are also detected. Low serum complement levels, a high ESR, and leucopenia or thrombocytopenia are also commonly present.

3. **C – Hashimoto's thyroiditis**
   This patient shows the typical symptoms, signs and thyroid function test profile of hypothyroidism. Hashimoto's thyroiditis is the commonest cause of hypothyroidism in the UK. As with other autoimmune diseases, it is much more common in women than in men (in a ratio of about 9 : 1) and is associated with other organ-specific autoimmune diseases. Several autoantibodies are detected in the serum, most commonly anti-thyroid peroxidase and antithyroglobulin. These lead to atrophy of the thyroid parenchyma and intense lymphoid infiltration of the gland. The anaemia seen in Hashimoto's thyroiditis is usually of normochromic normocytic type but can be megaloblastic if there is associated pernicious anaemia. In this patient, the raised serum creatine kinase is due to the myopathy.

4. **H – Sjögren's syndrome**
   Sjögren's syndrome is a disorder characterised by dry eyes and dry mouth which result from immune-mediated destruction of the lacrimal and salivary glands. It can occur as an isolated disorder (the primary form) or in association with other autoimmune diseases (the secondary form). Around 90% of cases occur in middle-aged women. Salivary gland enlargement is common and is due to lymphocytic infiltration. A number of autoantibodies are found in the serum, including antinuclear antibodies, rheumatoid factor and autoantibodies to the ribonucleoprotein antigens SS-A (Ro).

5. **E – Polymyositis**

Polymyositis is one of the inflammatory myopathies, a heterogeneous group of uncommon disorders characterised by immune-mediated muscle injury and inflammation. The main clinical feature is symmetrical muscle weakness that initially affects the large muscles of the trunk, neck and limbs. Tasks such as getting up from a chair and climbing stairs therefore become increasingly difficult. Muscle biopsy demonstrates chronic inflammation and myopathic features. Several autoantibodies are found in the serum, including antinuclear antibodies and rheumatoid factor. Jo-1 antibodies (to tRNA synthetase) are specific to this disorder and their presence is predictive of pulmonary involvement.

13. UROGENITAL ANATOMY

1. C – Left ureter

The ureter descends on the psoas muscle and common iliac vessels, over the sacroiliac joint, and on reaching the ischial spine it passes forwards to the bladder. It is crossed by the root of the sigmoid mesentery and in males by the vas deferens. In females it is crossed by the broad ligament and uterine artery and has a close relationship with the neck of the cervix.

2. F – Pelvis of the right kidney

The right kidney is capped by the adrenal gland, the hilum being covered by the descending part of the duodenum, and the lower pole by the right colic flexure laterally and the duodenum medially. The remainder of the surface is related to the visceral surface of the liver.

3. I – Right ureter

The right ureter descends on the psoas muscle and crosses the genitofemoral nerve. Anteriorly it is crossed by the descending part of the duodenum, the right colic, ileocolic and gonadal vessels, and the root of the small gut mesentery. Elsewhere, it is covered by adherent peritoneum. Its pelvic relations in males and females are as described in the answer to question 1 above.

4. G – Prostate

The prostate lies under the bladder, surrounding the prostatic urethra; it sits on the perineum. The prostatic urethra becomes the membranous urethra, passing through the deep perineal pouch to pierce the perineal membrane and become the bulbous urethra. The prostate is divided into a median lobe that lies posteriorly between the urethra and the ejaculatory ducts, and lateral lobes that are below and lateral. They are continuous anteriorly but separated posteriorly by a midline sulcus that is palpable on rectal examination.

5. E – Ovary

The posterior relations of the ovary are the internal iliac vessels and the ureter. Superiorly, the external iliac vessel completes the triangle of the ovarian fossa on the lateral wall of the pelvis. The ovary, however, is clasped by the infundibulum and lies on the posterior aspect of the broad ligament; the pelvic wall relationship described varies with changes in uterine size and position.

14. SURFACE MARKINGS OF THE HEART

1. **I – Mid-sternal at the level of fourth intercostal space**
    The optimal site for auscultation of the tricuspid valve is at the right sternal border in line with the fourth intercostal space.

2. **C – Left fifth intercostal space in the mid-clavicular line**
    This is also the marking for the apex of the heart and where the cardiac impulse can be seen and palpated. Murmurs from the mitral valve can radiate to the axilla and are accentuated by lying on the left side; the opening snap of mitral stenosis is heard more prominently over the fourth left costal cartilage when leaning forwards.

3. **J – Right sternal border**
    The maximum convexity of this line is opposite the fourth intercostal space, bulging beyond the sternal border and in line with the superior vena cava above and the inferior vena cava below.

4. **E – Medial end of the second right intercostal space**
    Aortic murmurs can radiate into the right-hand side of the neck and occasionally across towards the apex.

5. **F – Medial end of the sixth left intercostal space**
    At this site, and also at the medial end of the left fifth intercostal space, the pleura is reflected away from the midline in the cardiac notch. Agents (eg adrenaline after cardiac arrest) can be delivered directly into the ventricles at this site.

PAPER 10

Paper 10 Questions

1. THEME: THYROID FUNCTION TESTS

	TSH (mU/l)	fT$_4$ (pmol/l)	fT$_3$ (nmol/l)
A	48.9	3.2	0.4
B	<0.01	64.8	7.3
C	<0.01	15.9	8.8
D	7.3	14.3	1.8
E	3.2	18.7	2.4
F	0.71	7.0	1.2
G	18.9	14.3	2.8

The following patients all have abnormal thyroid function test results. Please match their presentations to the thyroid function test profiles in the above table. Each profile may be used once, more than once or not at all.

1. An 81-year-old woman on thyroxine for long-standing primary hypothyroidism is seen in Medical Out-patients for her 6-monthly check-up. She is clinically well and euthyroid but her AMTS is 6/10. Routine investigations show her to be poorly compliant with her thyroid medication.

2. A 19-year-old woman presents to her GP with palpitations and sweats. On examination, she appears to be agitated and tremulous and is tachycardic at 130 bpm in atrial fibrillation. She is admitted to hospital and improves with β-blockers and carbimazole.

3. A 69-year-old woman is admitted to the Emergency Department with fast atrial fibrillation and pulmonary oedema. On examination, she is thin and sweaty and has marked palmar erythema. Her initial investigations reveal normal cardiac enzymes and echocardiography but her thyroid function tests confirm T$_3$ thyrotoxicosis.

4. A 34-year-old woman presents to her GP with a 3-month history of worsening lethargy, malaise and amenorrhoea. Examination reveals her to have a pale complexion and postural hypotension and a capillary blood glucose is 3.1 mmol/l. Examination is otherwise unremarkable.

5. A 78-year-old woman presents in the Emergency Department with pneumonia and fast atrial fibrillation. Investigations reveal sick euthyroid syndrome.

2. THEME: MISCELLANEOUS RADIOGRAPHIC IMAGES – CLINICAL ABNORMALITIES

*Please match the radiographic images **A–J on pages 354–356** as causes for each of the clinical abnormalities listed below. Images may be used once, more than once or not at all. There may be more than one correct image for each of the abnormalities.*

1. Nausea and vomiting. ☐

2. Septic shock. ☐

3. Hypercalcaemia. ☐

4. Headache. ☐

5. Endocrine abnormality. ☐

3. THEME: PLEURAL EFFUSION

A   Alcoholic cirrhosis
B   Amyloidosis
C   Bronchogenic carcinoma
D   Chronic hepatitis B virus infection
E   Constrictive pericarditis
F   Diabetic nephropathy
G   Ischaemic cardiomyopathy
H   Pulmonary emboli
I   Renal-cell carcinoma
J   Tuberculous pericarditis

The following patients have all presented with a pleural effusion. Please choose the most appropriate cause from the above list. Each cause may be used once, more than once or not at all.

1. A 38-year-old man presents to his GP with increasing exertional dyspnoea and abdominal swelling. On examination, he has ascites and bilateral pleural effusions and is noted to have several spider naevi. An abdominal ultrasound scan shows a 'hypoechogenic mass in the liver, ?hepatoma'.

2. A 49-year-old smoker presents to his GP with increasing shortness of breath and peripheral oedema. On examination he has no clubbing or palpable lymphadenopathy but has a large right pleural effusion. An ECG shows sinus tachycardia, left axis deviation and poor anterior R-wave progression.

3. A 51-year-old smoker presents to his GP with increasing abdominal swelling and shortness of breath. On examination, he has tar-staining of the fingers and is clinically anaemic. His chest radiograph confirms a left pleural effusion with three large lesions spread throughout the two lung fields.

4. A 62-year-old woman is admitted to hospital with a 2-month history of insidious worsening of shortness of breath, which has worsened acutely in the last 10 days. On examination, she is tachycardic, tachypnoeic and unwell. She has signs consistent with a large right pleural effusion and a smaller left pleural effusion, a raised JVP and a third heart sound. Her ECG shows large dominant R-waves in V_1 and V_2 with associated T-wave inversion, right axis deviation and sinus tachycardia.

5. A 32-year-old man presents in the Emergency Department with weight loss, haemoptysis and exertional dyspnoea. Examination reveals a low-volume pulse, pulsus paradoxus and positive Kussmaul's sign. The heart sounds are poorly heard. His ECG shows low-voltage complexes but is otherwise unremarkable. The diagnosis is confirmed by pericardiocentesis, which drains 50 ml of bloodstained fluid.

4. THEME: NEUROLOGICAL DEFICIT/DISABILITY

A Agraphia
B Aphasia (global)
C Astereognosis
D Ataxia
E Dysarthria
F Dysdiadochokinesia
G Dyspraxic gait
H Expressive dysphasia
I Nystagmus
J Resting tremor

The following patients have all presented with neurological disability. Please choose the most appropriate cause from the above list. You may use each cause once, more than once, in combination or not at all.

1. A 31-year-old man with known epilepsy is placed on erythromycin for a chest infection. Ten days later he presents in the Emergency Department with phenytoin toxicity.

2. A 63-year-old man visits his GP complaining of falls. On examination he is bradykinetic with 'mask-like facies' and he improves with L-dopa therapy.

3. A right-handed, 71-year-old woman presents in the Emergency Department with symptoms suggestive of a dominant-hemisphere stroke. She is able to follow three-stage commands but is unable to produce any coherent words. Sensory examination is normal but she cannot recognise objects placed in her right hand when her eyes are closed.

4. A 61-year-old man with known type-2 diabetes mellitus attends his GP with worsening burning pains and numbness in his feet associated with falls. On examination, his gait is abnormal and he has a glove-and-stocking distribution of peripheral sensory neuropathy.

5. A 74-year-old man is admitted to hospital with worsening mobility, confusion and urinary incontinence. Routine investigations including FBC, U&Es, random blood glucose, LFTs, thyroid function tests and corrected Ca^{2+} are normal and his chest radiograph is unremarkable, as is his mid-stream urine. A CT head scan shows marked ventricular dilatation and he improves after placement of a ventriculoperitoneal shunt.

5. THEME: COLLAPSE

A Aortic stenosis
B Complete heart block
C Neurocardiogenic syncope
D Postural hypotension
E Sick sinus syndrome
F Tachy-brady syndrome
G Tonic–clonic seizure
H Transient ischaemic attack
I Ventricular tachycardia
J Vertebrobasilar insufficiency

The following patients have all presented with an episode of collapse. Please choose the most appropriate cause from the above list. Each cause may be used once, more than once or not at all.

1. A 76-year-old man with a known history of ischaemic heart disease presents in the Emergency Department with an episode of collapse, preceded by 'a feeling of light-headedness'. On examination, he is pale but is otherwise haemodynamically stable. The medical ST2 doctor in the Emergency Department thinks he can see cannon waves in the JVP. His ECG shows atrioventricular dissociation with a narrow-complex escape rhythm at a rate of 48 bpm.

2. An 83-year-old woman is sent for a tilt-table test after an episode of collapse in the street. Her routine blood tests, chest radiograph and ECG were within normal limits, as was her 24-hour tape. She becomes extremely hypotensive and bradycardic, associated with pre-syncope, sweating and clamminess within 2 minutes of carotid sinus massage and tilting to 70°.

3. A 74-year-old woman is seen in Medical Outpatients with a history of three episodes of collapse in the past 4 months related to washing the top shelves of her kitchen cabinets and, more recently, while looking up to watch an air display at her local airport.

4. A 71-year-old woman presents in the Medicine for the Elderly Out-patient Clinic with two episodes of collapse associated with dizziness while out playing golf. On examination, her blood pressure is 110/100 mmHg and there is an 'abnormal feel' to her carotid pulse. The ECG shows the voltage criteria of left ventricular hypertrophy.

5. An 87-year-old man with known ischaemic heart disease, cardiac failure and hypertension is admitted to hospital with an episode of collapse which has led to a fractured left neck of femur. On examination, he is well but in obvious distress, with a shortened, externally rotated left leg. His pulse is 60 bpm and regular and his BP is 100/70 mmHg. The admitting doctor notes that he is on bendroflumethiazide, atenolol, isosorbide mononitrate and ramipril. His ECG shows sinus rhythm, left axis deviation and an old anterior myocardial infarct but no acute changes. The subsequent 24-hour tape shows normal sinus rhythm throughout.

6. THEME: HAEMATOLOGICAL MALIGNANCIES

A   Acute lymphoblastic leukaemia (ALL)
B   Acute myeloid leukaemia (AML)
C   Chronic lymphocytic leukaemia (CLL)
D   Chronic myeloid leukaemia (CML)
E   Hairy-cell leukaemia
F   Hodgkin's lymphoma
G   Multiple myeloma
H   Myelofibrosis
I   Non-Hodgkin's lymphoma
J   Waldenström's macroglobulinaemia

The following patients have all presented with a haematological malignancy. Please choose the most appropriate disorder from the above list. Each diagnosis may be used once, more than once or not at all.

1. A 46-year-old man presents to his GP with a 2–month history of increasing lethargy, vague abdominal pains and recurrent chest infections. On examination, he is clinically anaemic and has multiple areas of bruising over his limbs and torso. He has a massively enlarged spleen which extends down into the right iliac fossa. His blood film shows 'pancytopenia with atypical B-cell lymphocytes with spiky projections'.

2. An 81-year-old man presents in Haematology Out-patients with a vague, non-specific systemic upset and an ESR of 129 mm/h. On examination, he is clinically anaemic but has no lymphadenopathy or organomegaly. Routine investigations reveal: haemoglobin 7.8 g/dl, MCV 89 fl, WCC 3.6 × 10⁹/l, platelets 17 × 10⁹/l; Na⁺ 137 mmol/l, K⁺ 4.7 mmol/l, urea 4.7 mmol/l, creatinine 86 μmol/l, corrected Ca²⁺ 2.45 mmol/l. The plasma electrophoresis shows 'an IgM monoclonal band with associated immunoparesis'.

3. A 38-year-old woman presents in the Emergency Department with a 1-month history of painful enlargement of her cervical and axillary lymph nodes, lethargy and severe oral ulceration. On examination, she has gross cervical, axillary and inguinal lymphadenopathy associated with splenomegaly. Her blood film shows 'occasional blast cells'. The diagnosis is subsequently confirmed on lymph node biopsy.

4. An 87-year-old man presents in the Emergency Department with a chest infection and malaise. Routine investigations reveal: haemoglobin 11.3 g/dl, MCV 80 fl, WCC 126 × 10⁹/l, platelets 347 × 10⁹/l. The blood film shows 'predominantly lymphocytes with no blast cells seen'. He is seen by the haematologist and started on chlorambucil.

5. A 41-year-old woman is seen by her GP with increasing neck swelling associated with night sweats and weight loss. Routine investigations reveal: haemoglobin 8.5 g/dl, MCV 84 fl, WCC 7.6 × 10⁹/l, platelets 216 × 10⁹/l; Na⁺ 135 mmol/l, K⁺ 4.9 mmol/l, urea 5.7 mmol/l, creatinine 91 μmol/l; ESR 109 mm/h. A subsequent lymph node biopsy confirms the presence of Reed–Sternberg cells.

7. THEME: DIARRHOEA

A   Amoebic dysentery
B   Autonomic neuropathy
C   Bacterial enteritis
D   Colorectal carcinoma
E   Crohn's disease
F   Diverticulitis
G   Irritable bowel syndrome
H   Overflow diarrhoea
I   Pseudomembranous colitis
J   Thyrotoxicosis
K   Ulcerative colitis
L   Viral gastroenteritis

The following patients have all presented with diarrhoea as a predominant symptom. Please select the most appropriate diagnosis from the above list. Each diagnosis may be used once, more than once or not at all.

1. A 67-year-old man presents with a history of several months of diarrhoea (loose stool, three times per day) and has now noticed rectal bleeding and passage of mucus. He previously opened his bowels once every 2 days with formed stool. He has lost approximately 1 stone in weight. He is afebrile with a pulse of 78 bpm. His haemoglobin is 9.1 g/dl.

2. A 1-year-old child is brought to the Emergency Department by his parents with diarrhoea, vomiting and fever. His siblings and several children at the nursery have had the same problem recently and one required admission for correction of dehydration. On examination, the child is listless, dehydrated and febrile (39.5 °C), pulse 120 bpm. Investigations show: haemoglobin 13.4 g/dl, WCC 6.2 × 10⁹/l.

3. An 80-year-old woman develops acute cholecystitis and is treated with intravenous cefuroxime. She is due to go home but then develops lower abdominal pain associated with severe diarrhoea (10–15 times per day). She is febrile (39.5 °C), pulse 100 bpm. Her haemoglobin is 10.2 g/dl and her WCC is 21.4 × 10⁹/l.

4. A 35-year-old patient with severe cerebral palsy has long-standing constipation for which he has a routine prescription of laxatives in his nursing home. He has been having increasing abdominal pain and the nurses say that the abdomen has become distended and that he has copious diarrhoea. He is afebrile, pulse 90 bpm. Investigations show: haemoglobin 14.2 g/dl, WCC 8.7 × 10⁹/l.

5. A 66-year-old woman presents in the Emergency Department with a 3–day history of increasing lower abdominal pain associated with diarrhoea. On examination, her temperature is 37.7 °C and she has tenderness and guarding in the left iliac fossa. Investigations show: haemoglobin 12.4 g/dl, WCC 15.6 × 10⁹/l.

8. THEME: EVIDENCE-BASED MEDICINE

A   Case–control series
B   Case series
C   Cohort study
D   Controlled clinical trial
E   Cross-sectional survey
F   Experimental research paper
G   Guidelines
H   Meta-analysis
I   Non-systematic review
J   Randomised controlled trial
K   Systematic review

The following are descriptions of types of medical study. Please select the most appropriate descriptive term from the above list. Each option may be used once, more than once or not at all.

1. The gold standard in medical research. Usually designed to prospectively assess the effects of an intervention.

2. An overview of primary studies that contains a statement of objectives, materials and methods and which has been conducted according to explicit and reproducible methodology.

3. A statistical synthesis of the numerical results of several trials which all addressed the same question.

4. A study in which two or more groups of people are selected on the basis of differences in exposure to a particular agent and followed up to observe differences in outcome between the groups.

5. A study in which medical histories of more than one patient with a particular condition are described to illustrate one interesting aspect of the condition or treatment.

9. THEME: MELANOTIC SKIN LESIONS

A   Acral melanoma
B   Amelanotic melanoma
C   Blue naevus
D   Café-au-lait patch
E   Compound naevus
F   Hutchinson's lentigo (malignant lentigo, lentigo maligna)
G   Intradermal naevus
H   Junctional naevus
I   Nodular melanoma
J   Superficial spreading melanoma

The following are descriptions of pigmented lesions of the skin. Please select the most appropriate descriptive term from the above list. Each option may be used once, more than once or not at all.

1.   A 50-year-old Afro-Caribbean man presents with a 2-cm, irregular pigmented lesion on the palm of his hand.

2.   A 75-year-old man presents with a slowly growing, irregular area of brown/dark-brown pigmentation on the face. He consults a dermatologist who informs him that while the lesion is potentially malignant, it should be completely cured by local excision.

3.   A pathology report describes a benign pigmented lesion in which melanocyte proliferation is observed within the basal epithelial layer.

4.   A 60-year-old patient presents with anal pain and bleeding. On examination, there is a tumour at the anal verge which is suspected to be an anal carcinoma. Biopsies under anaesthesia are reported as showing undifferentiated anaplastic cells of unknown origin. Subsequent immunostaining is positive for S100.

5.   A large (3 cm × 4 cm), irregular melanotic lesion with varying degrees of pigmentation is widely excised from the leg of a 25-year-old woman who has been resident in Australia for the last 2 years. The pathologist reports that the thickness of the lesion is 1 mm and that the lesion is confined to the epidermis.

10. THEME: PERINATAL AND NEONATAL MORTALITY

A Birth asphyxia
B Congenital abnormality
C Early pregnancy complications, eg ectopic pregnancy
D Hypertensive disorders
E Maternal genital tract sepsis
F Maternal medical conditions
G Maternal obstetric haemorrhage
H Neonatal sepsis
I Prematurity
J Thromboembolic disease

From the above list please choose the condition most likely to fit the following statements. The options may be used once, more than once or not at all.

1. This condition is the biggest contributor to perinatal mortality. ☐

2. This is the single biggest cause of indirect maternal mortality. ☐

3. This condition is the single biggest contributor to direct maternal mortality. ☐

4. This condition is a cause of direct maternal death, usually due to pulmonary oedema associated with inappropriate fluid balance management. ☐

5. This condition is only a small contributor to perinatal mortality but is the commonest cause of complaint in cases that reach litigation. ☐

11. THEME: DISEASES OF THE UPPER GASTROINTESTINAL TRACT

A Acute erosive gastritis
B Adenocarcinoma
C Adenoma
D Barrett's oesophagus
E Chronic peptic ulcer
F Coeliac disease
G Crohn's disease
H Giardiasis
I Lymphoma of mucosa-associated lymphoid tissue (MALT)
J Squamous-cell carcinoma

From the above list, please select the disease that each of the following patients is most likely to have. Each disease may be used once, more than once or not at all.

1. A 63-year-old man presents with a 3-month history of 'acid heartburn'. Endoscopy shows red, velvety patches in the lower oesophagus, extending 5 cm above the oesophagogastric junction. Biopsies of the red patches show gastric-type glandular epithelium with foci of intestinal metaplasia.

2. A 27-year-old woman presents with a 9-month history of weight loss, abdominal pain and diarrhoea. A barium follow-through reveals a stricture and mucosal cobblestoning in the mid-ileum. Endoscopy reveals several small ulcers in the stomach and duodenum. Gastric and duodenal biopsies show non-necrotising granulomas.

3. A 51-year-old man presents with a 3-month history of burning epigastric pain that is relieved by antacids and food. He has recently had two episodes of vomiting coffee grounds. Endoscopy reveals a 3-cm antral ulcer with 'punched-out' edges. Biopsies of the ulcer reveal inflammatory debris and granulation tissue only. Biopsies of the gastric mucosa adjacent to the ulcer show an infiltrate of lymphocytes, plasma cells and neutrophils. None of the lymphocytes are atypical and there is no evidence of epithelial malignancy.

4. A 25-year-old man presents with a 6-month history of abdominal discomfort and, more recently, steatorrhoea. He has also felt tired in the past few weeks and has been taking iron supplements. Blood tests show a megaloblastic anaemia. Vitamin B_{12} levels are normal but serum and red-cell folate concentrations are low. Anti-endomysial antibodies are present in the serum. A duodenal biopsy shows subtotal villous atrophy with an increased number of intraepithelial lymphocytes.

5. A 75-year-old man presents with a 2-month history of anorexia, weight loss and epigastric pain. Blood tests done by his GP reveal an iron-deficiency anaemia. Endoscopy shows a polypoid mass in the gastric antrum. Biopsies show sheets of atypical glands infiltrating into the submucosa, with clusters of signet-ring cells.

12. THEME: 12-LEAD ECG (ST-SEGMENT AND T-WAVE CHANGES)

A

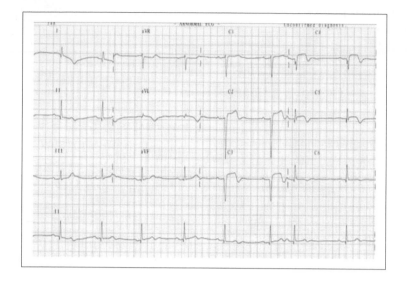

B

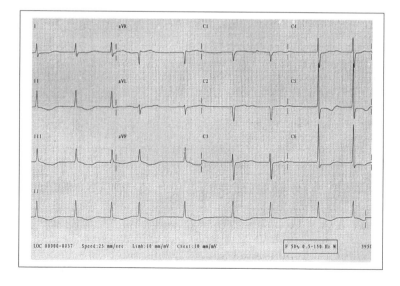

C

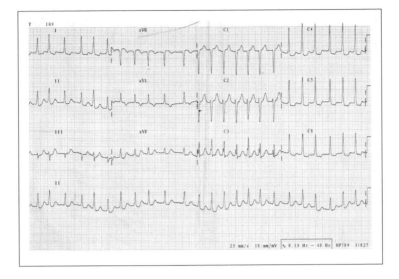

D

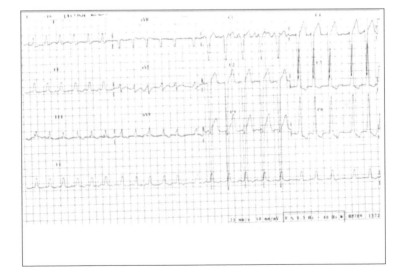

E

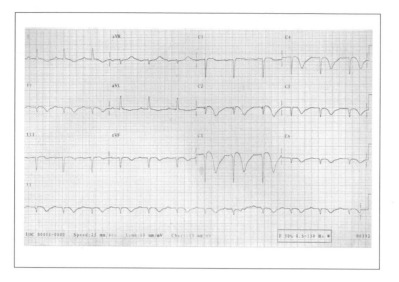

F

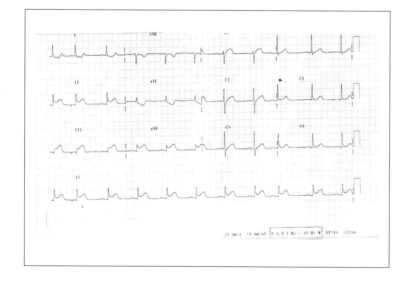

G

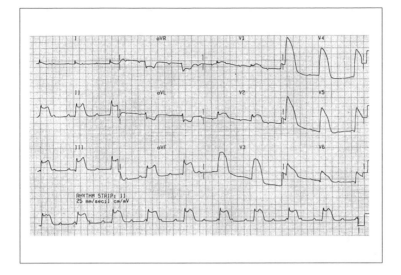

H

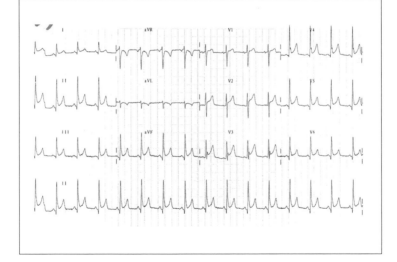

I

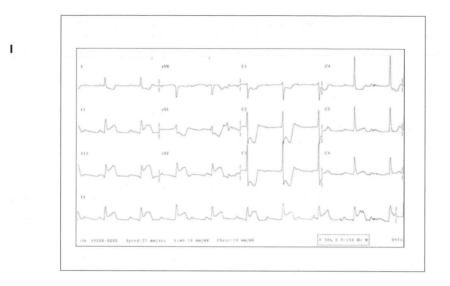

J

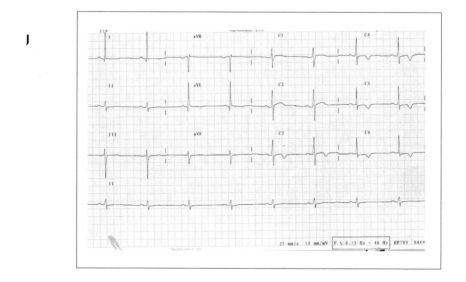

The following patients have all presented with conditions leading to ST-segment or T-wave changes on their ECG. Please choose the most appropriate ECG from those shown above. You may use each ECG once, more than once or not at all.

1. A 28-year-old Asian man is referred to the medical team on call with sharp central chest pain. The pain is eased when he leans forwards and has been associated with night sweats and, more recently, with large tender swollen lymph nodes in his neck.

2. A 39-year-old 'heavy smoker' presents to the Emergency Department with a 3–hour history of worsening central chest pain. The pain is radiating across the left side of his chest through to his back. The ECG confirms posterior, as well as inferolateral ST-segment changes.

3. A 51-year-old man with known angina presents to his GP with a 30-minute history of severe central chest pain. His ECG shows a possible septolateral non-STEMI, left axis deviation, and inferior Q-waves. A paramedic ambulance is called for immediately.

4. A 71-year-old man is referred to the medical team on-call with atypical chest pain and an ECG showing an 'anterior STEMI'. On review of the patient he has very definite dyspepsia (probably due to the aspirin he is taking) and an ECG demonstrating a left bundle branch block pattern with 'high take off' in the anterior leads.

5. A 61-year-old woman with known ischaemic heart disease presents to the Emergency Department with severe central chest pain and 'fluttering' in her chest. Her ECG confirms her to be in fast atrial fibrillation with probable rate-related ischaemia in the inferoseptolateral leads.

13. THEME: ANATOMY OF THE LIVER

A   Bare area of the liver
B   Caudate lobe
C   Caudate process
D   Coronary ligament
E   Falciform ligament
F   Gallbladder
G   Left lobe
H   Left triangular ligament
I   Porta hepatis
J   Right lobe

For each of the following descriptions, please choose the most appropriate structure from the above list. Each structure may be used once, more than once or not at all
.

1. Lies on the lateral side of the quadrate lobe.   ☐

2. Is the superior relation of the aditus of the lesser sac.   ☐

3. Site of the entry of the hepatic artery into the liver.   ☐

4. Anterior relation of the upper pole of the right kidney.   ☐

5. Forms the upper limit of the lesser sac.   ☐

14. THEME: BLOOD SUPPLY OF THE HEART

A   Anterior interventricular artery
B   Circumflex artery
C   Coronary sinus
D   Diagonal artery
E   Great cardiac vein
F   Left coronary artery
G   Left marginal artery
H   Posterior interventricular artery
I   Right coronary artery
J   Right marginal artery

For each of the following descriptions, please choose the most appropriate vessel from the above list. Each vessel may be used once, more than once or not at all.

1. Has its origin in the anterior aortic sinus.

2. Gives rise to the diagonal artery.

3. Supplies the apex of the heart.

4. Supplies the sinoatrial node.

5. Lies between the left auricular appendage and the pulmonary trunk.

Paper 10 Answers

1. THYROID FUNCTION TESTS

1. **G – TSH 18.9 mU/l, fT$_4$ 14.3 pmol/l, fT$_3$ 2.8 nmol/l**
    Patients with cognitive impairment often take their medication intermittently, so their TSH is raised but their fT$_4$ and fT$_3$ levels are within normal limits. This is because they have often taken several thyroxine tablets over the preceding week prior to their thyroid function tests being checked. A dosset box might improve things but, failing this, a carer or district nurse should be instructed to help the patient take their medications regularly.

2. **B – TSH < 0.01 mU/l, fT$_4$ 64.8 pmol/l, fT$_3$ 7.3 nmol/l**
    This young woman has developed signs and symptoms consistent with primary thyrotoxicosis, the most likely cause of which is autoimmune thyroid disease. She can be treated with carbimazole or propylthiouracil to block her thyroid hormone production, and with β-blockers for the systemic symptoms.

3. **C – TSH < 0.01 mU/l, fT$_4$ 15.9 pmol/l, fT$_3$ 8.8 nmol/l**
    This woman has signs and symptoms of thyrotoxicosis but her T$_4$ is normal. She has therefore developed the less common T$_3$ thyrotoxicosis which can present with similar signs and symptoms.

4. **F – TSH 0.71 mU/l, fT$_4$ 7.0 pmol/l, fT$_3$ 1.2 nmol/l**
    This woman has developed secondary hypothyroidism due to pituitary failure. She has signs consistent with Addison's disease (low blood pressure and a low blood glucose) as well as amenorrhoea. Causes include post-partum infarction (Sheehan's syndrome), stroke, and infiltration (eg sarcoid, amyloid or haemochromatosis).

5. **D – TSH 7.3 mU/l, fT$_4$ 14.3 pmol/l, fT$_3$ 1.8 nmol/l**
    Patients who are acutely unwell with severe systemic illness often have abnormal thyroid function tests which do not fit into any 'obvious' pattern. This is because the thyroid stops hormone synthesis, more T$_3$ is converted peripherally to rT$_3$ than to T$_4$, and less T$_3$ and T$_4$ are bound to albumin.

2. MISCELLANEOUS RADIOGRAPHIC IMAGES – CLINICAL ABNORMALITIES

1. **(P8–10) G, H – Small-bowel obstruction and left-hemisphere ring-enhancing lesion**
   Radiograph **G** is a supine abdominal film showing dilated small-bowel loops. Small-bowel obstruction commonly presents with severe abdominal pain and profuse vomiting. Radiograph **H** is a contract-enhanced CT head scan which shows a ring-enhancing lesion associated with surrounding cerebral oedema. This can present with symptoms of raised intracranial pressure, including blurred vision, nausea and vomiting.

2. **(P8–10) A, G – Osteomyelitis and small-bowel obstruction**
   Radiograph **A** shows features suggestive of osteomyelitis and radiograph **G** shows features of small-bowel obstruction. Both conditions can be associated with bacteraemia and subsequent septicaemia.

3. **(P8–10) B, H, I – Paget's disease of bone, left-hemisphere ring-enhancing lesion, cannon-ball metastases**
   Although Paget's bone disease (radiograph **B**) classically does not affect the serum calcium it can be associated with hypercalcaemia due to prolonged immobilisation or other concomitant causes of hypercalcaemia (eg primary hyperparathyroidism or bony metastases). Radiographs **H** and **I** both show metastases, and malignancy can be associated with hypercalcaemia due to bony metastases or to the production of parathyroid hormone-like peptide.

4. **(P8–10) C, H, J – Cervical spondylosis, left-hemisphere ring-enhancing lesion and skull fracture**
   All three of these conditions can present with headache. Radiograph **C** shows cervical spondylosis, which commonly presents with neck and shoulder pain and occipital headache. The contrast-enhanced CT head scan shows a ring-enhancing lesion. Clearly, blunt trauma to the head (causing the large frontoparietal fracture in radiograph **J**) will be associated with a severe headache.

5. **(P8–10) A, B, D, F – Osteomyelitis, Paget's disease of bone, calcified thyroid nodule and acromegaly**
   The endocrine abnormalities represented here are diabetes mellitus, Paget's bone disease, thyroid disease and acromegaly.

IMAGES: pages 354–356

3. PLEURAL EFFUSION

1. **D – Chronic hepatitis B virus infection**
   The three major metabolic 'failures' – hepatic, cardiac and renal – all lead to fluid overload, peripheral oedema, ascites and transudative pleural effusions. This patient has signs of chronic liver disease and a possible hepatoma. (This picture is primarily associated with chronic viral hepatitis but can also occur with any condition leading to cirrhosis.)

2. **G – Ischaemic cardiomyopathy**
   This man has signs of old ischaemic heart disease on his ECG, including left axis deviation and poor anterior R-wave progression. Common causes of cardiomyopathy include ischaemic heart disease, hypertension, alcohol, post-viral and idiopathic.

3. **I – Renal-cell carcinoma**
   Although this man initially presents with the signs and symptoms of bronchogenic carcinoma, the radiographic findings are more in keeping with cannon-ball metastases of renal-cell carcinoma. Primary and secondary carcinomas can produce an exudative effusion.

4. **H – Pulmonary emboli**
   This woman has a history suggestive of multiple pulmonary emboli, which have led to right heart strain and cardiac failure. Her ECG confirms signs of right ventricular strain (dominant R-waves with T-wave inversion in leads V_1 and V_2 and right axis deviation). The diagnosis should be confirmed (after initiating anticoagulation with low-molecular-weight heparin) by V/Q scan or spiral CT scan of the chest with angiography. Pulmonary emboli classically produce an exudative effusion.

5. **J – Tuberculous pericarditis**
   This patient has signs consistent with a significant pericardial effusion/tamponade. The most likely cause is a tuberculous infection; others include ischaemic heart disease, malignant infiltration, pericarditis, rheumatic fever and uraemia.

4. NEUROLOGICAL DEFICIT/DISABILITY

1. **D, E, F, I – Ataxia, dysarthria, dysdiadochokinesia and nystagmus**
    This man has been placed on erythromycin, which is a liver enzyme inhibitor. This will reduce the metabolism of phenytoin and lead to toxicity. Phenytoin toxicity is manifest as cerebellar syndrome and paradoxically causes seizures. The phenytoin should be stopped until the levels are back in the therapeutic range and the patient should be told about future antibiotics and other medications that could affect his phenytoin therapy.

2. **J – Resting tremor**
    This man has parkinsonism, as evidenced by his bradykinesia, his 'frozen' facial expression and falls. This is classically associated with a resting tremor and rigidity (hypertonia) leading to 'cogwheeling' of the upper limbs.

3. **C, H – Astereognosis and expressive dysphasia**
    This patient has had a left cerebral hemisphere stroke, leading to expressive dysphasia and astereognosis. Other features of a middle cerebral artery stroke include visuospatial problems and motor/sensory deficit of the contralateral limbs.

4. **D – Ataxia**
    This patient has a peripheral sensory neuropathy, which can lead to a sensory ataxia, which is characterised by a high-stepping, foot-slapping gait.

5. **G – Dyspraxic gait**
    This man has signs and symptoms suggestive of normal-pressure hydrocephalus. The classic triad of signs in this condition is cognitive impairment, gait dyspraxia and urinary incontinence. Patients with a good history of the triad and CT head scan findings in keeping with the disorder should benefit from the insertion of a ventriculoperitoneal shunt.

5. COLLAPSE

1. B – Complete heart block

This patient has developed symptomatic complete heart block. He has characteristic cannon waves in his JVP due to the associated atrioventricular dissociation, which means that his right atrium is contracting against a closed tricuspid valve. He needs to have a permanent pacemaker inserted.

2. C – Neurocardiogenic syncope

This patient has developed symptomatic bradycardia and hypotension 2 minutes after tilting her to 70° and carotid sinus massage. This is known as 'neurocardiogenic syncope' and is thought to be a result of an abnormal response to venous pooling in the legs. The pooling leads to a reduction in the cardiac filling pressure which in turn leads to an increased, 'vigorous' ventricular contraction. This response stimulates mechanoreceptors which send afferent messages to medullary centres which in turn send out efferent messages leading to increased vagus-mediated hypotension and bradycardia. This is known as the 'Bezold–Jarisch reflex'. It is unclear how to treat this syndrome successfully and several therapeutic interventions might be required. Paradoxically, β-blockers are used, which block the afferent part of the pathway and lead to an improved vasomotor response. Permanent pacemakers might also have a role.

3. J – Vertebrobasilar insufficiency

This patient has symptoms suggestive of vertebrobasilar insufficiency. This is caused by compression of the vertebrobasilar arteries by bone (cervical spondylosis) or through atherosclerosis. Unlike similar disease in the carotid arteries, operative intervention carries excessive risks and supportive therapy is the only treatment at present. The appropriate management of coexisting severe carotid artery disease might improve her symptoms.

4. A – Aortic stenosis

This patient has significant aortic stenosis, as evidenced by her narrow pulse pressure, slow-rising pulse and the voltage criteria of left ventricular hypertrophy on her ECG. She needs an echocardiogram to estimate the degree of stenosis, the pressure gradient across the valve and her left ventricular function. Subsequent management (which could include cardiac catheterisation and possible valve replacement) depends on the patient's wishes, her co-morbidity and the left ventricular function.

5. D – Postural hypotension

Patients presenting with a fractured neck of femur should have the reason for their fall investigated. Common causes include mechanical falls due to poorly fitting footwear, loose fitting fixtures in the home and accidental falls which may happen to anyone. However pathological falls due principally to cardiovascular and neurological conditions must be excluded by history and investigation, particularly in the presence of loss of consciousness or amnesia with regard to the fall. Postural hypotension may occur as a result of degenerate autonomic responses but is principally iatrogenic induced by antihypertensive agents, as in this case. The patient should have all possible hypotensive agents stopped and his anti-anginal therapy reconsidered.

6. HAEMATOLOGICAL MALIGNANCIES

1. **E – Hairy-cell leukaemia**
    This man has developed hairy-cell leukaemia, so called because of the appearance of the abnormal B cells. It is a disease of middle age and is more common in men than in women, usually presenting with clinical features of pancytopenia and splenomegaly.

2. **J – Waldenström's macroglobulinaemia**
    This man has a pancytopenia, and ESR of more than 100 mm/h and has evidence of a monoclonal gammopathy with associated immunoparesis. However, he has a normal serum calcium, no evidence of renal impairment and no symptoms suggestive of bony lesions. These features differentiate the patient with Waldenström's macroglobulinaemia from the patient with multiple myeloma. Waldenström's is generally a more benign condition but requires similar supportive treatment with blood transfusions and rapid treatment of sepsis.

3. **B – Acute myeloid leukaemia (AML)**
    Acute myeloid leukaemia (AML) is the principal leukaemia of adults. It presents in middle to late middle age with symptoms of pancytopenia (anaemia, recurrent infection and spontaneous bruising and bleeding), lymphadenopathy and splenomegaly. AML is differentiated by the predominant cell morphology of the abnormal leukaemic blast cells and these dictate the various treatment options, which include chemotherapy, bone marrow transplantation and supportive treatment with blood transfusion, blood products and rapid treatment of sepsis.

4. **C – Chronic lymphocytic leukaemia (CLL)**
    Chronic lymphocytic leukaemia (CLL) is the predominant leukaemia of older people. It is often discovered as an incidental finding when the patient has a routine full blood count or can present insidiously with non-specific symptoms such as malaise, weight loss and fever. The peripheral blood film shows anaemia and a leucocytosis with a lymphocytosis of abnormal B cells. Most patients only require observation and regular blood transfusion but the more symptomatic and those with higher white cell counts are put on hydroxyurea. Patients are very susceptible to severe sepsis as the abnormal B cells cause an immunoparesis and thus patients can not mount an effective immune response.

5. **F – Hodgkin's lymphoma**
    This middle-aged woman has developed painless lymphadenopathy, night sweats and weight loss. Her lymph node biopsy confirms the presence of Reed–Sternberg cells, which are pathognomonic of Hodgkin's lymphoma. These are malignant giant cells which are characterised by their binuclear, bilobed appearance or multilobed, polypoid mononucleus containing inclusion-like 'owl's eye' nucleoli surrounded by a clear halo. Hodgkin's lymphoma has a bimodal distribution of incidence, the first peak occurring in young adults and the second in middle age. Patients present with gross lymphadenopathy, particularly of the cervical region, and systemic features, known as 'B symptoms', which include weight loss, fever and night sweats. Patients can also complain of pain in the enlarged lymph nodes on drinking alcohol and of tobacco intolerance. Treatment depends on the patient's wishes, staging, site and bulk of the disease, and includes chemotherapy, radiotherapy and supportive haematological treatments.

7. DIARRHOEA

1. **D – Colorectal carcinoma**
    This gentleman has the commonest clinical presentation of colorectal carcinoma, with a change in bowel habit (usually to diarrhoea), rectal bleeding and weight loss. This particular case is typical of a rectal or left-sided colonic cancer. Caecal carcinomas present more commonly present with diarrhoea and anaemia, but no evident bleeding.

2. **L – Viral gastroenteritis**
    This is a very common condition in infants and children and typically occurs in outbreaks as described. Common enteroviruses are RNA viruses such as rotavirus and Norwalk virus. Treatment is supportive.

3. **I – Pseudomembranous colitis**
    This is caused by overgrowth of the bacteria *Clostridium difficile* following treatment with oral or intravenous broad-spectrum antibiotics. Diagnosis is confirmed by stool culture. Treatment involves stopping the causative agents and starting metronidazole or vancomycin. The disorder takes its name from the pseudomembrane observed if the colonic mucosa is examined endoscopically. In an 80-year-old in-patient, overflow diarrhoea and incontinence caused by faecal impaction should be excluded by rectal examination.

4. **H – Overflow diarrhoea**
    Overflow occurs as a consequence of faecal impaction, which prevents the normal anorectal mechanisms of defaecation and continence from functioning. While severe impaction can be manifest as large-bowel obstruction, liquid faeces and air more commonly circumnavigate the impacted bolus periodically, presenting as diarrhoea. In this case the cause of constipation is neurogenic, and this is a serious management problem in many patients with degenerative central neurological disorders or spinal cord injuries.

5. **F – Diverticulitis**
    Diverticular disease of the colon can manifest itself in many ways: constipation, diarrhoea, bleeding, obstruction and perforation. When a diverticulum becomes inflamed the condition is described as diverticulitis, some of the findings of which are described in this case. With increasing severity there may be localised perforation and abscess formation or free perforation with purulent or even faecal peritonitis. Treatment of diverticulitis is principally intravenous antibiotics and bowel rest.

8. EVIDENCE-BASED MEDICINE

1. **J – Randomised controlled trial**
   Such trials, which are by necessity prospective, evaluate by randomisation the effect of a single variable in a precisely defined patient group. They potentially eradicate bias and should use hypothetico-deductive reasoning (ie aim to falsify rather than confirm a specific hypothesis).

2. **K – Systematic review**
   Overview-type studies include systematic reviews, meta-analyses and non-systematic reviews. The former two types of overview have a much higher relative weighting in the traditional hierarchy of evidence when making decisions about clinical interventions. The Cochrane Database is a database of systematic reviews and meta-analyses.

3. **H – Meta-analysis**
   When reviewing the impact of new therapies, evidence can come from several studies of modest size and with slightly differing conclusions. One solution might be to carry out a definitive randomised controlled trial but this might require considerable time, effort and expense. An alternative is to combine data from several modest studies into a meta-analysis. By combining studies in a coherent (and statistically robust) way, conclusions can be reached that are based on a larger pool of study subjects.

4. **C – Cohort study**
   This differs slightly from a randomised controlled trial in that it generally takes two or more large cohorts of subjects (rather than a specific sample size of patients) and follows them up long-term to assess the effects of a certain agent (eg an environmental factor) on the basis of which they are selected. An example is the work of Sir Richard Doll in which he studied the association of lung cancer with smoking by observing a cohort of 40 000 doctors in four cohorts according to the number of cigarettes they smoked over a period of 10 years.

5. **B – Case series**
   This is really just a series of case reports that together illustrate an interesting aspect of a condition or a treatment. Although they are not randomised and rarely prospective, and represent a low relative weight in the traditional hierarchy of evidence, they are easy for the less scientifically minded to digest and can still convey very important information rapidly before a definitive trial can be performed. An example is McBride's 1961 *Case series of two infants with limb absence born to mothers taking Thalidomide*, which first alerted the world to this terrible drug complication.

9. MELANOTIC SKIN LESIONS

1. **A – Acral melanoma**
   This is one of the five classically described clinicopathological types of malignant melanoma, which are: Hutchinson's lentigo, acral lentiginous, mucosal, superficial spreading, and nodular. The diagnosis is suggested by the ethnic origin of the patient and site of the lesion (the latter giving its name). It is the only type to affect black people and occurs on the palms or soles or under the nail bed. It is the rarest form in white people (0.5–1%). The two commonest types are superficial spreading melanoma (65%) and nodular melanoma (25%).

2. **F – Hutchinson's lentigo (malignant lentigo, lentigo maligna)**
   The clues to the diagnosis are in the clinical description and the prognosis given to the patient. This is considered to be a type of malignant melanoma *in situ* by some pathologists and a pre-malignant lesion by others. Regardless of this debate, the tumour is confined to the epidermis. Slow-growing, it carries an excellent prognosis after local excision. If left, however, it can progress to the more aggressive invasive form, that of superficial spreading melanoma.

3. **H – Junctional naevus**
   Proliferating benign melanocytic lesions are pathologically classified into intradermal (proliferation deep to the basal layer of the epidermis, ie confined within the dermis), junctional (as described in this question) and compound (which has both junctional and intradermal elements). The importance of this classification lies in the increased risk of malignant change in lesions with junctional proliferation. A specific variant that is the exception to this rule is the juvenile naevus (pre-pubertal).

4. **B – Amelanotic melanoma**
   This is usually a variant of nodular melanoma, in which the cell of origin is the melanocyte but melanin production is not evident (had this been the case, the diagnosis of mucosal melanoma would have been obvious). The diagnosis is finally made by staining for the neural marker, S100, which stains melanocytes because they share a common tissue of origin embryologically with some neural tissues (the neural crest). Mucosal melanoma carries the worst prognosis of all melanomas because of its late presentation and early lymphatic spread. (Other melanoma sites, apart from the skin, include ocular and subungual tumours.)

5. **J – Superficial spreading melanoma**
   The clinical and pathological descriptions fit with this diagnosis, which has the best prognosis of the melanoma variants because of the late vertical invasion (compared with nodular melanoma) and therefore decreased risk of tumour spread. There are two local microstaging systems for melanoma which are complementary and reliable indicators of prognosis: Breslow's system measures the depth of invasion in mm whereas Clark's system defines the depth of invasion by histological level, from the epidermis (I) through to subcutaneous fat (V).

10. PERINATAL AND NEONATAL MORTALITY

1. **I – Prematurity**
    Complications of prematurity (respiratory distress syndrome or RDS, intraventricular haemorrhage, sepsis, necrotising enterocolitis) are by far the greatest contributors to perinatal mortality (death after 24 weeks' gestation and up to 28 days post-delivery) as reported by the Confidential Enquiry into Stillbirths and Deaths in Infancy (CESDI). Not surprisingly, the mortality rate decreases with increasing gestation.

2. **F – Maternal medical conditions**
    Indirect maternal deaths are defined as deaths due to previously existing conditions that might have been exacerbated by the physiological effects of pregnancy but which are not directly due to obstetric causes. The only cause of indirect maternal death in the list is 'maternal medical conditions'. Important examples are maternal congenital cardiac disease resulting in high-output heart failure due to the increased cardiac output (40%) and epilepsy leading to status epilepticus due to the altered handling of antiepileptic medication in pregnancy.

3. **J – Thromboembolic disease**
    Direct maternal deaths are defined as deaths during pregnancy and up to 42 days after delivery due to causes directly related to pregnancy or its management, including omissions and incorrect management. Thromboembolic disease, particularly pulmonary embolism, has repeatedly been by far the leading cause of direct maternal death in the triennial Confidential Enquiries into Maternal Death (CEMD). There are often multiple risk factors for thromboembolic disease, and guidelines for the use of thromboprophylaxis in pregnancy and the puerperium aiming to reduce the occurrence of thromboembolic disease and thus maternal mortality are used nationally.

4. **D – Hypertensive disorders**
    Hypertensive disorders of pregnancy (pre-eclampsia) cause a number of maternal deaths each year. Unfortunately, the commonest mode of death is iatrogenic failure to manage fluid balance appropriately, resulting in fluid overload and pulmonary oedema. Pre-eclampsia (particularly if severe) causes a small-vessel angiopathy which results in a tendency for fluid to shift to the extravascular space, with renal dysfunction, leading to an inability to excrete excess fluid. On this pathophysiological background, a relatively small amount of fluid overload can cause overwhelming pulmonary oedema. Pulmonary oedema can also occur in obstetric haemorrhage and maternal sepsis but the mode of death in these conditions is usually hypovolaemia and multiorgan failure, respectively.

5. **A – Birth asphyxia**
    Deaths due to birth asphyxia are actually rare and therefore only a small contributor to perinatal mortality. Recent Australian epidemiological studies have shown that the majority of deaths in which birth asphyxia can be implicated are in fact probably due to pre-existing intrinsic fetal problems. However, the public perception is that it is much more common and as such is the commonest complaint in obstetric litigation in relation to perinatal death.

11. DISEASES OF THE UPPER GASTROINTESTINAL TRACT

1. **D – Barrett's oesophagus**
    The most common cause of 'acid heartburn' is gastro-oesophageal reflux, during which gastric acid refluxes from the stomach into the lower oesophagus. The oesophagus is normally lined by stratified squamous epithelium. This type of epithelium cannot easily withstand the damage caused by gastric acid, so metaplasia occurs to gastric-type glandular epithelium, which is better able to withstand the damage. Endoscopically, the metaplastic mucosa has a red, velvety appearance, in contrast to the smooth, white appearance of normal oesophageal epithelium. This condition is known as 'Barrett's oesophagus'. Like many other metaplastic conditions, Barrett's oesophagus is associated with an increased risk of malignancy, particularly when there is associated intestinal metaplasia.

2. **G – Crohn's disease**
    The only granulomatous disease on this list is Crohn's disease. This can affect any part of the alimentary tract from the mouth to the anus, and there is often microscopic involvement of the stomach and duodenum, even in the absence of referrable symptoms or macroscopic disease. In this patient, the barium meal findings of cobblestoning and stricture formation are typical of Crohn's disease.

3. **E – Chronic peptic ulcer**
    The main differential diagnosis of a gastric ulcer lies between a chronic peptic ulcer and an ulcerating malignant tumour. Chronic peptic ulcers have sharply defined, punched-out borders, in contrast to ulcerating malignancies, which tend to have raised, rolled, everted edges. The floor of a peptic ulcer is composed of fibrous scar tissue overlaid by granulation tissue, inflammatory exudate and necrotic slough. The endoscopic and histological findings in this patient therefore support a diagnosis of chronic peptic ulcer. The mucosa adjacent to a chronic peptic ulcer often shows chronic gastritis, particularly when *Helicobacter pylori* infection is the underlying cause.

4. **F – Coeliac disease**
    This patient has symptoms and signs of fat malabsorption, suggestive of small-intestinal disease. The fact that the duodenal biopsy shows subtotal villous atrophy confirms an enteropathy, so the differential diagnosis lies between coeliac disease and Crohn's disease. The presence of anti-endomysial antibodies in the serum and the intraepithelial lymphocytosis are diagnostic of coeliac disease, as is positivity for the more recently characterised anti-tissue transglutaminase antibodies. This is an immune-mediated disorder in which there is sensitivity to the α-gliadin component of gluten. Anaemia is common in coeliac disease and is due to malabsorption of iron and/or folic acid. The dietary iron supplements have probably prevented significant iron deficiency and the most likely cause of this patient`s anaemia is therefore folate deficiency. Management of coeliac disease with a gluten-free diet usually brings about a rapid clinical and histological response.

5. **B – Adenocarcinoma**
    Epigastric pain is a non-specific symptom of upper gastrointestinal pathology, but the weight loss and anorexia are more sinister, and the anaemia suggests chronic gastrointestinal bleeding. The endoscopic appearance of a polypoid mass is suspicious of malignancy and the differential diagnosis lies between an adenocarcinoma and a lymphoma. The finding on biopsy of atypical glands that infiltrate the submucosa, together with signet-ring cells, confirms an adenocarcinoma.

12. 12 LEAD ECG (ST-SEGMENT AND T-WAVE CHANGES)

Whenever one looks at a set of clinical investigations they need to be placed in the context of the clinical history and wellbeing of the patient (ie whether they are sick or not). ECGs are no different and one should always treat the patient and not the findings on the ECG! The ten ECGs shown are not simple and you need a good and reliable method for dealing with each part of the ECG. If you have difficulties with these ECGs, perhaps you can use them as the basis for a tutorial with a friendly junior or senior doctor.

The ECGs show:

A – Acute anterolateral myocardial infarction with high lateral ischaemia (sinus rhythm, normal axis, Q-waves and ST elevation in V_2–V_5; ST depression with T-wave inversion in I and aVL).

B – Slow atrial fibrillation secondary to digoxin toxicity (slow atrial fibrillation with slurred ST depression in the inferior and lateral leads).

C – Fast atrial fibrillation with global rate-related ischaemia (fast atrial fibrillation with ST depression in inferior and septolateral leads; T-wave inversion in high lateral leads).

D – Fast atrial fibrillation with left bundle branch block.

E – Evolving global ST-elevation myocardial infarction (STEMI) (Q-waves and T-wave inversion in inferior and anterolateral leads; high lateral T-wave inversion).

F – Inferior STEMI.

G – Global, massive STEMI, including changes in the inferior, anterior and lateral leads.

H – Acute pericarditis (concave ST elevation in leads I, II, III, aVF, V_3–V_6).

I – Acute inferoposterolateral myocardial infarction with complete heart block (inferolateral ST elevation with acute posterior changes; ST depression V_1–V_3).

J – Acute T-wave changes in septolateral leads – possible non-STEMI (sinus bradycardia, left axis deviation and T-wave inversion in V_3–V_6, I and aVL).

The answers are:

1. H – Acute pericarditis.
2. I – Acute inferoposterolateral myocardial infarction with complete heart block.
3. E – Evolving global STEMI.
4. D – Fast atrial fibrillation with left bundle branch block.
5. C – Fast atrial fibrillation with global rate-related ischaemia.

13. ANATOMY OF THE LIVER

1. **F – Gallbladder**
    The gallbladder descends along the lateral border of the quadrate lobe. The falciform ligament with the ligamentum teres in its lower border lies on the medial side.

2. **C – Caudate process**
    The opening of the lesser sac from the peritoneal cavity passes anterior to the inferior vena cava and behind the free margin of the lesser omentum, above the first part of the duodenum.

3. **I – Porta hepatis**
    The hepatic artery lies medial to the common bile duct, both lying in front of the portal vein within the free margin of the lesser omentum. The three structures enter the porta hepatis and divide into right and left branches, which then ramify within the right and left lobes of the liver.

4. **A – Bare area of the liver**
    The upper pole of the right kidney and adjacent adrenal gland and a part of the inferior vena cava are surrounded by the coronary ligament within the bare area on the posterior aspect of the liver.

5. **B – Caudate lobe**
    The lesser omentum extends upwards into the liver and surrounds the caudate lobe, the reflections from the posterior abdominal wall peritoneum completing the surround. The sac extends downwards behind the stomach within the greater omentum and across to the left into the hilum of the spleen, behind the stomach.

14. BLOOD SUPPLY OF THE HEART

1. I – Right coronary artery
From its origin in the anterior aortic sinus, the artery lies between the right auricular appendage and the pulmonary trunk, before descending in the anterior atrioventricular groove. It passes around the inferior margin of the heart, giving off the right marginal artery, and becomes the posterior interventricular artery.

2. A – Anterior interventricular artery
The diagonal artery is a prominent branch of the anterior interventricular artery.

3. A – Anterior interventricular artery
The artery has two to nine branches that supply the anterior surface of the left ventricle as it passes to the apex of the heart. It often passes onto the posterior surface as well as supplying the left ventricle through its prominent diagonal branch.

4. B – Circumflex artery
The sinoatrial node is usually supplied by a branch of the circumflex artery. In 80–90% of people the atrioventricular node is supplied by the first septal branch of the posterior interventricular artery.

5. F – Left coronary artery
The left coronary artery lies between the left auricular appendage and the pulmonary trunk, and gives off the anterior interventricular artery to become the circumflex artery. This passes around the upper border of the heart to lie in the posterior atrioventricular groove.

RADIOLOGY IMAGES

Paper 1   THEME: CHEST RADIOGRAPHS – CLINICAL SCENARIOS
Paper 2   THEME: CHEST RADIOGRAPHS – CLINICAL SCENARIOS

P1–P2 A

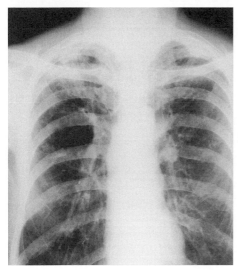

P1–P2 B

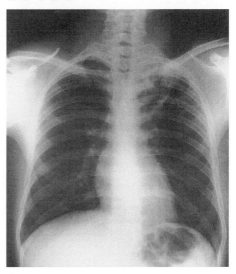

P1–P2 C

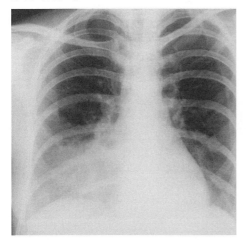

P1–P2 D

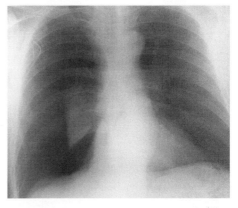

THEMES: P1 (14), P2 (13), pages 17, 48

Paper 1 THEME: CHEST RADIOGRAPHS – CLINICAL SCENARIOS
Paper 2 THEME: CHEST RADIOGRAPHS – CLINICAL SCENARIOS

P1–P2 E

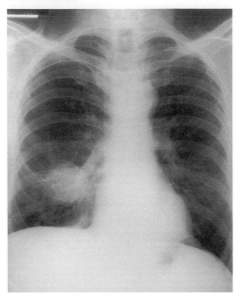

P1–P2 F

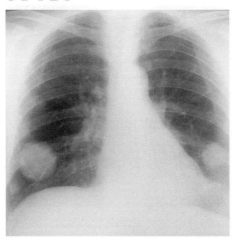

P1–P2 G

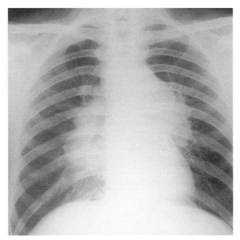

P1–P2 H

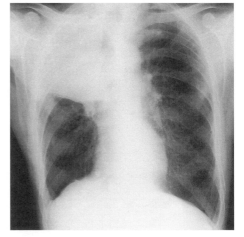

THEMES: P1 (14), P2 (13), pages 17, 48

Paper 1 THEME: CHEST RADIOGRAPHS – CLINICAL SCENARIOS
Paper 2 THEME: CHEST RADIOGRAPHS – CLINICAL SCENARIOS

P1–P2 I

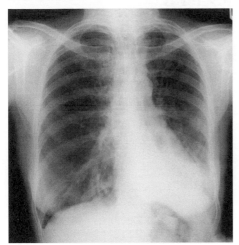

P1–P2 J

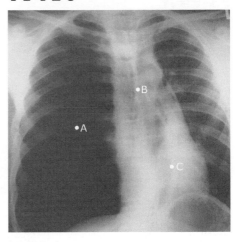

THEMES: P1 (14), P2 (13), pages 17, 48

347

Paper 3 THEME: CHEST RADIOGRAPHS – ASSOCIATED DISORDERS
Paper 4 THEME: CHEST RADIOGRAPHS – CLINICAL SIGNS

P3–P4 A

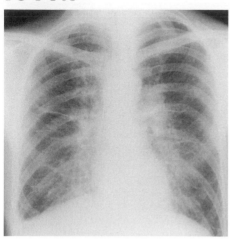

P3–P4 B

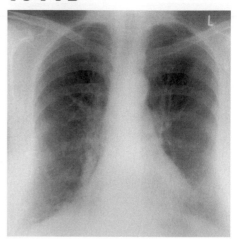

P3–P4 C

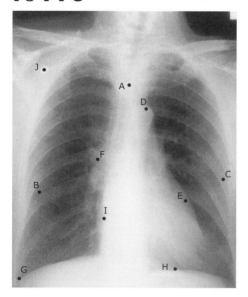

P3–P4 D

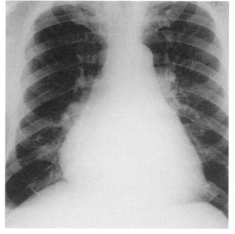

THEMES: P3 (12), P4 (11), pages 81, 114

Paper 3 THEME: CHEST RADIOGRAPHS – ASSOCIATED DISORDERS
Paper 4 THEME: CHEST RADIOGRAPHS – CLINICAL SIGNS

P3–P4 E

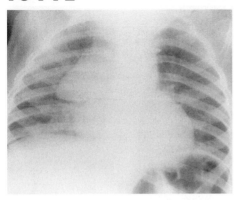

P3–P4 F

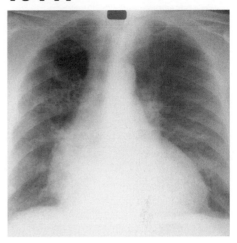

P3–P4 G

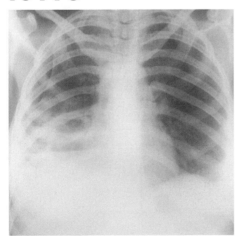

P3–P4 H

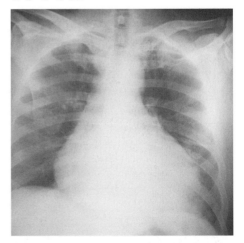

THEMES: P3 (12), P4 (11), pages 81, 114

Paper 3 THEME: CHEST RADIOGRAPHS – ASSOCIATED DISORDERS
Paper 4 THEME: CHEST RADIOGRAPHS – CLINICAL SIGNS

P3–P4 I

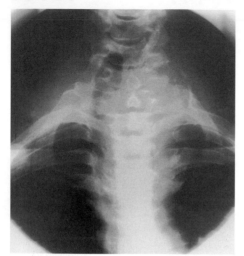

P3–P4 J

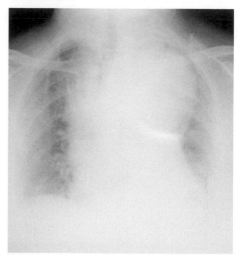

THEMES: P3 (12), P4 (11), pages 81, 114

Paper 5 **THEME 10: UROGENITAL RADIOLOGY – RADIOLOGICAL DIAGNOSIS**
Paper 6 **THEME 9: UROGENITAL RADIOLOGY – RENAL TRACT ABNORMALITIES**
Paper 7 **THEME 8: UROGENITAL RADIOLOGY – CLINICAL SCENARIOS**

P5–P7 A

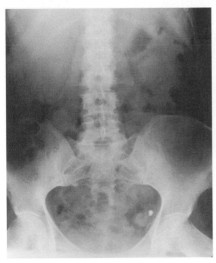

P5–P7 B

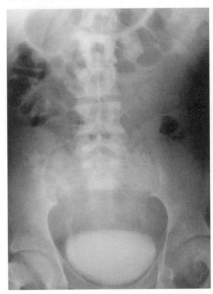

P5–P7 C

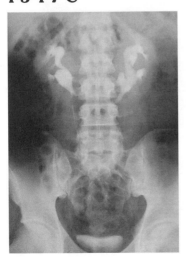

P5–P7 D

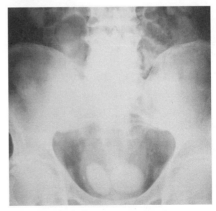

THEMES: P5 (10), P6 (9), P7 (8) pages 147, 181, 215

Paper 5 THEME 10: UROGENITAL RADIOLOGY – RADIOLOGICAL
        DIAGNOSIS
Paper 6 THEME 9: UROGENITAL RADIOLOGY – RENAL TRACT
        ABNORMALITIES
Paper 7 THEME 8: UROGENITAL RADIOLOGY – CLINICAL
        SCENARIOS

P5–P7 E

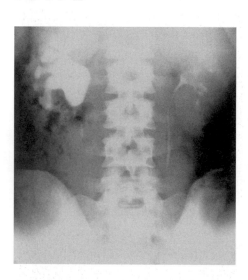

P5–P7 F

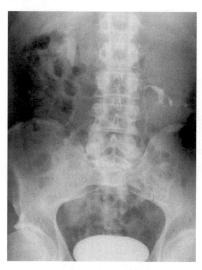

P5–P7 G

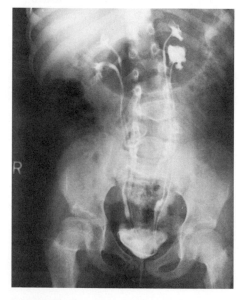

P5–P7 H

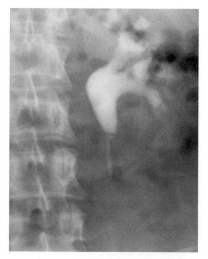

THEMES: P5 (10), P6 (9), P7 (8) pages 147, 181, 215

Paper 5 THEME 10: UROGENITAL RADIOLOGY – RADIOLOGICAL DIAGNOSIS
Paper 6 THEME 9: UROGENITAL RADIOLOGY – RENAL TRACT ABNORMALITIES
Paper 7 THEME 8: UROGENITAL RADIOLOGY – CLINICAL SCENARIOS

P5–P7 I

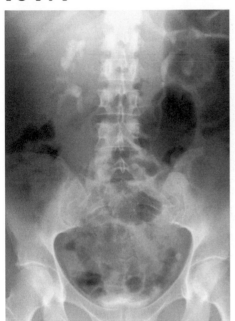

P5–P7 J

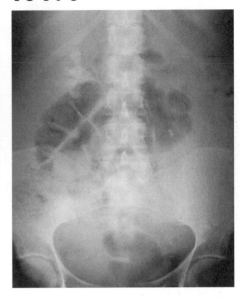

THEMES: P5 (10), P6 (9), P7 (8) pages 147, 181, 215

Paper   8   **THEME 8: MISCELLANEOUS RADIOGRAPHIC IMAGES – RADIOLOGICAL DIAGNOSIS**
Paper   9   **THEME 6: MISCELLANEOUS RADIOGRAPHIC IMAGES – CLINICAL DIAGNOSIS**
Paper 10   **THEME 2: MISCELLANEOUS RADIOGRAPHIC IMAGES – CLINICAL ABNORMALITIES**

P8–P10 A

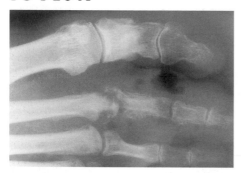

P8–P10 B

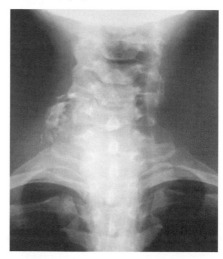

P8–P10 C

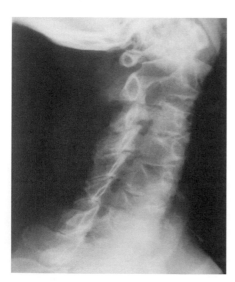

P8–P10 D

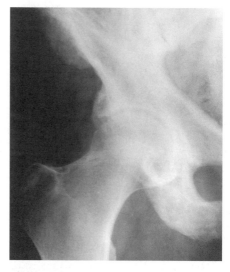

THEMES: P8 (8), P9 (6), P10 (2) pages 249, 280, 310

Paper 8 THEME 8: MISCELLANEOUS RADIOGRAPHIC IMAGES –
              RADIOLOGICAL DIAGNOSIS
Paper 9 THEME 6: MISCELLANEOUS RADIOGRAPHIC IMAGES –
              CLINICAL DIAGNOSIS
Paper 10 THEME 2: MISCELLANEOUS RADIOGRAPHIC IMAGES –
              CLINICAL ABNORMALITIES

P8–P10 E

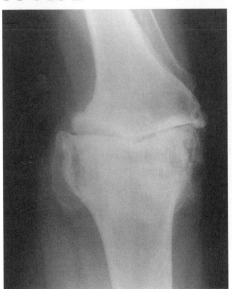

P8–P10 F

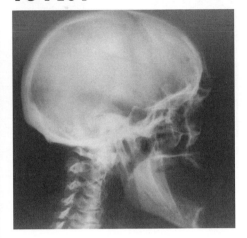

THEMES: P8 (8), P9 (6), P10 (2) pages 249, 280, 310

Paper 8 **THEME 8: MISCELLANEOUS RADIOGRAPHIC IMAGES –
         RADIOLOGICAL DIAGNOSIS**
Paper 9 **THEME 6: MISCELLANEOUS RADIOGRAPHIC IMAGES –
         CLINICAL DIAGNOSIS**
Paper 10 **THEME 2: MISCELLANEOUS RADIOGRAPHIC IMAGES –
         CLINICAL ABNORMALITIES**

P8–P10 G

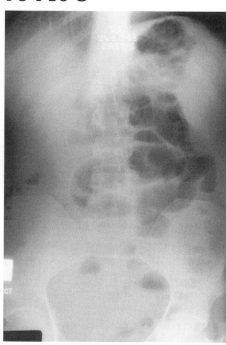

P8–P10 H

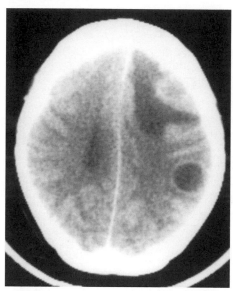

P8–P10 I

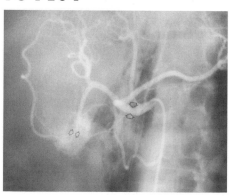

P8–P10 J

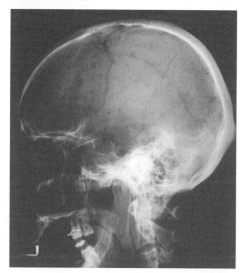

THEMES: P8 (8), P9 (6), P10 (2) pages 249, 280, 310

Index

Numbers refer to papers, and questions within each paper

abciximab 3.1, 5.6
abdominal aortic aneurysm 8.6
abdominal pain 3.4, 7.6
abducent nerve 3.13
abruptio placentae 6.11
acetylcholine-receptor antibody 8.5
achalasia 5.3
acidosis 7.7
acoustic neuroma 2.8
acral melanoma 10.9
acromegaly 7.1, 9.6, 10.2
acute abdomen 8.6
acute epididymo-orchitis 8.7
acute epiglottitis 7.10
acute inferior ST-elevation myocardial
    infarction 4.1
acute inferoposterolateral myocardial
    infarction 10.12
acute intermittent porphyria 3.4
acute middle ear effusion 2.8
acute myeloid leukaemia 9.3, 10.6
acute pancreatitis 4.7, 8.6
acute pericarditis 10.12
acute renal failure 9.5
acute viral hepatitis 5.7
Addison's disease 8.1
adductor longus 7.14
adductor magnus 7.14
adenocarcinoma 1.11, 10.11
adenoid cystic carcinoma 3.9
adenoma 5.12
adenomatous polyposis 9.8
adhesions 5.8
albumin 3.3
alimentary tract 6.13
alkaline phosphatase 3.3
alkalosis 7.7
alpha-fetoprotein 4.4
alpha-interferon 5.6

alveolitis 8.2
Alzheimer's disease 6.4
amelanotic melanoma 10.9
amiodarone 7.4
amoebiasis 5.12
amyloidosis 7.4
amyotrophy 5.4
anaemia 1.2
anal carcinoma 3.7
anal fissure 3.7
anastomotic dehiscence 5.9
aneurysm
    aortic 2.13, 3.12, 8.6
    ventricular 8.12
angiodysplasia 3.7
angioneurotic oedema 7.10
ankylosing spondylitis 3.2
antalgic gait 2.5
anterior condylar canal 6.14
anterior interventricular artery 10.14
anterior vaginal repair 7.11
anthrax 8.10
anti-ACH receptor 6.6
anti-dsDNA antibody 5.2
anti-endomysial antibody 8.5
anti-GBM disease 9.5
anti-glomerular basement membrane
    antibody 5.2
anti-Hu 6.6
anti-Jo-1 antibody 6.6, 8.5
anti-proteinase-3 (cANCA) 6.6
anti-Ri 6.6
anti-tissue-transglutaminase (anti-tTG)
    6.6
antibiotics 6.5
anticoagulant therapy 1.9
antihypertensive agents 6.1
antimitochondrial antibody 8.5
aortic aneurysm 2.13, 3.12, 8.6

aortic arch 1.12
aortic disruption 4.8
aortic regurgitation 5.1
aortic stenosis 10.5
aphthous ulceration 2.4
apical fibrosis 4.11
aplastic anaemia 1.2
appendix mass 1.7
Argyll Robertson pupil 8.4
arm *see* upper limb
arterial blood gases 7.7, 8.9
arteriovenous (AV) nipping 9.1
arthritis 4.2
   rheumatoid 7.9
arytenoid cartilage 5.13
asbestosis 1.3
ascites 1.4
astereognosis 10.4
asthma 8.2
ataxia 10.4
atenolol 6.1
atonic uterus 6.11
atrial fibrillation 9.9, 10.12
atrophic glossitis 2.4
atrophy 2.12
atypical pneumonia 3.5, 8.2
auditory conditions 2.8
autoantibodies 6.6, 8.5
autoimmune diseases 9.12
autoimmune haemolytic anaemia 1.2
autoimmune hepatitis 6.3
autosomal dominant disorders 7.2
AV nipping 9.1
axillary nerve 1.13

Bacillus cereus 7.3
back pain 3.2
   musculoskeletal causes 6.10
bacterial infections 3.11
bacterial peritonitis 3.4
bacterial sialedenitis 3.9
bacterial vaginosis 1.10
Barrett's oesophagus 10.11
basal atelectasis 5.9
basal-cell carcinoma 8.10
benign intracranial hypertension 1.5
Bennett's fracture 3.8
benzylpenicillin 6.5, 9.5

beta-interferon 5.6
bilateral hilar lymphadenopathy 1.14,
   9.2
biliary colic 4.7
bilirubin 3.3
birth asphyxia 10.10
bisoprolol 3.1
bladder: transitional-cell carcinoma 1.9
bleeding per vagina in pregnancy 6.11
blood count 2.2
blood gases 7.7, 8.9
blot haemorrhage 9.1
brachialis 4.14
breast
   disorders 6.8
      abscess 6.8
      carcinoma 1.8, 6.8
      fibrocystic disease 1.8
breathlessness 8.2
bronchielectasis 2.13, 3.12
bronchus: carcinoma 6.12
bubble-contrast transoesophageal
   echocardiogram 5.5
buccinator 3.14
bursitis 7.9

^{13}C urea breath test 5.5
CA-15.3 4.4
CA-19.9 4.4
CA-27.29 4.4
caecum
   carcinoma 1.7
   perforated 8.6
calcified thyroid nodule 8.8, 10.2
calculi 5.10, 6.9, 7.8
Campylobacter jejuni 7.3
cANCA (anti-proteinase-3) 6.6
cancer
   colorectal 9.8
   ovarian 1.7
   see also neoplasms; tumours
Candida albicans 2.11
candidiasis: oesophageal 5.3
cannon-ball metastases 1.14, 9.6, 10.2
carcinoma of the breast 6.8
cardiac chest pain 4.1
cardiac tamponade 4.8, 5.1
cardiac therapies 3.1

cardiomegaly 9.2
cardiomyopathy 1.4, 5.1, 8.12, 10.3
carotid artery 8.14
case series 10.8
caudate lobe 10.13
caudate process 10.13
cefoxatime 6.5
cerebellar ataxia 2.5
cerebellar stroke 4.5
cerebral abscess 9.4
cervical lymphadenopathy 9.10
cervical spondylitis 8.8, 9.6, 10.2
Chagas' disease 9.7
chancroid sexually transmitted disease
    4.6
    chancrous ulcer 8.10
chest pathology 2.3
chest radiographs
    abnormal findings 9.2
    associated disorders 3.12
    clinical scenarios 1.14, 2.13
    clinical signs 4.11
chest trauma 4.8
chiropedists 6.2
Chlamydia trachomatis 1.10
cholangitis 5.7, 6.3
chondromalacia patellae 7.9
chronic cholecystitis 4.7
chronic granulocytic leukaemia 9.3
chronic hepatitis virus infection 10.3
chronic lymphocytic leukaemia 10.6
chronic peptic ulcer 10.11
chronic serous middle ear effusion (glue
    ear) 2.8
Chvostek's sign 1.6
circumflex artery 10.14
cirrhosis 5.7, 8.3
clarithromycin 6.5
clopidogrel 3.1
Clostridium difficile 3.11, 7.3
coagulation disorders 7.12
coeliac disease 10.11
cohort study 10.8
colitis 5.12, 9.8, 10.7
collapse 101.5
colon 6.13
colonic carcinoma 4.3, 5.8
colorectal cancer 9.8, 10.7

colposcopy 7.11
colposuspension 7.11
combined oral contraceptive pill 4.10
community psychiatric nurses 6.2
complete heart block 9.9, 10.5, 10.12
complete miscarriage 8.11
Conn's syndrome 7.1
constipation 6.7
contraceptive pill 4.10
Cooper's ligament 7.13
cor pulmonale 8.12
cord prolapse 3.10
coronary artery 10.14
coronavirus 4.12
cranial nerves 3.13
creatinine 1.1
cricoid cartilage 5.13
Crohn's disease 1.6, 9.8, 10.11
Cryptosporidium parvum 2.11
Cullen's sign 1.6
cyproterone acetate 4.10
cystocoele 5.11
cytomegalovirus 2.11, 9.3

de Musset's sign 1.6
deep inguinal ring 8.13
deep peroneal (anterior tibial) nerve 5.14
delayed miscarriage 8.11
delirium 3.5
dementia 6.4
demyelination 7.4
detrusor overactivity 5.11
diarrhoea 7.3, 10.7
diastolic murmurs 2.1
dieticians 6.2
digoxin effect 9.9
displaced left-sided kidney 5.10, 7.8
disseminated intravascular coagulation
    (DIC) 6.11, 7.12
district nurses 6.2
diverticular disease 3.7, 4.3, 5.12, 6.7,
    10.7
    Zenker's diverticulum 9.7
donovanosis 4.6
dot haemorrhage 9.1
doxazosin 6.1
doxycycline 6.5
duct papilloma 6.8

duodenal ulcer 4.3
  perforated 8.6
duodenojejunal flexure 6.13
duodenum 6.13
duplex kidneys 5.10, 6.9, 7.8
Duroziez's sign 1.6
dysarthria 10.4
dysdiadochokinesia 10.4
dysphagia 5.3, 9.7, 10.4
dyspraxic gait 10.4
dystrophia myotonica 7.2

early diastolic murmur 2.1
early pregnancy 8.11
early systolic murmur 2.1
ECG rhythm strips 9.9
  ST-segment and T-wave changes 10.12
ectopic pregnancy 8.11
ejection systolic click 2.1
electrolytes 1.1
empyema 2.3
  gallbladder 4.7
encephalitis 8.1
endocarditis 8.12, 9.3
endometriosis 2.10
epididymo-orchitis 8.7
epiglottis 5.13, 7.10
eponymous signs 1.6
Epstein-Barr virus 2.6, 4.12, 7.5
erythema multiforme 3.6
erythema nodosum 3.6
Escherichia coli 3.11, 7.3
evidence-based medicine 10.8
evolving global STEMI 10.12
expressive dysphasia 10.4
extensor carpi radialis longus 4.14

facial nerve 3.13
familial adenomatous polyposis 9.8
familial hypercholesterolaemia 7.2
fast atrial fibrillation 9.9, 10.12
femoral hernia 3.4, 5.8
femoral nerve 7.13
femoral region 7.13
festinating gait 2.5
α-fetoprotein (αFP) 4.4
fibrillation 9.9, 10.12
fibrinous pericarditis 8.12

fibroadenoma 1.11, 6.8
fibroadenosis 1.8, 6.8
fibrocystic disease of the breast 1.8, 6.8
fibrosing alveolitis 8.2
fixed dilated pupil 8.4
flail chest 4.8
flexor digitorum profundus 4.14
flucloxacillin 6.5
foramen ovale 6.14
αFP (α-fetoprotein) 4.4
fractures 3.8
  skull 8.8, 10.2
full blood count 2.2

gait disturbance 2.5, 10.4
gallbladder 10.13
  empyema 4.7
gallstone ileus 4.7
gallstones 3.4, 5.7, 6.3
  complications of disease 4.7
Garden II fracture 3.8
gastric outflow obstruction 2.7
gastro-oesophageal reflux disease 9.7
gastrocnemius 7.14
gastroenteritis 2.7, 10.7
gastrointestinal blood loss 4.3
gastrointestinal tract 10.11
genital tract agenesis/dysgenesis 2.10
genital tract infections 1.10
genital ulceration 4.6
genuine stress incontinence 5.11
giant-cell arteritis 1.5
Gilbert's syndrome 7.2
Glasgow Coma Scale (GCS) 2.9
globular heart 2.13, 3.12
glomerulonephritis 1.9
glossal lesions 2.4
glossopharyngeal nerve 3.13
glue ear 2.8
GnRH analogues 4.10
goitre 3.12
gonadotrophin-releasing hormone
  analogues 4.10
gonococcal arthritis 4.2
goserelin (GnRH analogue) 4.10
granulocyte colony-stimulating factor 5.6
Grey Turner's sign 1.6
Guillain-Barré syndrome 5.4

gynaecological procedures 7.11
gynaecological therapeutic agents 4.10

haematocoele 8.7
haematocrit 2.2
haematological malignancies 10.6
haematuria 1.9
haemochromatosis 6.3, 8.3
haemoglobin 2.2
haemolytic anaemia 1.2
haemophilia A 7.12
   induced haemarthrosis 4.2
haemophilia B 7.12
haemothorax 4.8
hairy-cell leukaemia 10.6
hard exudates 9.1
Hashimoto's thyroiditis 9.12
head injury 2.9
headache 1.5
heart
   blood supply 10.14
   diseases 8.12
   surface markings 9.14
heart block 9.9, 10.5, 10.12
heart failure 5.1
heart sounds 2.1
Helicobacter pylori 3.11
hemiscrotal pain 8.7
hepatic flexure of the colon 6.13
hepatitis 5.7
   autoimmune 6.3
hepatitis A virus 6.3, 8.3
hepatitis B virus 10.3
hepatitis C virus 4.12
hepatomegaly 8.3
hereditary non-polyposis colorectal cancer
   (HNPCC) 9.8
hernia: femoral 3.4, 5.8
herpes encephalitis 8.1
herpes simplex virus 1.10, 4.6
hilar lymphadenopathy 1.14, 9.2
histoplasmosis 7.5
HIV 2.6, 9.11
   associated sialadenitis 3.9
Hodgkin's lymphoma 9.3, 10.6
Holmes-Adie pupil 8.4
Horner's syndrome 8.4
horseshoe kidney 5.10, 6.9

human papillomavirus 2.11, 4.12
Huntington's disease 6.4
Hutchinson's lentigo 10.9
hydatidiform mole 8.11
hydrocephalus 6.4
hyoglossus 3.14
hypercholesterolaemia 7.2
hyperplasia 2.12
hypertension 10.10
   intracranial 1.5
   secondary 7.1
hypertrophic cardiomyopathy 8.12
hypertrophy 2.12
hypocalcaemia 9.4
hypoglycaemia 3.5
hypokalaemia 5.4
hyponatraemia 3.5, 9.4, 8.1
hypothalamic dysfunction 2.10
hypothyroidism 7.4, 8.1
hysteroscopy 7.11

iatrogenic constipation 6.7
idiopathic megacolon 6.7
idiopathic pulmonary fibrosis 1.3
IF antibody 8.5
IgA nephropathy 9.5
iliac fossa masses 1.7
iliac lymphadenopathy 1.7
iliopsoas 7.14
immunocompromise 2.11
incarcerated femoral hernia 3.4
incomplete miscarriage 8.11
incontinence 5.11
infarction 2.12
infective diarrhoea 7.3
infective endocarditis 8.12, 9.3
infective gastroenteritis 2.7
inferior constrictor 4.13
inferior epigastric vessels 8.13
inferior orbital fissure 6.14
inferior ST-elevation myocardial infarction
   4.1
infertility 2.10
infliximab 5.6
ingested irritants 7.10
inguinal ligament 7.13, 8.13
inguinal region 8.13
inhaled irritants 7.10

α-interferon 5.6
β-interferon 5.6
internal carotid artery 8.14
internal jugular vein 8.14
internal oblique muscle 8.13
interventricular artery 10.14
intestinal obstruction 2.7, 5.8, 10.2
intracranial hypertension 1.5
intraduct papilloma 1.8
intrapartum complications 3.10
intussusception 5.8
investigations
    less common diagnostic tests 5.5
    urological 5.2
iron deficiency 1.2
irritable bowel syndrome 7.6
ischaemic cardiomyopathy 1.4, 5.1, 10.3,
        10.12

jaundice 5.7, 6.3
jejunum 6.13
jugular foramen 6.14
jugular vein 8.14
junctional naevus 10.9

Kaposi's sarcoma 2.4
kidneys
    displaced 5.10, 7.8
    duplex kidneys 5.10, 6.10, 7.8
    horseshoe kidney 6.9
    obstructed 5.10, 7.8
    polycystic disease 5.10, 7.1, 7.8, 8.3
    radiological diagnosis 5.10
knee
    osteoarthritis 8.8
    pain 7.9
Kocher's incision 4.9

laparoscopy 7.11
large intestine
    diseases 5.12
    obstruction 2.7
larynx 5.13
    fracture 7.10
late systolic murmur 2.1
lateral cutaneous nerve of forearm 1.13
lateral pterygoid 3.14
left coronary artery 10.14

left vagus nerve 1.12
left ventricular failure 2.13, 3.12
leg see lower limb
Legionella pneumonia 1.3, 8.1, 9.5
lentigo maligna 10.9
leukaemia
    acute myeloid 9.3, 10.6
    chronic granulocytic 9.3
    chronic lymphocytic 10.6
    hairy-cell leukaemia 10.6
lichen planus 2.4
liver anatomy 10.13
liver tests 3.3
lobar pneumonia 6.12
long midline incision 4.9
long thoracic nerve 2.14
losartan 6.1
lower limb
    knee pain 7.9
    muscle attachments 7.14
    nerve supply of the muscles 5.14
lower midline incision 4.9
lung 6.12
lupus vulgaris 3.6
Lyme disease 7.5
lymphadenopathy 2.6, 9.2, 9.10
    hilar 1.14
    iliac 1.7
lymphocytes 2.2
lymphogranuloma venereum 4.6
lytic metastases 3.2

macroglobulinaemia 10.6
maculopathy 9.1
malignant lentigo 10.9
malignant mesothelioma 1.11
malposition of the occiput 3.10
mammary duct ectasia 1.8
Marjolin's ulcer 8.10
masseter 3.14
mastication 3.14
maternal medical conditions 10.10
Meckel's diverticulum 4.3
meconium-stained liquor 3.10
medial cutaneous nerve of forearm 1.13
median nerve 1.13, 2.14
mediastinum 1.12
medullary strokes 4.5

mefanamic acid 4.10
megacolon 6.7
melanotic skin lesions 10.9
Ménière's disease 2.8
meningitis: viral 1.5
meniscal tear 7.9
mesenteric adenitis 7.6
mesenteric ischaemia 3.4
mesentery of the sigmoid colon 6.13
mesothelioma 1.11
meta-analysis 10.8
metabolic acidosis 7.7
metabolic alkalosis 7.7
metaplasia 2.12
metastases
    cannon-ball metastases 1.14, 9.6, 10.2
    multiple 8.3
metastatic carcinoma 6.10
methyldopa 6.1
metronidazole 6.5
mid-diastolic murmur 2.1
mid-systolic click 2.1
middle constrictor 4.13
middle ear effusion 2.8
middle lobe pneumonia 1.14, 4.11
miscarriage 8.11
mitral stenosis 5.1
mitralised left heart border 2.13, 3.12
monoarthritis 4.2
Monteggia fracture dislocation 3.8
motor neurone disease 5.3, 5.4
multidisciplinary team 6.2
multiple metastases 8.3
multiple myeloma 1.2, 3.2
murmurs 2.1
muscle weakness 5.4
musculocutaneous nerve 2.14
musculoskeletal causes of back pain 6.10
myeloma 1.2, 3.2
mylohyoid 3.14
myocardial infarction 4.1, 10.12

naevus 10.9
nausea 2.7
neck
    lumps 9.10
    vessels 8.14
Neisseria gonorrhoeae 1.10

Neisseria meningitidis 3.11
neonatal mortality 10.10
neoplasms 1.11
    see also cancer; tumours
nephrocalcinosis 5.10
neurocardiogenic syncope 10.5
neurofibromatosis 7.2
neurological disability 10.4
neuropathy: peripheral sensory 7.4
neurosyphilis 6.4
neutrophils 2.2
new therapeutic interventions 5.6
nicorandil 3.1
Nikolsky's sign 1.6
nipple discharge 1.8
non-Hodgkin's lymphoma 2.6
non-specific abdominal pain 7.6
non-ST-elevation myocardial infarction
    4.1
normal-pressure hydrocephalus 6.4
nurses 6.2
nystagmus 10.4

obstructed kidneys 5.10, 7.8
occipital strokes 4.5
occupational therapists 6.2
oesophageal candidiasis 5.3
oesophageal carcinoma 5.3, 9.7
oesophageal varices 4.3
oesophagus 1.12
oestrogen-only HRT 4.10
ophthalmoscopy 9.1
oral contraceptive pill 4.10
oral hairy leukoplakia 2.4
oral lesions 2.4
orthotists 6.2
Osgood-Schlatter's disease 7.9
osteoarthritis 8.8, 9.6
osteomyelitis 8.8, 9.6, 10.2
osteosarcoma 1.11
ovarian carcinoma 1.4, 1.7
ovary 9.13
overflow diarrhoea 10.7

paced rhythm 9.9
Paget's disease of bone 3.2, 8.8, 9.6,
    10.2
palatoglossus 4.13

pancreatic carcinoma 5.7
pancreatitis 2.7, 8.6
pancytopaenia 1.2
papilloedema 9.1
papilloma 1.8
paraoesophageal hernia 9.7
pathogenic viruses 4.12
pathological processes 2.12
pectineal ligament 7.13
pelvic abscess 5.9
pelvic inflammatory disease 7.6
pelvic-nerve injury 6.7
pelvic renal transplant 6.9
pelvis of the right kidney 9.13
pemphigus 3.6
peptic ulcer 10.11
perforated caecum 8.6
perforated duodenal ulcer 8.6
perforated sigmoid disease 8.6
pericarditis 4.1, 10.3, 8.12, 10.12
perifollicular haemorrhages 2.4
perinatal mortality 10.10
peripheral sensory neuropathy 7.4
peritoneal mesothelioma 1.4
peritonitis 3.4
pernicious anaemia 9.12
peroneus longus 7.14
Peutz-Jeghers syndrome 9.8
Pfannenstiel incision 4.9
phaeochromocytoma 7.1
pharyngeal muscles 4.13
pharyngeal pouch 9.7
pharyngobasilar fascia 4.13
phrenic nerve 1.12
physiotherapists 6.2
Pick's disease 6.4
Pickwickian syndrome 1.3
pinpoint pupils 8.4
plasma electrophoresis 5.2
platelets 2.2
pleomorphic adenoma 3.9
pleura 6.12
pleural effusion 2.3, 9.2, 10.3
Pneumocystis carinii 2.11, 6.12
pneumonia 1.14, 4.11, 6.12
  atypical 3.5, 8.2
  Legionella 1.3, 8.1, 9.5
pneumothorax 1.14, 2.3, 4.8, 4.11

polycystic kidney disease 5.10, 7.1, 7.8,
  8.3
polycystic ovary syndrome (PCOS) 2.10
polymyositis 9.12
polyposis 9.8
pontine strokes 4.5
porphyria 3.4
porta hepatis 10.13
post-operative pyrexia 5.9
posterior myocardial infarction 4.1
postural hypotension 10.5
Pott's disease of the spine 3.2
Pott's fracture 3.8
pre-patellar bursitis 7.9
pregnancy
  ectopic 8.11
  infections 9.11
  vaginal bleeding 6.11
prematurity 10.10
presbyoesophagus 5.3
primary biliary cirhosis 5.7, 8.3
prolactinoma 1.8
prolapsed intervertebral disc 6.10
pronator teres 4.14
prostate 9.13
prostatic-specific antigen (PSA) 4.4, 5.2
pseudohyponatraemia 8.1
pseudomembranous colitis 5.12, 10.7
pubic tubercle 7.13
pulmonary consolidation 2.3
pulmonary embolism 8.2, 10.3
pulmonary fibrosis 1.3, 2.3, 5.1
pulmonary oedema 1.3
pupillary defects 8.4
pyoderma gangrenosum 3.6
pyrexia 5.9
  of unknown origin (PUO) 7.5
pyrophosphate arthropathy 4.2

Quinke's sign 1.6

radial nerve 2.14
radiology
  chest
    abnormal findings 9.2
    associated disorders 3.12
    clinical scenarios 1.14, 2.13
    clinical signs 4.11

miscellaneous images 8.8, 9.6, 10.2
  urogenital 5.10
    clinical scenarios 7.8
    renal tract abnormalities 6.9
ramipril 6.1
randomised controlled trials 10.8
rashes 3.6
rectal biopsy 5.5
rectal bleeding 3.7
recurrent laryngeal nerve 5.13
referred pain 2.8
Reiter's syndrome 4.2
renal artery stenosis 7.1
renal-cell carcinoma 1.4, 1.9, 7.5, 10.3
renal failure 9.5
renal tract
  abnormalities 6.9
  ultrasound scans 5.2
respiratory acidosis 7.7
respiratory alkalosis 7.7
respiratory failure 1.3, 7.7
resting tremor 10.4
retinitis 9.1
rheumatoid arthritis 7.9
right coronary artery 10.14
right iliac fossa pain 7.6
right middle lobe pneumonia 1.14, 4.11
right phrenic nerve 1.12
right-sided pneumothorax 1.14, 4.11
right upper lobe collapse 4.11
ring-enhancing lesion 9.6, 10.2
Romano-Ward syndrome 7.2
rooftop/gable incision 4.9
rubella 9.11
ruptured abdominal aortic aneurysm 8.6

sagittal sinus thrombosis 1.5
sail sign 3.12
salivary duct stones 3.9
salivary gland disease 3.9
Salter-Harris fracture 3.8
saphenous opening 7.13
sarcoidosis 2.6, 6.12, 7.5, 8.2
Scheuermann's disease 6.10
sciatic nerve 5.14
sclerosing cholangitis 5.7, 6.3
secondary hypertension 7.1
seizures 9.4

sensory ataxia 2.5
sensory neuropathy 7.4
serous middle ear effusion 2.8
sexual dysfunction 2.10
Shigella flexneri 7.3
shortness of breath 8.2
sialadenitis 3.9
sialolithiasis 3.9
sigmoid colon 6.13
  perforated 8.6
silver wiring 9.1
Sjögren's syndrome 9.12
skin lesions 10.9
skin rashes 3.6
skin ulceration 8.10
skull-base openings 6.14
skull fracture 8.9, 10.2
slow atrial fibrillation 9.9
small-cell carcinoma of the bronchus
  6.12
small intestine obstruction 2.7, 10.2
social workers 6.2
soft exudates 9.1
specialist nurses 6.2
spinal-cord injury 6.7
spinal stenosis 6.10
splenomegaly 9.3
spondylosis 6.10
spontaneous bacterial peritonitis 3.4
squamous-cell carcinoma 1.11
  bronchus 6.12
ST-elevation myocardial infarction (STEMI)
  10.12
staghorn calculus 5.10, 6.9, 7.8
sternomastoid tumour 9.10
Streptococcus
  group B β-haemolytic 9.11
  S. pneumoniae 3.11
stress incontinence 5.11
stroke 4.5
Sturge-Weber syndrome 9.4
subarachnoid haemorrhage 9.4
subclavian artery 8.14
subdural haemorrhage 1.5, 3.5
subphrenic abscess 5.9
superficial peroneal (musculocutaneous)
  nerve 5.14
superficial spreading melanoma 10.9

superficial temporal artery 8.14
superior gluteal nerve 5.14
superior orbital fissure 6.14
supraclavicular lymphadenopathy 9.10
supraventricular tachycardia (SVT) 9.9
surgical incisions 4.9
syndrome X 4.1
syphilis 9.11
syphilitic chancre 4.6, 8.10
systematic reviews 10.8
systemic lupus erythematosus 9.12
systolic murmur 2.1

technetium-99-labelled red cell scan 5.5
temporal artery 8.14
tension pneumothorax 1.14, 4.8, 4.11
tensor palatini 4.13
testicular seminoma 8.7
testicular torsion 8.7
thalamic strokes 4.5
thalassaemia trait 1.2
thoracic aortic aneurysm 2.13, 3.12
thoracic vertebrae 1.12
thromboembolic disease 10.10
thrombosis: sagittal sinus 1.5
thyroid carcinoma 7.10
thyroid cartilage 5.13
thyroid disease 9.10
thyroid function tests 10.1
thyroid nodule 8.8, 10.2
thyrotoxic proximal myopathy 5.4
tibial (posterior tibial) nerve 5.14
tibialis posterior 7.14
torsion of an ovarian cyst 7.6
toxoplasmosis 2.6
tPA 3.1
tracheal deviation 3.12, 9.2
transitional-cell carcinoma of the bladder
    1.9
transversalis fascia 8.13
traumatic aortic disruption 4.8
tremor 10.4
Trendelenburg gait 2.5
triceps 4.14
Trichomonas vaginalis 1.10
trigeminal nerve 3.13
Troisier's sign 1.6
Trousseau's sign 1.6

true posterior myocardial infarction 4.1
tuberculosis 1.4
tuberculous arthritis 4.2
tuberculous pericarditis 10.3
tumour markers 4.4
tyrosinase 4.4

ulcerative colitis 3.7, 5.12, 9.8
ulnar nerve 1.13, 2.14
ultrasound scans: renal tract 5.2
upper airways obstruction 7.10
upper limb
    cutaneous innervation 1.13
    innervation of the muscles 2.14
    muscle attachments 4.14
upper lobe collapse 4.11
uraemia 3.5
urea 1.1
ureter 9.13
urinary tract infection 5.9, 5.11, 9.11
urogenital anatomy 9.13
urogenital radiology 5.10
    clinical scenarios 7.8
    renal tract abnormalities 6.9
urogynaecological disorders 5.11
urological investigations 5.2
urolithiasis 1.9
uterine hyperstimulation 3.10
uterine inertia 3.10
uterine rupture 6.11

vaginal bleeding in pregnancy 6.11
vaginal repair 7.11
vaginosis 1.10
vagus nerve 1.12, 3.13
vancomycin 6.5
varicella zoster virus 4.12
varicocoele 8.7
vasa praevia 6.11
vastus lateralis 7.14
venous ulcer 8.10
ventricular aneurysm 8.12
ventricular failure 2.13, 3.12
vertebral artery 8.14
vertebrobasilar insufficiency 10.5
vesical calculus 5.10, 6.9, 7.8
vesicovaginal fistula 5.11
viral gastroenteritis 10.7

viral hepatitis 5.7
viral meningitis 1.5
viruses 4.12
visual-evoked reponses 5.5
vitamin B12 deficiency 7.4
vitamin K deficiency 7.12
volvulus 5.8
vomiting 2.7
von Willebrand's disease 7.12

waddling gait 2.5
Waldenström's macroglobulinaemia
    10.6
weakness 5.4
Wegener's granulomatosis 9.5

Zenker's diverticulum 9.7